Davis's Pocket Guide to Herbs and Supplements

Davis's
Pocket Guide
to Herbs and Supplements

Catherine Ulbricht, PharmD, MBA(c)
Founder, Natural Standard Research Collaboration
Senior Attending Pharmacist
Massachusetts General Hospital
Chief Editor, *Journal of Dietary Supplements*

F.A. Davis Company • Philadelphia

F. A. Davis Company
1915 Arch Street
Philadelphia, PA 19103
www.fadavis.com

Printed in the United States of America

Last digit indicates print number: 10 9 8 7 6 5 4 3 2 1

Senior Acquisitions Editor: Thomas A. Ciavarella
Director of Content Development: Darlene D. Pedersen
Senior Project Editor: Meghan K. Ziegler
Assistant Editor: Maria Z. Price
Cover Design: Liz DiFebo
Design and Illustration Manager: Carolyn O' Brien

ISBN 10: 0-8036-2303-8
ISBN 13: 978-0-8036-2303-3

Reviewers

Mary Fabick, MSN, MEd, RN-BC, CEN
Associate Professor of Nursing
Milligan College
Milligan College, Tennessee

Lisa Garsman, MS, FNP-BC
Director of BSN Program
Saint Peter's College School of Nursing
Jersey City, New Jersey

Dawn K. Kochara, RN, BSN, MHSc
Medical Assisting Program Director
Orange County Public Schools
Winter Park, Florida

Nora M. Lee, MSN, RN, CEN
Instructor of Nursing
Charleston Southern University
Charleston, South Carolina

Linda Lipstate, MD
Associate Professor
University of Louisiana
Lafayette, Louisiana

Christie Maranto, MSN, APRN, FNP-BC
Assistant Professor
Northern State University
Shreveport, Louisiana

Barbara Marchelletta, CMA, CPC, CPT
Director
Allied Health
Bangor, Maine

Libba Reed McMillan, RN, MSN, PhD
Assistant Professor
Auburn School of Nursing
Auburn University
Auburn, Alabama

Joseph Monaco, PA-C, MSJ
Assistant Professor
Seton Hall University Physician Assistant Program
South Orange, New Jersey

Lisa Quinn, PhD, CRNP, MSN
Assistant Professor of Nursing
Gannon University, Villa Maria School of Nursing
Erie, Pennsylvania

Sandra Saucier, DNP, NP-C, CSC
Assistant Professor
Eastern Michigan University
Ypsilanti, Michigan

Stacey Singer-Leshinsky, PA, MS, Ed
Physician Assistant Instructor
St. John's University
Fresh Meadows, New York

Marilyn M. Turner, RN, CMA
Program Director, Medical Assisting
Ogeechee Technical College
Statesboro, Georgia

Linda S. Weaver, RN, MSN
Clinical Nursing Instructor
University of Colorado
Colorado Springs, Colorado

Acknowledgments

We are sincerely grateful for the ongoing contributions of Natural Standard's authors, peer reviewers, and editors since the founding of our international research collaboration. The hard work and dedication of Wendy Chao and Erica Seamon deserve special recognition for helping make this particular book available. Additionally, we thank our operational, outreach, member services, and technical support teams, along with our Board of Directors for their support of evidence-based integrative medicine research.

Please visit www.naturalstandard.com to learn more about our work. We welcome additional members, including students, to participate in our academic research programs.

Natural Standard was founded by clinicians and researchers to provide high quality, evidence-based information about complementary and alternative therapies. This international multidisciplinary collaboration now includes contributors from more than 100 eminent academic institutions.

For each therapy covered by Natural Standard, a research team systematically gathers scientific data and expert opinions. Validated rating scales are used to evaluate the quality of available evidence. Information is incorporated into comprehensive monographs which are designed to facilitate clinical decision making. All monographs undergo blinded editorial and peer review prior to inclusion in Natural Standard databases.

Natural Standard is impartial; not supported by any interest group, professional organization, product manufacturer. Institutional subscriptions, custom content and licensing are available.

Systematic Aggregation, Analysis, and Review of the Literature

Search Strategy

To prepare each Natural Standard monograph, electronic searches are conducted in many databases, including AMED, CANCERLIT, CINAHL, CISCOM, the Cochrane Library, EMBASE, HerbMed, International Pharmaceutical Abstracts, Medline, and NAPRALERT. Search terms include the common name(s), scientific name(s), and all listed synonyms for each topic. Hand searches are conducted of 20 additional journals (not indexed in common databases), and of bibliographies from 50 selected secondary references. No restrictions are placed on language or quality of publications. Researchers in the field of complementary and alternative medicine (CAM) are consulted for access to additional references or ongoing research.

Selection Criteria

All literature is collected pertaining to efficacy in humans (regardless of study design, quality, or language), dosing, precautions, adverse effects, use in pregnancy/lactation, interactions, alteration of laboratory assays, and mechanism of action (in vitro, animal research, human data). Standardized inclusion/exclusion criteria are utilized for selection.

Data Analysis

Data extraction and analysis are performed by health care professionals conducting clinical work and/or research at academic centers, using standardized instruments that pertain to each monograph section (defining inclusion/exclusion criteria and analytic techniques, including validated measures of study quality). Data are verified by a second reviewer.

Review Process

Blinded review of content is conducted by multidisciplinary research-clinical faculty at major academic centers with expertise in epidemiology and biostatistics, pharmacology, toxicology, complementary and alternative medicine (CAM) research, and clinical practice. In cases of editorial disagreement, a three-member panel of the Editorial Board addresses conflicts, and consults experts when applicable. Authors of studies are contacted when clarification is required.

Update Process

Natural Standard regularly monitors scientific literature and industry warnings. When clinically relevant new data emerge, best efforts are made to update content immediately. In addition, regular updates with renewed searches occur every 3-18 months, variable by topic.

Contents

List of Abbreviations

↑ increase
↓ decrease
AAMI age-associated memory impairment
ACE angiotensin-converting enzyme
ACTH adrenocorticotropic hormone
ADHD attention-deficit hyperactivity disorder
ADR adverse drug reaction
AHCC active hexose correlated compound
AI adequate intake
AIDS acquired immune deficiency syndrome
AKG alpha-ketoglutarate
ALA omega-3 alpha-linolenic acid
ALP alkaline phosphatase
ANP atrial natriuretic peptide
ARDS adult respiratory distress syndrome
BCAAs branched-chain amino acids
BCG bacille Calmette-Guérin
BCNU carmustine (bis-chloronitrosurea)
BMI body mass index
BPH benign prostatic hyperplasia
BSE bovine spongiform encephalopathy
BUN blood urea nitrogen
CA cancer
CABG coronary artery bypass grafting
CAD coronary artery disease
CAPD central auditory processing disorders
CBC complete blood count
CFU colony-forming unit
CHD coronary heart disease
CHF congestive heart failure
CI contraindication
CNS central nervous system
COPD chronic obstructive pulmonary disease
COX cyclooxygenase
CPR cardiopulmonary resuscitation
CRP C-reactive protein
CSF cerebrospinal fluid
CVI chronic venous insufficiency
D2 dopamine
DIC disseminated intravascular coagulation
DMARDs disease-modifying antirheumatic drugs
DSPS delayed sleep phase syndrome
DVT deep vein thrombosis
EBV Epstein-Barr virus
EDTA ethylenediaminete-traacetic acid
EEG electroencephalogram
EKG electrocardiogram
FDA US Food and Drug Administration
FMF familial Mediterranean fever
FPIA fluorescence polarization immunoassay
5-FU fluorouracil

FSH follicle-stimulating hormone

FT4 free thyroxine

g gram(s)

G6PD glucose-6-phosphate dehydrogenase deficiency

GAMT guanidinoactetate methyltransferase

GBF germinated barley foodstuff

GERD gastroesphageal reflux disease

GH growth hormone

GHB gamma hydroxybutyrate

GI gastrointestinal

GLA omega-6 gamma-linolenic acid

GnRH gonadotropin releasing hormone

GRAS generally recognized as safe

h hour

H2 histamine-2

HCSE horse chestnut seed extract

HDL high-density lipoprotein

HIV human immunodeficiency virus

HMB hydroxymethylbutyrate

HMG-CoA 3-hydroxy-3-methylglutaryl-coenzyme A

HTN hypertension

IBS irritable bowel syndrome

IGF-1 insulin-like growth factor 1

INR international normalized ratio

IOP intraocular pressure

ITP idiopathic thrombocytopenic purpurea

IUD intrauterine device

IV intravenous

LDH lactate dehydrogenase

LDL low-density lipoprotein

LFT liver function test

MAOI monoamine oxidase inhibitor

MB methylene blue

MCAD acyl-CoAdehydrogenase

MCV mean corpuscular volume

mg milligram(s)

MI myocardial infarction

min minute

mL milliliter(s)

MRSA methicillin-resistant *Staphylococcus aureus* infection

MSM methylsulfonylmethane

MTHFR methylenetetrahydro-folate reductase

N/A not applicable

NAC N-acetyl cysteine

NCI National Cancer Institute

NDGA Nordihydroguaiaretic acid

NMDA *N*-methyl-D-aspartic acid

NNRTI non-nucleoside reverse transcriptase inhibitor

NSAID nonsteroidal anti-inflammatory drug

N/V nausea and vomiting

OCD obsessive-compulsive disorder

ODTS organic dust toxic syndrome

OKG ornithine alpha-ketoglutarate

OPCs oligomeric proanthocyanidins

OTC over the counter

oz ounce(s)

PCOS polycystic ovary disease

PKU phenylketonuria

PMDD premenstrual dysphoric disorder

PMS premenstrual syndrome

PO by mouth, orally

PPI proton pump inhibitor

Preg pregnancy category

PSA prostate-specific antigen

PT prothrombin time

PTH parathyroid hormone

PTCA percutaneous transluminal angioplasty

PUD peptic ulcer disease

q every

RA rheumatoid arthritis

RBC red blood cell

RDA U.S. Recommended Dietary Allowance

RPGN rapidly progressive glomerulonephritis

RPIS renal pelvic instillation sclerotherapy

SAD seasonal affective disorder

SCFA short-chain fatty acid

SIDS sudden infant death syndrome

SLE systemic lupus erythematosus

SLS sodium lauryl sulfate

S/S signs and symptoms

SSRI selective serotonin reuptake inhibitor

TCA trichloroacetic acid

TCM traditional Chinese medicine

TMJ temporomandibular joint

TPN total parenteral nutrition

TSH thyroid-stimulating hormone

tsp teaspoon(s)

TTP thrombotic thrombocytopenic purpura

URI upper respiratory infection

USDA United States Department of Agriculture

UTI urinary tract infection

UV ultraviolet

WBC white blood cell

yr year

absinthe | **Uses:** Insufficient evidence; | **Preg:** Possibly unsafe because some products may contain thujone (a neurotoxin); | **CIs:** Allergy/hypersensitivity, Seizure disorders, Concurrent use of other thujone-containing herbs (e.g., sage, tansy, yarrow); | **ADRs:** absinthism (chronic use; characterized by brain damage, epilepsy, gastrointestinal distress, hallucinations, paralysis, tremors), muscle ache, nausea/vomiting, renal toxicity, rhabdomyolysis, seizures; | **Interactions:** Anticonvulsants (interfere with effects), drugs that lower seizure threshold (↑ risk of seizures); | **Dose:** Insufficient evidence; | **Monitor:** Neurological function; kidney function; | **Notes:** Wormwood or *Artemisia absinthum* is found in various foods and drinks. It has a high alcohol content. The active ingredient in wormwood, responsible for the additional effects, is thujone, a neurotoxin.

abuta *(Cissampelos pareira)* | **Uses:** Menstrual cramps; | **Preg:** Avoid use due to possible abortifacient properties; | **CIs:** Allergy/hypersensitivity, Pregnancy, Lactation; | **ADRs:** no side effects have been reported; | **Interactions:** Insufficient available evidence; | **Dose:** 1 or 2 g of powdered abuta bark have been taken by mouth twice daily. Abuta has also been used as a 4:1 tincture in a dose of 2–4 mL twice daily; | **Monitor:** Insufficient available evidence; | **Notes:** Be aware that many plants related to abuta look alike. Some abuta products may be contaminated with similar plants

acacia *(Acacia arabica, Acacia senegal)* | **Uses:** Plaque; | **Preg:** Not recommended due to lack of sufficient data; | **CIs:** Allergy/hypersensitivity; | **ADRs:** asthma, bloating, contact dermatitis, diarrhea, flatulence, gastrointestinal upset, HEMOLYTIC ANEMIA, rhinitis, urticaria; | **Interactions:** ↓ the absorption of amoxicillin, antineoplastic agents, ethanol (alcohol), iron, oral drugs, tannin-containing herbs and supplements and other herbs or supplements with similar effects; | **Dose:** For plaque, *Acacia arabica* chewing stick has been used daily; | **Monitor:** Insufficient available evidence; | **Notes:** Acacia may reduce the absorption of amoxicillin. Dose times should be separated by at least 4 hours.

acai *(Euterpe oleracea)* | **Uses:** There are no scientific studies on the use of acai for medical conditions; | **Preg:** Not recommended due to lack of sufficient data; | **CIs:** Allergy/hypersensitivity; | **ADRs:** edema, hypertension, ulcers or intestinal bleeding; | **Interactions:** Insufficient available evidence; | **Dose:** Insufficient available evidence; | **Monitor:** Blood pressure; | **Notes:** N/A.

A

acerola *(Malpighia glabra, Malpighia punicifolia)* | **Uses:** There are no scientific studies on the use of acerola for medical conditions; | **Preg:** Not recommended due to lack of sufficient data; | **CIs:** Allergy/hypersensitivity; | **ADRs:** abdominal cramps, fatigue, insomnia, nausea, sleepiness; | **Interactions:** acidic or basic drugs (may alter excretion), anticoagulants (↓ anticoagulant activity of warfarin), estrogen, fluphenazine, alfalfa, ↑ absorption of iron, soy, vitamin C, herbs or supplements with similar effects; | **Dose:** Insufficient available evidence; | **Monitor:** Insufficient available evidence; | **Notes:** Doses of 1 g or more of acerola may cause diarrhea. Large doses may cause kidney stones.

ackee *(Blighia sapida)* | **Uses:** There are no scientific studies on the use of ackee for medical conditions; | **Preg:** Not recommended due to lack of sufficient data; | **CIs:** Allergy/hypersensitivity; | **ADRs:** abdominal pain, cholestatic jaundice, coma, confusion, convulsions, diarrhea, dizziness, encephalopathy, fatty degeneration of the liver, fever, headache, hypoglycemia, hypotonia, Jamaican vomiting sickness, liver centrilobular zonal necrosis, nausea, neutropenia, pruritus, pulmonary toxicities, right upper quadrant pain, stupor, sweating, tachycardia, tachypnea, thirst, thrombocytosis (without anemia), tonic-clonic convulsions, toxic hypoglycemic syndrome, vomiting, weakness; | **Interactions:** Antidiabetic drugs, methylene blue (MB), herbs and supplements with similar effects; | **Dose:** Insufficient available evidence; | **Monitor:** Blood glucose, CBC, S/S of hypoglyemia; | **Notes:** Hypoglycin A (the causative toxic substance in ackee) is contained in the aril, seeds, and husks of ackee fruit at various stages of ripeness. Unripe ackee fruit is unsafe for ingestion.

aconite *(Aconitum napellus)* | **Uses:** Arrhythmia, heart failure, postoperative pain in infants (homeopathic dilutions); | **Preg:** Avoid use; | **CIs:** Allergy/hypersensitivity; | **ADRs:** agitation, arrhythmia, blurred vision, cardiovascular dysfunctions, coma, convulsions, diarrhea, dimness of vision, dizziness, dyspnea, hypersalivation, hypoglycemia, hypokalemia, hypotension, hypothermia, leukocytosis, muscle cramps, nausea, paresthesia, renal damage, stiff muscles, throat constriction, ventricular tachyarrhythmias, vomiting; | **Interactions:** Antiarrhythmics, antihypertensives, anesthetics, digoxin, diuretics, and herbs or supplements with similar effects (like foxglove and Siberian ginseng); | **Dose:** Aconite homeopathic preparations of 6–30 C have been used; Tincture, pain: 1–5 drops 4 times per day; | **Monitor:** Toxic symptoms (vomiting, dizziness, muscle spasms, throat constriction, tingling of mouth, fingers, or toes, ventricular tachycardia, and possibly death); **Notes:** Aconite is known for being toxic and is UNSAFE when used orally or topically. Poisoning may cause severe adverse effects to the heart and CNS.

activated charcoal **Uses:** Poisoning, cholestasis (pregnancy), diarrhea, diuresis, hypercholesterolemia, gastric cancer, neonatal jaundice, wound healing; **Preg:** In cases of acute poisoning, activated charcoal can be administered to women who are pregnant or lactating. Birth defects have not been reported in women who have ingested activated charcoal; moreover, no problems have been reported in nursing infants of mothers who have ingested activated charcoal. Some anecdotal information recommends avoidance during pregnancy and lactation; therefore, potential benefits during risk must be weighed before activated charcoal administration; **CIs:** Allergy/hypersensitivity, Variegate porphyria, Severe gastrointestinal obstruction, Paralytic ileus, Unconsciousness, Prolonged use (more than 3–4 days); **ADRs:** abdominal fullness, aspiration, black stools, constipation, DIARRHEA (with sorbitol-containing products), dizziness, drowsiness, fluid/electrolyte abnormalities, gastrointestinal obstruction, headache, nausea/vomiting, nutrient/drug depletion; **Interactions:** ↑ antibiotics, anticholinergics (↑ activated charcoal effectiveness), N-acetyl cysteine, ↓ beta blockers, ↓ oral contraceptives, ipecac (↓ activated charcoal effectiveness), oral agents (↓ absorption), sorbitol (↑ activated charcoal effectiveness), may interact with agents with similar effects or related mechanisms of action (antilipemic); **Dose:** Oral: 25- to 100-g single dose, then give additional doses at 12.5 g given every hour, 25 g given every 2 hours, or 50 g given every 4 hours; may be given in a slurry with sorbitol; **Monitor:** LFTs, lipid profile, renal function tests; **Notes:** Activated charcoal interferes with the absorption of many drugs, herbs, foods, and vitamin supplements.

active hexose correlated compound (AHCC) **Uses:** Antioxidant, immune function, cancer, diabetes; **Preg:** Not recommended due to insufficient evidence; **CIs:** Allergy /hypersensitivity; **ADRs:** bloating, ↓ blood glucose, diarrhea, fatigue, foot cramps, headache, nausea; **Interactions:** May ↓ chemotherapy-induced side effects, may interact with agents with similar effects or related mechanisms of action (immunomodulatory, antidiabetic); **Dose:** Oral: 3 g daily; **Monitor:** Blood glucose, immune parameters, LFTs, renal function tests; **Notes:** Extracted from the mycelia of Basidiomycota mushrooms, including shiitake (*Lentinula edodes*);

A

contains a mix of oligosaccharides (74% of AHCC, 20% 1,4-glucan type), amino acids, lipids, and minerals.

adder's tongue | **Uses:** Insufficient evidence; | **Preg:** Not recommended due to insufficient evidence; | **CIs:** Allergy/hypersensitivity; | **ADRs:** insufficient evidence; | **Interactions:** Antiviral agents (altered effects); | **Dose:** Insufficient evidence; | **Monitor:** N/A; | **Notes:** Adder's tongue ferns make up the family Ophioglossaceae and have been used in folk medicine as a poultice for treating wounds.

adrenal extract | **Uses:** There are no scientific studies on the use of adrenal extract for medical conditions; | **Preg:** Not recommended due to lack of sufficient data; | **CIs:** Allergy/hypersensitivity; | **ADRs:** insufficient available evidence; | **Interactions:** Hypophysis extract, minerals; | **Dose:** Insufficient available evidence; | **Monitor:** Insufficient available evidence; | **Notes:** Avoid using adrenal extract parenterally because bacterial infections have been reported. Adrenal extracts are derived from raw cow, pig, or sheep adrenal glands, so there is concern about contamination with diseased animal parts.

African wild potato ***(Hypoxis hemerocallidea)*** | **Uses:** Benign prostatic hyperplasia (BPH); | **Preg:** Not recommended due to lack of sufficient data; | **CIs:** Allergy/hypersensitivity; | **ADRs:** anxiety, diarrhea, erectile dysfunction, hepatotoxicity, ↓ libido, nausea, renal dysfunction, skin rash, stomach cramps, ↓ urine output, vomiting; | **Interactions:** Antidiabetic agents, antiretroviral drugs, CYP450 3A4 substrates, diuretics, nephrotoxic agents, carotene, vitamin E, herbs or supplements with similar effects; | **Dose:** For BPH, 60–130 mg of beta-sitosterol (a constituent of African wild potato) divided into 2–3 doses daily has been used; | **Monitor:** Blood glucose, S/S of hypoglycemia; | **Notes:** African wild potato contains beta-sitosterol; may alter insulin requirements.

agar | **Uses:** Hyperglycemia/glucose intolerance, neonatal hyperbilirubinemia; | **Preg:** Not recommended due to insufficient evidence; | **CIs:** Allergy/hypersensitivity; | **ADRs:** diarrhea, irritation, pain, phytobezoars; | **Interactions:** May interact with agents with similar effects or related mechanisms of action (antilipemic, antidiabetic, hepatotoxic, laxative); | **Dose:** Oral: 4–16 g daily, powder, 1–2 tsp with 8 oz water; 180 g agar gel; | **Monitor:** Bilirubin, lipid profile; | **Notes:** Although no specific studies of the carcinogenicity or other long-term investigations of agar have been made, agar has a long history of use as a gelling agent and bulk component of experimental animal diets. Therefore, it is reasonable to conclude that it produces no significant chronic effects. Take each dose with 8 oz of water. Agar fiber may impair the absorption of oral drugs and supplements. Separate administration times from agar to minimize potential interactions (e.g., 1 hour before or a few hours after taking agar).

agaric *(Amanita muscaria)* | **Uses:** There are no scientific studies on the use of agaric for medical conditions; | **Preg:** Avoid use; | **CIs:** Allergy/hypersensitivity to agaric or basidiomycetes; | **ADRs:** deep sleep, diarrhea, excitement, flushing, gastrointestinal symptoms, hallucination, hepatotoxicity, hypo-/hypertension, mania, nausea, nervous system dysfunction, transient ↑ followed by ↓ in respiratory rate, sinusitis, vomiting; | **Interactions:** Nephrotoxic agents; | **Dose:** Insufficient available evidence; | **Monitor:** Toxic symptoms; | **Notes:** Agaric has been traditionally used in rituals as a hallucinogen. Based on several case reports and accidental toxicity reports, consumption of agaric is not recommended.

agave *(Agave americana)* | **Uses:** There are no scientific studies on the use of agave for medical conditions; | **Preg:** Caution due to contraceptive properties; | **CIs:** Allergy/hypersensitivity; | **ADRs:** hyperglycemia, liver disease, skin rash, vascular damage; | **Interactions:** Antidiabetic agents, contraceptives, steroids; | **Dose:** Insufficient available evidence; | **Monitor:** Insufficient available evidence; | **Notes:** Agave is useful as a sugar alternative because with a 90% fructose, it has a low glycemic index. Steroid hormone precursors are obtained from the leaves.

agrimony *(Agrimonia eupatoria, Agrimonia procera)* | **Uses:** Cutaneous disorders, gastrointestinal disorders; | **Preg:** Caution due to the risk of increased bleeding; | **CIs:** Allergy/hypersensitivity; | **ADRs:** cyanosis, esophageal cancer, gastrointestinal upset, hepatotoxicity, hypotension, nausea, necrosis, nephrotoxicity, photosensitivity; | **Interactions:** ↑ risk of bleeding with anticoagulants/antiplatelets, ↓ blood glucose levels with antidiabetic agents, antihypertensives, estrogens, nephrotoxic agents; | **Dose:** Liquid extract (1:1 in 25% alcohol): 1–3 mL has been used 3 times daily. Tincture (1:5 in 45% alcohol): 1–4 mL has been used 3 times daily. 3–5 mL has been used every 2–3 hours for mild symptoms. Agrimony leaf: 1 cup or 3–5 mL of tincture has been used every 2–3 hours; then

A

decreased as symptoms decrease. Tea: 1 tsp has been used in 8 oz of water every 2–3 hours for acute symptoms. Dried herb: 2–4 g has been used by infusion (injected) 3 times daily. A typical dose of agrimony is 3 g daily. Poultice (medical dressing): A poultice is typically applied several times daily using approximately 10% water extract, which is prepared by boiling agrimony at low heat for 10–20 minutes; | **Monitor:** PT/INR, blood glucose, S/S of hypoglycemia, blood pressure; | **Notes:** May alter insulin requirements.

albizia | **Uses:** Insufficient evidence; | **Preg:** Not recommended due to insufficient evidence; | **CIs:** Allergy/hypersensitivity; | **ADRs:** asthma, sedation; | **Interactions:** antidepressants (↑ risk of serotonin syndrome), chloroquine (synergistic effects), CNS depressants (additive sedation); dopamine agonists (altered effects), fertility agents (interferes with effects), GABAergic drugs (altered effects), immunosuppressants (altered effects); | **Dose:** Liquid extract (1:2): 1.25–6.25 mL PO qd; | **Monitor:** N/A; | **Notes:** *Albizia* is an Asian herb native to Southern and Eastern Asia, from Iran to China and Korea, which is known to many by its more common name of mimosa, or silk tree. It is an ornamental tree producing fine red filamentous flowers during the summer.

alfalfa ***(Medicago sativa)*** | **Uses:** Atherosclerosis, diabetes, hyperlipidemia; | **Preg:** Avoid use due to possible uterine stimulating effects; | **CIs:** Allergy/hypersensitivity to alfalfa, clover, grass, lupus; Surgery; Hormone-sensitive conditions; | **ADRs:** abnormal immune system function, dermatitis, diarrhea, estrogen-like effects, fatigue, flatulence, gastrointestinal upset and discomfort, gout flares, hypoglycemia, hypokalemia, larger/more frequent stools, lupus-like reactions, muscle pain, pancytopenia, photosensitivity, renal dysfunction, ↑ thyroid hormone levels; | **Interactions:** Alcohol, anticoagulants (contains large amounts of vitamin K), antidiabetic agents, antilipemic agents, azathioprine, calcium, contraceptives, cyclosporine, disulfiram, immunosuppressants, photosensitizing agents, prednisone, thyroid hormones, vitamin K, herbs and supplements with similar effects; | **Dose:** For hyperlipidemia, 40 g of heated prepared seeds 3 times daily with food has been used. Cholestaid (esterin processed alfalfa), 2 tablets (1 g each) orally 3 times daily for up to 2 months have been used; | **Monitor:** PT/INR; blood glucose, S/S of hypoglycemia, lipid profile, serum antinuclear antibodies; | **Notes:** Monitor INR in individuals using warfarin and alfalfa. Adjust dose, if necessary.

A

algin *(Ascophyllum nodosum)* | **Uses:** There are no scientific studies on the use of algin for medical conditions; | **Preg:** Avoid use due to possible cervical dilation; | **CIs:** Allergy/hypersensitivity; | **ADRs:** cervical dilation; | **Interactions:** The fiber in algin may reduce the body's ability to absorb drugs, herbs, or supplements taken by mouth; antihypertensives (additive effects), antilipemic agents (additive effects); | **Dose:** Insufficient available evidence; | **Monitor:** Blood pressure, lipid profile; | **Notes:** N/A.

alizarin | **Uses:** Viral infections; | **Preg:** Avoid use; | **CIs:** Allergy/hypersensitivity; | **ADRs:** discolored urine, dyspnea, insomnia, muscle rigidity, nausea, rash, vomiting, weakness; | **Interactions:** Tetracyclines; | **Dose:** As a tea, 1 to 2 cups madder bark tea (prepared by using 1 tsp madder bark boiled in a covered container with 3 cups of water for 30 min, then cooled slowly and taken cold) has been taken daily. Topically, 0.2%–0.5% ointment has been used; | **Monitor:** Insufficient available evidence; | **Notes:** N/A.

alkanna *(Alkanna tinctoria)* | **Uses:** Anti-inflammatory, wound healing; | **Preg:** Not recommended due to lack of sufficient available evidence; | **CIs:** Allergy/hypersensitivity; Liver disease; | **ADRs:** HEPATOTOXICITY; | **Interactions:** CYP450 3A4 substrates, hepatotoxic agents; | **Dose:** Insufficient available evidence; | **Monitor:** LFTs; | **Notes:** Pyrrolizidine alkaloids found in alkanna may be potentially hepatotoxic.

allspice *(Pimenta dioica)* | **Uses:** There are no human studies for the use of allspice; | **Preg:** Not recommended due to lack of sufficient data; | **CIs:** Allergy/hypersensitivity to allspice, Balsam of Peru, tomatoes, lettuce, or carrots; | **ADRs:** skin rash; | **Interactions:** Antineoplastic agents, CYP450 substrates, immunosuppressants; | **Dose:** Insufficient available evidence; | **Monitor:** WBC count; | **Notes:** Allspice is sold either as whole dried fruits or in powdered form. The spice has a complex, peppery taste that resembles a mix of cinnamon, juniper, clove, and nutmeg. Historically, allspice was used to treat indigestion and flatulence.

aloe *(Aloe vera)* | **Uses:** Constipation, seborrheic dermatitis, genital herpes, psoriasis, cancer prevention, aphthous stomatitis, type 2 diabetes, dry skin, HIV infection, lichen planus,

A

skin burns, skin ulcers, ulcerative colitis, wound healing; | **Preg:** Avoid oral use; | **CIs:** Allergy/hypersensitivity; Ileus; | **ADRs:** abdominal cramps, dehydration, delayed wound healing, diarrhea, electrolyte imbalances, hepatitis, hypoglycemia, HYPOKALEMIA, laxative dependency, muscle spasms, palpitations, rash, redness or burning to skin (topical use); | **Interactions:** Antidiabetic agents (↓ blood glucose), antihypertensives, antineoplastic agents, antiretroviral agents, cardiac glycosides (↑ risk of adverse effect due to potassium depletion), contraceptives, corticosteroids, diuretics (↑ risk of electrolyte imbalances), hormone replacement therapy, licorice, and herbs or supplements with similar effects; | **Dose:** Orally, 40–70 mg capsules of aloe latex (dried inner lining of the leaf) have been taken by mouth daily for up to 7 days; diabetes (type 2): 5–15 mL aloe juice twice daily; HIV: 400 mg acemannan (polysaccharide constituent of aloe) 4 times daily. Topically, pure *Aloe vera* gel is used liberally on the skin 3–4 times per day; | **Monitor:** Blood glucose, S/S of hypoglycemia, electrolytes; | **Notes:** Anthroquinones found in aloe may be toxic; excessive laxative use may cause electrolyte imbalances and dependency.

alpha-hydroxy acids | **Uses:** Acne, dry skin, melasma, psoriasis, UV damage, wrinkled skin; | **Preg:** Topical use is likely safe; | **CIs:** Allergy/hypersensitivity; | **ADRs:** topical: blistering, burns, irritation, stinging; | **Interactions:** 5-FU (additive effects), corticosteroids (altered effects), retinoids (additive effects); | **Dose:** General: facial peels of 12%, 15%, 20%, 35%, 50%, and 70% applied twice weekly; | **Monitor:** Damaged skin; | **Notes:** Alpha hydroxy acids include glycolic acid, lactic acid, citric acid, and malic acid, among others. These compounds are derived from fruit, sugarcane, or milk sugars. Over-the-counter topical preparations are available, as are prescription products. In general, over-the-counter preparations contain approximately 5%–8% AHA.

alpha-ketoglutarate (AKG) | **Uses:** Burns, childhood growth, dialysis, hepatic encephalopathy, liver cirrhosis, myocardial protection (in heart surgery), postsurgical recovery, trauma; | **Preg:** Not recommended due to insufficient evidence; | **CIs:** Allergy/hypersensitivity; | **ADRs:** abdominal pain, bloating, diarrhea, nausea/vomiting, thiamine-dependent sideroblastic anemia; | **Interactions:** Lipofundin (fat emulsion) (alters AKG concentrations); | **Dose:** Burn and wound healing, enteral tube: 10 g (as a single bolus), 20 g (10 g, 2 boluses), or 30 g (10 g, 3 boluses) of ornithine alpha-ketoglutarate (OKG) (10 g OKG, dissolved in 200 mL water and administered directly through enteral tube); topical: 1%. Postsurgical recovery, IV infusion: 25–30 g AKG/hour after the operation. Children, growth development: 15 g OKG added to parenteral nutrition; | **Monitor:** N/A; | **Notes:** According to most experts, alpha-ketoglutarate likely is safe to be used as an enteral nutritional supplement for burn injuries and other trauma. Ornithine alpha-ketoglutarate (OAKG or OKG) is a common subtype of AKG and a salt formed of two molecules of ornithine and one molecule of AKG.

alpha-lipoic acid (1,2-dithiolane-3-pentanoic acid) | **Uses:** Diabetes, nerve pain/damage, alcoholic liver disease, cognitive function, glaucoma, burning mouth syndrome, pancreatic cancer, postoperative tissue injury prevention, radiation injuries, renal disease, skin aging, wound healing; | **Preg:** Not recommended due to lack of sufficient data; | **CIs:** Allergy/hypersensitivity; | **ADRs:** altered thyroid hormones, bleeding, bruising, dizziness, dyspnea, hypoglycemia, liver damage, nausea, paresthesia, pruritus, skin rash, vomiting; | **Interactions:** Antidiabetic agents, anti-inflammatory agents, antineoplastic agents, CNS depressants, CYP450 substrates, thyroid hormones, vasodilators, vitamin C, herbs and supplements with similar effects; | **Dose:** 100–1,800 mg have been taken by mouth daily for up to 2 yr; | **Monitor:** Blood glucose, S/S of hypoglycemia, blood pressure, thyroid hormones; | **Notes:** May alter insulin requirements.

alpinia *(Alpinia galanga)* | **Uses:** Fungal infections; | **Preg:** Not recommended due to lack of sufficient available data; | **CIs:** Allergy/hypersensitivity; | **ADRs:** diuresis, drowsiness/prolonged sleep, gastrointestinal complaints, hypoglycemia, hypotension, pruritus, psychomotor excitation and writhing, ↑ RBCs, slow movement, ↑ weight of sexual organs; | **Interactions:** Antacids, antidiabetic agents, antihypertensives, diuretics, H2-blockers, proton pump inhibitors (PPIs), herbs and supplements with similar effects; | **Dose:** 2–4 g of the herb per day or 1 cup of the tea (prepared by steeping 0.5–1 g alpinia in 150 mL of hot water for 10 min and then straining), 30 min before meals, has been taken; | **Monitor:** Blood pressure, blood glucose, S/S of hypoglycemia; | **Notes:** May alter insulin requirements.

amaranth (*Amaranthus* spp.) | **Uses:** Antioxidant; cardiovascular disease; immune system function; night vision; | **Preg:** Not recommended due to lack of sufficient and conflicting evidence; | **CIs:** Allergy/hypersensitivity; | **ADRs:** clinical side effects have not been reported; may contain heavy

A

metals and nitrates; high doses have shown toxicity in rats; | **Interactions:** Antidiabetic agents (↓ blood glucose), antihistamines, antihypertensive agents (↓ blood pressure), antilipemic agents (additive effects), may ↑ nephrotoxic agents (due to oxalic acid); | **Dose:** Tea: 1 tsp in 1 cup water, 1–2 cups daily; 200–600 mg squalene (amaranth constituent) daily; 18 mg amaranth oil daily for 3 weeks; 850 mcg of retinol equivalents given to pregnant women daily; | **Monitor:** Blood glucose, blood pressure, lipid profile, renal function tests; | **Notes:** Amaranth has been historically used as a food. It is cultivated primarily for its grain.

ambrette *(Abelmoschus moschatus)* | **Uses:** Insufficient evidence; | **Preg:** Not recommended due to insufficient evidence; | **CIs:** Allergy/hypersensitivity; | **ADRs:** contact dermatitis, photosensitivity; | **Interactions:** Antidiabetic agents (↑ risk of hypoglycemia), photosensitizers (↑ risk of photosensitivity); | **Dose:** Insufficient evidence; | **Monitor:** Blood glucose; | **Notes:** Ambrette seeds are commonly used medicinally in India and throughout the Caribbean as a tea or tincture.

American (false) hellebore (*Veratrum* spp.) | **Uses:** Cancer, cardiovascular dysfunction, pre-eclampsia, renal dysfunction; | **Preg:** AVOID USE due to known toxicity and teratogenicity; | **CIs:** Allergy/hypersensitivity; Extreme caution with cardiovascular disease and renal dysfunction; | **ADRs:** arrhythmias, birth defects, bradycardia, DEATH, depressed mental status, headache, hypotension, nausea/vomiting, vertigo; | **Interactions:** Antihypertensive agents (↓ blood pressure), beta-adrenergic agents (may ↓ beta-adrenergic activity), diuretics (may ↓ glomerular filtration rate); | **Dose:** 20–60 Craw units of Vertavis, 0.2 mL of Veratrone for pre-eclampsia, 1.2–1.6 mcg/kg of the jervine alkaloid protoveratrine, 5–15 minims daily of American hellebore tincture, 0.2–1.0 mL of Veratrone jervine alkaloids; | **Monitor:** Heart rate, blood pressure, renal function tests (BUN and creatinine); | **Notes:** Plants of the genus *Veratrum* (including American hellebore) are commonly confused with the true hellebores (genus *Helleborus*). Thus, *Vertarum* species are commonly referred to as "false" hellebores. The plant is HIGHLY TOXIC.

American pawpaw *(Asimina triloba)* | **Uses:** Cancer, lice; | **Preg:** Contraindicated due to cytotoxic effects; | **CIs:** Hypersensitivity, Pregnancy; | **ADRs:** nausea, pruritus, urticaria, vomiting; | **Interactions:** May ↓ antioxidants (due to oxidative effects), may ↓ coenzyme Q10 (↓ electron transfer), may ↓ 7-ketosteroid; | **Dose:** Cancer: 12.5–50 mg extract 4 times daily with food for up to 18 months. Lice: 40 mL Paw Paw Lice Remover Shampoo (0.5% pawpaw extract, 1% thymol, and 0.5% tea tree oil) applied 3 times to dry hair, once every 8 days for up to 24 days; | **Monitor:** Insufficient available evidence; | **Notes:** Pawpaw fruit has been used traditionally as a food. Pawpaw extracts are made from twigs, which are high in acetogenins; American pawpaw extracts were determined to be nonmutagenic (Ames test), nonsensitizing (guinea pig skin), and tolerable (up to 1% of mouse diet).

American wormseed | **Uses:** Parasitic infection; | **Preg:** Avoid use; | **CIs:** Allergy/hypersensitivity; Oral use; | **ADRs:** toxic symptoms: epileptiform spasms, fasciculation, gastroenteritis, kidney irritation (eg, flank pain, painful urination), stupor, visual disorders; | **Interactions:** Antibiotics (synergistic effects), antifungals (additive effects); | **Dose:** Decoctions (a preparation in which plant matter is boiled in water to made a concentrated extract): containing up to 300 mg of dry plant material per kilogram of body weight; electuary (a form of medicine made of conserves and powders, in the consistence of honey) of bruised fruit: 20 grains (1,300 mg); fluid extract: prepared with 0.5–1 drachm (1.78–3.55 mL); | **Monitor:** Toxic effects; | **Notes:** American wormseed is TOXIC and cross-allergy exists with Asteraceae/Compositae family (ragweed, chrysanthemums, marigolds, daisies).

amylase inhibitors | **Uses:** Diabetes, obesity/weight loss; | **Preg:** Not recommended due to insufficient evidence; | **CIs:** Allergy/hypersensitivity; Pregnancy; | **ADRs:** abdominal discomfort, diarrhea; | **Interactions:** May ↑ antidiabetic agents (due to ↓ postprandial glucose), weight loss agents (additive effects); | **Dose:** General: 1,500–6,000 mg before meals. Diabetes: 4–6 g daily up to 7 days. Weight loss: 3,000 amylase inhibitor units (AIU) from Phase 2 dietary supplement, for 30 days; 1,500 mg Phase 2 twice daily for 8 weeks (no evidence of benefit); | **Monitor:** Blood glucose; | **Notes:** Commercially available amylase inhibitors are extracted from white kidney bean (*Phaseolus vulgaris*) or wheat. In humans, use of amylase inhibitor has been shown to reduce intestinal amylase activity and decrease absorption of carbohydrates by the intestine.

andiroba (*Carapa* spp.) | **Uses:** Insect repellent; | **Preg:** Not recommended due to insufficient evidence; | **CIs:** Allergy/hypersensitivity, Infants; | **ADRs:** case report of severe burns

A

following pediatric topical application of andiroba; contains cyclic terpenes known to induce dermatological inflammation; | **Interactions:** Insufficient available evidence; | **Dose:** Insect repellent: andiroba oil (100% or 15%) applied topically to the forearm; | **Monitor:** Contact dermatitis or inflammation; | **Notes:** As an insect repellent, andiroba oil has been shown to be slightly superior to soy oil control but significantly inferior to N,N-diethyl-3-methylbenzamide (DEET).

andrographis *(Andrographis paniculata)* | **Uses:** Upper respiratory infection (treatment and prevention), familial Mediterranean fever, influenza; | **Preg:** Not recommended during pregnancy due to possible contraceptive effects observed in animal studies; | **CIs:** Allergy/hypersensitivity, Pregnancy, Fertility disorders, Those attempting to conceive; | **ADRs:** generally mild, infrequent, and self-limiting; abdominal discomfort, ↓ blood pressure, ↓ blood glucose, diarrhea, fatigue, headache, nausea, vomiting, ↓ spermatogenesis (observed in animal studies); | **Interactions:** Antidiabetic agents (↑ risk of hypoglycemia), anticoagulants/antiplatelets (↑ risk of bleeding), antihypertensives (↑ risk of hypotension); | **Dose:** General: 500–3,000 mg leaf 3 times daily. Digestive disorders: tea (1 tsp herb per 8 oz water) taken with meals; | **Monitor:** Blood glucose, blood pressure, coagulation panel; | **Notes:** Based on available research, andrographis appears to be safe and well tolerated at recommended doses; long-term safety remains unclear.

androstenediol | **Uses:** Athletic enhancement; | **Preg:** Not recommended due to hormonal effects and insufficient evidence; | **CIs:** Allergy/hypersensitivity, Pregnancy; Lactation; Hormone-sensitive cancers, Pediatric use; | **ADRs:** ↑ estrogen levels, ↓ HDL, ↑ testosterone levels, ↑ risk of tendon ruptures; possible ADRs from contaminants (e.g., ephedrine, caffeine, steroids); | **Interactions:** Estrogens (↑ risk of adverse effects of estrogens), testosterone (↑ risk of adverse effects of testosterone); androgenic effects not blocked by two potent antiandrogens—hydroxyflutamide (Eulexin) and bicalutamide (Casodex); | **Dose:** Insufficient available information; | **Monitor:** Estrogen levels, lipid profile, testosterone levels; | **Notes:** Sales of androstenediols and other proandrogen hormones are prohibited without a prescription in the United States.

androstenedione | **Uses:** Insufficient evidence; | **Preg:** Avoid use; | **CIs:** Allergy/hypersensitivity; Pregnancy; | **ADRs:** acne, amenorrhea, clitoromegaly, coarse skin, depression, early development of secondary sex characteristics (boys), early closure of the growth plates, ↑ estrogen, excess hair growth,

A

↓ HDL, hirsutism, infertility, male-pattern baldness, menorrhea, psychosis, ↑ risk of cardiovascular disease, virilization; | **Interactions:** Alcohol (alters metabolism of androstenedione), androgens (additive effects); antidiabetic agents (alters metabolism of androstenedione), antilipemic agents (altered effects), aromatase inhibitors (alters metabolism of androstenedione), cabergoline (alters metabolism of androstenedione), dexamethasone (alters plasma concentrations of androstenedione), estrogens (↑ estrogenic effects), GnRH agonists (↓ androstenedione levels), ketoconazole (alters metabolism of androstenedione), octreotide (↓ androstenedione levels); | **Dose:** 100–200 mg PO qd; | **Monitor:** Estrogens, lipid profile, testosterone levels; | **Notes:** Androstenedione, or "andro," is a testosterone prohormone. Testosterone prohormones are marketed as testosterone-enhancing and muscle-building nutritional supplements. Androstenedione has been banned by the International Olympics Committee, the National Collegiate Athletic Association, the National Basketball Association, the National Football League, the World Natural Body Building Federation, and the World Anti-Doping Agency.

angel's trumpet (*Brugmansia* and *Datura* spp.) | **Uses:** There are no scientific studies on the use of angel's trumpet for medical conditions; | **Preg:** Avoid use; | **CIs:** Allergy/hypersensitivity, Narrow-angle glaucoma, Obstructive bowel disease, Oral use (TOXIC tropane alkaloids), Pregnancy and lactation, (tropane alkaloids TOXIC), Ulcerative colitis, Urinary retention; | **ADRs:** ANTICHOLINERGIC POISONING: agitation, altered mental status, ataxia, ↓ bowel sounds, cardiovascular collapse, coma, confusion, DEATH, delirium, disorientation, dry skin and mucous membranes, fever, flushing, functional ileus, hallucination, hypertension, memory loss, mydriasis, myoclonic jerking, psychosis, respiratory failure, seizures, tachycardia, urinary retention; | **Interactions:** ANTICHOLINERGICS (↑ risk of adverse effects), anticoagulants/antiplatelets (↑ risk of bleeding), CNS depressants (additive effects); | **Dose:** Traditionally used as an enema, tea, or smoked to induce visions, any dosage is not recommended based on known toxicity; | **Monitor:** Blood pressure, coagulation panel, LFTs, renal function tests; | **Notes:** Angel's trumpet contains poisonous tropane alkaloids, particularly in the seeds and foliage. Ingestion can result in severe toxicity presenting as anticholinergic poisoning.

angostura (*Galipea officinalis*, syn. *Angostura trifoliata*) | **Uses:** There are no scientific studies on the use of angostura for medical conditions; | **Preg:** Not recommended

A

due to insufficient evidence; | **CIs:** Allergy/hypersensitivity; | **ADRs:** very little information regarding potential adverse effects; | **Interactions:** May ↑ antibiotics, antimalarials, antineoplastics, and antiparasitics due to in vitro activity against pathogens and tumor cells; | **Dose:** Insufficient available information, extracts and pure tetrahydroquinoline alkaloids showed in vitro cytotoxic activity at concentrations ranging from 5.8 to higher than 50 mcg/mL; | **Monitor:** Insufficient available evidence; | **Notes:** Angostura has Generally Regarded as Safe (GRAS) status according to the FDA, and is approved as a food additive.

anhydrous crystalline maltose | **Uses:** Dry mouth (Sjögren's syndrome); | **Preg:** Not recommended due to lack of sufficient data; | **CIs:** Allergy/hypersensitivity; | **ADRs:** no significant adverse events were reported; | **Interactions:** Insufficient available evidence; | **Dose:** For dry mouth (Sjögren's syndrome), 200-mg lozenges 3 times daily for up to 24 weeks; | **Monitor:** Insufficient available evidence; | **Notes:** Anhydrous crystalline maltose has been used as a food stabilizer and a desiccant for use in foods, cosmetics, and pharmaceuticals.

anise ***(Pimpinella anisum)*** | **Uses:** There are no scientific studies on the use of anise for medical conditions; | **Preg:** Not recommended due to traditional use as an abortifacient; | **CIs:** Allergy/hypersensitivity, Hormone-dependent cancers; | **ADRs:** an anise-flavored beverage was associated with cardiorespiratory arrest, hypermineralocorticism, hypertension, hypokalemia, weakness; ↑ bleeding risk, estrogenic effects, photosensitivity; | **Interactions:** Anticoagulants/antiplatelets (↑ risk of bleeding), antidiabetic agents (↑ risk of hypoglycemia), diuretics (antagonistic effects); | **Dose:** Colic: 10–30 grains of bruised (lightly ground) or powdered seeds steeped in distilled hot water, taken in wineglassful doses; 4–20 drops of anise essential oil on sugar. Digestive aid: essence of aniseed in hot water at bedtime. Runny nose: tea made with 2 tsp bruised seed in 8 oz water; | **Monitor:** Blood glucose, coagulation panel, electrolytes, estrogen levels; | **Notes:** Anise is used both for medicinal purposes and for cooking in many cultures. Many anise-flavored beverages also contain licorice root, which has been associated with cardiovascular adverse effects. It is not to be confused with Chinese star anise *(Illicium verum)*.

annatto ***(Bixa orellana)*** | **Uses:** There are no scientific studies on the use of annatto for medical conditions; | **Preg:** Likely safe when used in amounts commonly found in food;

possibly safe in medicinal amounts/lack of sufficient information; | **CIs:** Allergy/hypersensitivity; | **ADRs:** anaphylaxis (rare), angioedema, ↑/↓ blood glucose, hypotension (severe), urticaria; | **Interactions:** Antidiabetic agents (↑/↓ blood glucose), antihypertensives (↑ risk of hypotension), anti-inflammatory agents (additive effects), CNS depressants (↑ risk of sedation); CYP1A1 and 2B substrates (altered drug levels); | **Dose:** General: 1–2 g of powdered leaf in tablets or capsules twice daily. 4:1 tincture: 2–4 mL twice daily. Ground annatto seed powder: 10–20 mg daily; | **Monitor:** Blood glucose; | **Notes:** Annatto's history of use as a food coloring is well established worldwide, and current trends show that it is being used increasingly in body care products.

antineoplastons | **Uses:** Cancer, HIV, sickle cell anemia/thalassemia; | **Preg:** Not recommended due to risk of fetal toxicity; | **CIs:** Allergy/hypersensitivity, Pregnancy, Lactation; | **ADRs:** abdominal pain, abdominal upset, agranulocytosis, cerebral edema, chills, DEATH, dizziness, eosinophilia, fever, finger rigidity, flatulence, granulocytopenia, headache, hypernatremia, hypotension, leukocytosis, metabolic/electrolyte abnormalities, myelosuppression, nausea/vomiting, numbness, palpitations, peripheral edema, rash, somnolence, sore throat, thrombocytosis, vertigo; | **Interactions:** Antidiabetic agents (↑ risk of hypoglycemia), antineoplastic agents (altered effects), diuretics (↑ risk of hypokalemia); | **Dose:** General: Antineoplaston A10 doses range from 10–40 g PO daily or 100–288 mg/kg body weight IV daily for varying duration. Antineoplaston AS2-1 has been studied at doses from 12–30 g PO daily or 97–130 mg/kg of body weight IV daily for 425 days. Topical: Antineoplaston A 0.6–33 U/m^2/24 hr; | **Monitor:** Albumin, amylase levels, blood glucose, blood pressure, coagulation panel, electrolytes, WBCs; | **Notes:** Antineoplastons are generally used by those with serious illnesses such as advanced cancers. It is not clear if these effects may be from the illnesses themselves or caused by antineoplastons.

aortic acid | **Uses:** Chronic venous ulcers, intermittent claudication, atherosclerosis, cerebral ischemia, deep vein thrombosis, venous disorders; | **Preg:** Not recommended due to insufficient evidence; | **CIs:** Allergy/hypersensitivity; | **ADRs:** diarrhea (minor), headache (minor); | **Interactions:** Anticoagulants/antiplatelets (↑ risk of bleeding), antidiabetic agents (↑ risk of hypoglycemia), arginine (↓ levels of arginine), estrogens (altered effects), thyroid hormones (altered effects); vasopressors (antagonistic effects); | **Dose:** General: Mesoglycan (a constituent of aortic acid) up to 200 mg daily for up to 18 months; | **Monitor:** ALP, blood glucose, coagulation panel, creatinine, LFTs, lipid profile, urea; | **Notes:** The FDA cautions

A

against dietary supplements made from animal glands or organs, especially from cows and sheep from countries with known cases of bovine spongiform encephalitis (BSE, or "mad cow" disease) or scrapie. Currently, there are no available reports of transmission of BSE through aortic acid.

apple *(Malus domestica)* | **Uses:** Allergic rhinitis, antioxidant, burn wounds, cancer, diabetes, diarrhea (children), duodenal ulcers, enteritis (chronic), exercise recovery, hair growth, hypercholesterolemia, mercury poisoning, preoperative, radiation side effects (adjunct); | **Preg:** Likely safe in food amounts in pregnant or breastfeeding patients based on traditional use. Other uses are not recommended due to lack of sufficient evidence; | **CIs:** Allergy/hypersensitivity; | **ADRs:** abdominal discomfort, abdominal fullness, ↑ blood pressure, colic, dental caries, dental erosion, diarrhea, flatulence, nausea, oral lesions; | **Interactions:** Fexofenadine (↓ levels of fexofenadine), oral agents (↓ bioavailability), omeprazole (↓ gastric acid), quazepam (↓ absorption), ramipril (altered effects), theophylline (delayed absorption); may interact with agents with similar effects or related mechanisms of action (antibiotic, antilipemic, anticoagulant, antidiabetic, hypotensive); | **Dose:** Oral: apple pectin, 500 mg daily; juice, up to 1 L daily; apple pectin powder, 10 g twice daily for 6 months; | **Monitor:** Blood glucose, folate level, lipid profile, inflammatory markers; | **Notes:** Apple juice taken to soften gallstones, per unconfirmed sources.

apple cider vinegar | **Uses:** There are no scientific studies on the use of apple cider vinegar for medical conditions; | **Preg:** Not recommended in medicinal amounts due to lack of sufficient data; | **CIs:** Allergy/hypersensitivity; | **ADRs:** hypokalemia, osteoporosis, urinary disorders, weakened tooth enamel; | **Interactions:** Antacids (↓ effects), cardiac glycosides (↑ risk of toxicity, ↑ risk of hypokalemia), diuretics (↑ risk of hypokalemia), insulin (↑ risk of hypokalemia); | **Dose:** General: up to 1 oz apple cider vinegar in 4–8 oz water 3 times daily. Digestion aid: one 285-mg tablet daily with meals. Vaginitis: 3 cups of apple cider vinegar added to a hot bath. Viral hepatitis: retention enema containing chlorophyll, water, and apple cider vinegar; | **Monitor:** Potassium levels, renin levels, urinary ion gap; | **Notes:** Likely safe when used orally as a food flavoring and when used topically, diluted. Apple cider vinegar for food is standardized based on acidity content, usually 4%–8% acidity.

apricot *(Prunus armeniaca)* | **Uses:** Cancer; | **Preg:** Fruit likely safe when used as a food; kernel ingestion not recommended due to risk of cyanide poisoning and fetal malformations induced by Laetrile in hamsters; **CIs:** Allergy/hypersensitivity, Pregnancy, Lactation; **ADRs:** apricot kernels may cause chronic poisoning: ataxia, blindness, ↑ blood thiocyanate, cretinism, cyanosis, coma, demyelinating lesions and neuromyopathies, dizziness, drowsiness, dyspnea, headache, hypertonia, hypotension, hypothermia, lactic acidosis, mydriasis, nausea/vomiting, optic nerve lesions, paralysis, pulmonary edema, small bowel obstruction, tachypnea, urticaria, weakness; **Interactions:** antihypertensives (↑ risk of hypotension), laetrile (↑ amygdalin levels); **Dose:** 3–9 g kernel daily in divided doses (may be toxic); **Monitor:** Serum glucose, blood pressure; **Notes:** Apricot fruit is likely safe when ingested in food amounts. Apricot pit contains amygdalin, a plant compound that contains sugar and produces cyanide. Laetrile, an alternative cancer drug marketed in Mexico and other countries outside of the United States, is derived from amygdalin. Based on a phase II trial in 1982, the United States National Cancer Institute concluded that Laetrile, an acronym for levorotatory and mandelonitrile, is not an effective chemotherapeutic agent. Nonetheless, many people still travel to international clinics offering this therapy. Multiple cases of cyanide poisoning, including deaths, have been associated with Laetrile therapy. Laetrile remains unapproved by the United States Food and Drug Administration (FDA), which is also seeking a permanent injunction against three corporations for unlawfully promoting and marketing on their web sites injectable and oral formulations of Laetrile and apricot kernels for treating cancer.

arabinogalactan **Uses:** Hyperglycemia, hyperlipidemia, immune stimulation, renal disease (chronic renal failure); **Preg:** Supplemental use not recommended due to lack of sufficient evidence; **CIs:** Allergy/hypersensitivity to larch (*Larix sp.*); Not known to cross-react with arabinogalactans from ragweed or mugwort; **ADRs:** occupational exposure to larch dust may occur (larch arabinogalactan not implicated in allergic reactions); bloating, flatulence; **Interactions:** Amphotericin B (altered effects), andrographis (additive effects), antibiotics (additive effects), antidiabetic agents (↑ risk of hypoglycemia), antifungal agents (additive effects), antiviral/antiretroviral agents (additive effects), immunosuppressants (interfere with effects), oral agents (↓ absorption); **Dose:** General: 1–5 g daily for immune and prebiotic effects. Hyperglycemia: 8.4–50 g daily for up to 6 months (no evidence of benefit). Immune stimulation: 1,500 mg larch arabinogalactan daily (no evidence of benefit). Hyperlipidemia (cholesterol and triglycerides):

A

8.4–30 g daily for up to 6 months (no evidence of benefit); | **Monitor:** Blood glucose, fecal measurements, lipid profile; | **Notes:** Arabinogalactan (derived from *Larix occidentalis* or *Larix laricina*) has Generally Recognized as Safe (GRAS) status from the FDA as a dietary fiber in food.

arabinoxylan | **Uses:** Cancer, diabetes (type 2); | **Preg:** Not recommended due to lack of sufficient evidence; | **CIs:** Allergy/hypersensitivity, Pregnancy, Lactation (due to lack of safety data); | **ADRs:** no notable side effects reported in clinical studies; | **Interactions:** Antidiabetic agents (↑ risk of hypoglycemia), chemotherapy (may ↑ cytotoxic effects, ↓ adverse side effects); | **Dose:** General: 600 mg daily in divided doses for health maintenance. Cancer: 3 g MGN-3 daily for up to 6 months; 15, 30, and 45 mg/kg of MGN-3 daily for 2 months. Diabetes: 1–12 g of arabinoxylan-rich fiber daily; | **Monitor:** Blood glucose, LFTs, lipid profile; | **Notes:** Arabinoxylan compound is produced by enzymatically hydrolyzing the outer shell of rice bran using enzymes from *Hyphomycetes mycelia* mushroom extract. MGN-3 (or BioBran in Japan) is a hemicellulose complex containing arabinoxylan as a major component. The FDA ordered a permanent injunction against the marketing of MGN-3, charging that it has been promoted as a drug treatment for cancer, diabetes, and HIV.

arginine (L-arginine) | **Uses:** Adrenoleukodystrophy, altitude sickness, anal fissures, angina, autonomic failure, breast cancer, burns, CAD, chemotherapy (adjuvant), chest pain (noncardiac), critical illness, critical limb ischemia, dental pain, diabetes, diabetes (complications), diagnosis (pituitary disorder/growth hormone reserve test), erectile dysfunction, gastrointestinal surgery (recovery), heart failure, hyperlipidemia, HTN, immunomodulation, inborn errors of urea synthesis, intrauterine growth retardation, MELAS syndrome, migraine, peripheral vascular disease, pre-eclampsia, pressure ulcers, Raynaud's phenomenon, renal disorders, respiratory infections, restenosis prevention (after coronary angioplasty), senile dementia, sickle cell anemia, surgery (recovery), transplants (↓ rejection rates), would healing; | **Preg:** L-arginine has been used in pregnant women with pregnancy-induced HTN (pre-eclampsia) until 10 days after birth; 12 g of L-arginine PO daily between 28 and 36 weeks' gestation was used safely for pre-eclampsia; should be used only during pregnancy or lactation under medical supervision; | **CIs:** Allergy/hypersensitivity; | **ADRs:** abdominal bloating and cramps, anaphylaxis (associated with arginine injections; including rash, itching, shortness of breath; stomach discomfort), ↑/↓ blood glucose, ↑/↓ blood pressure, DEATH, diarrhea, electrolyte disturbances, gout, headache, hematuria, irritation, metabolic acidosis, nausea, numbness, periorbital edema, ↑ potassium (hyperkalemia), pruritus, restless leg, tissue necrosis, venous irritation; | **Interactions:** Analgesics (additive effects), antacids (antagonistic effects), anticoagulants/antiplatelets (↑ risk of bleeding), antihypertensives (additive effects/↑ risk of hypotension), diuretics (additive effects), lysine (↓ effects, particularly on cold sores), nitrates (additive vasodilation), potassium (altered effects), sildenafil (additive vasodilation and ↑ risk of hypotension); | **Dose:** General: 2–3 g 3 times daily PO. Clinical studies: 0.5–16 g of arginine daily PO for up to 6 months. Topical: arginine applied to the skin in order to improve wound healing; | **Monitor:** Blood pressure, blood glucose, BUN, coagulation panel, creatinine, electrolytes, hormone panel, potassium; | **Notes:** Arginine is considered a semiessential amino acid. Supplementation is needed in certain conditions (e.g., protein malnutrition, excessive ammonia production, excessive lysine intake, burns, infections, peritoneal dialysis, rapid growth, urea synthesis disorders, and sepsis). Patients who have had a recent myocardial infarction should avoid arginine supplements.

aristolochia (*Aristolochia* spp.) | **Uses:** There are no scientific studies on the use of aristolochia for medical conditions; | **Preg:** Not recommended due to known toxicity; | **CIs:** Aristolochia not recommended for any use due to known toxicity; | **ADRs:** hepatoxicity, nephrotoxicity (failure, tubulointerstitial fibrosis, Fanconi's syndrome, nephropathy, chronic renal insufficiency, urothelial cancer); | **Interactions:** Anticoagulants/antiplatelets (↑ risk of bleeding), CYP450 substrates (altered drug levels), nephrotoxic agents (↑ risk of nephrotoxicity), opiates (↓ effects); | **Dose:** Insufficient evidence; | **Monitor:** Coagulation panel, blood smear, CSF, hematocrit, LFTs, renal function tests, WBCs; | **Notes:** The FDA advises against the use of aristolochia and products containing aristolochic acid. In Britain, aristolochia is available by prescription only.

arnica (*Arnica* spp.) | **Uses:** Bruising, coagulation, diabetic retinopathy, diarrhea (acute, in children), osteoarthritis, pain (postoperative), postoperative ileus, stroke, trauma; | **Preg:** Avoid use due to known toxicity and potential uterine-stimulant effects; | **CIs:** Allergy/hypersensitivity, Inflammatory bowel conditions, Oral use or nonhomeopathic concentrations; | **ADRs:** abdominal pain, altered blood pressure, bleeding, coma, DEATH, diarrhea, drowsiness, dry mouth, eczema, hepatotoxicity,

A

myocardial infarction, miscarriage, mouth ulcers/blisters, muscle weakness, nausea/vomiting, nephrotoxicity, nervousness, pruritus, severe gastroenteritis Sweet's syndrome, swelling of lips/mouth/throat, tachycardia, ↓ urine flow, urticaria; | **Interactions:** Analgesics (additive effects), anti-inflammatory agents (additive effects), antihypertensives (additive effects/↑ risk of hypotension), antilipemic agents (additive effects); | **Dose:** Arnica is toxic if taken by mouth unless extremely diluted (homeopathic). Tincture, topical: 1:10 tincture prepared with 70% ethanol, 2–3 times per day. Cream/ointment, topical: 20%–25% tincture or a maximum of 15% arnica oil made from one part dried arnica flower head and five parts vegetable oil, applied 2–3 times per day; | **Monitor:** Blood pressure, coagulation panel, lipid profile; | **Notes:** The FDA has declared arnica an unsafe herb due to adverse effects when ingested orally. In contrast, the German market offers more than 100 preparations of arnica to its consumers.

arrowroot ***(Maranta arundinacea)*** | **Uses:** Diarrhea; | **Preg:** Medicinal amounts not recommended due to a lack of sufficient evidence; | **Cls:** Allergy/hypersensitivity; | **ADRs:** constipation, dyspepsia; | **Interactions:** Antidiarrheal agents (additive effects), laxatives (↓ effects); | **Dose:** 2 tsp powdered arrowroot 3 times daily PO with meals for 1 month; | **Monitor:** Insufficient evidence; | **Notes:** Arrowroot is likely safe when used in amounts commonly found in foods. Arrowroot may be sold as a flour.

arsenicum album | **Uses:** Insufficient evidence; | **Preg:** Organic arsenic (possibly safe), inorganic arsenic (avoid use); | **Cls:** Allergy/hypersensitivity, Inorganic arsenic, Long QT interval syndrome; | **ADRs:** anemia, bruising, coma, convulsions, DEATH, depression, encephalopathy, hepatotoxicity, peripheral neuropathy, PROLONGED QT INTERVAL; inorganic arsenic toxicity: alopecia, anorexia, arrhythmias, cancer, gastrointestinal disturbances, hyperkeratosis, hyperpigmentation; | **Interactions:** DRUGS THAT PROLONG QT INTERVAL (↑ risk of ventricular arrhythmias); | **Dose:** Arsenicum album 30 C and 200 C; arsenic trioxide, IV infusion: 0.15 mg/kg daily over 1–2 hours until bone marrow remission; do not exceed 60 doses; | **Monitor:** Toxic symptoms: abdominal pain, headache, lightheadedness, nausea/vomiting, numbness, thirst, weakness; | **Notes:** Arsenicum album is derived from arsenic. Arsenic may be highly diluted in homeopathic remedies for digestive and psychiatric problems, alcohol withdrawal, and allergies. Arsenic trioxide (Trisenox), an inorganic compound, is an FDA-approved drug. Inorganic arsenic has been associated with fatal toxicity.

arum | **Uses:** Insufficient evidence; | **Preg:** AVOID USE; | **CIs:** Allergy/hypersensitivity; Oral use; | **ADRs:** TOXIC effects: mucosal membrane irritation indicated by swelling of the lips, tongue, and palate; | **Interactions:** Calcium (interferes with mineral absorption), iron (interferes with mineral absorption); | **Dose:** Insufficient evidence; | **Monitor:** Toxic symptoms: swelling of tongue and throat; | **Notes:** Avoid use in all patients as *Arum* species are considered toxic with a lack of medicinal value. Significant levels of arsenic have been found in *Arum* species grown and exported from regions of India. Calcium oxalate, a constituent of *Arum*, is the most common constituent of kidney stones in humans.

asafoetida *(Ferula assafoetida)* | **Uses:** There are no scientific studies on the use of asafoetida for medical conditions; | **Preg:** Not recommended due to insufficient evidence and traditional use as an abortifacient; | **CIs:** Allergy/hypersensitivity, Pregnancy; | **ADRs:** insufficient evidence; | **Interactions:** Anticoagulants/antiplatelets (↑ risk of bleeding); anti-inflammatory agents (additive effects), antispasmodic agents (additive effects), antihypertensive agents (↑ risk of hypotension); | **Dose:** Insufficient evidence; | **Monitor:** Blood pressure, bone density, coagulation panel; | **Notes:** Asafoetida or asafetida is native to Iran; frequently used as a flavoring in Indian and Middle Eastern cuisine.

asarum (*Asarum* spp.) | **Uses:** There are no scientific studies on the use of asarum for medical conditions; | **Preg:** Not recommended due to known toxicity and insufficient evidence; | **CIs:** Allergy/hypersensitivity, Pregnancy, Renal dysfunction; | **ADRs:** contact dermatitis, DEATH, diarrhea, renal failure, skin rash; | **Interactions:** Nephrotoxic agents (↑ risk of nephrotoxicity), zinc (may ↓ blood levels); | **Dose:** General: 20–30 grains of asarum powder or 0.5 oz powdered root in 1 pint boiling water 2–3 times daily for short duration. Emesis: 0.5–1 drachms as an individual dose. Topical, premature ejaculation: 0.2% tincture (Indian God Lotion) sprayed on male genitalia, 30–60 minutes before sexual intercourse; homeopathic preparations have been used; | **Monitor:** Renal function tests; | **Notes:** Commonly known as snakeroot; not to be confused with bitter milkwort *(Polygala amara)* or senega *(Polygala senega)*, both also known as snakeroot.

ash (*Fraxinus* spp.) | **Uses:** Arthritis (gouty); | **Preg:** Not recommended due to lack of insufficient evidence; | **CIs:** Allergy/hypersensitivity, Autoimmune disease,

A

Immunocompromised, Renal dysfunction; | **ADRs:** insufficient evidence; | **Interactions:** Anticoagulants/antiplatelets (↑ risk of bleeding), anti-inflammatories/analgesics (additive effects), immunosuppressants (additive effects); | **Dose:** Insufficient evidence; | **Monitor:** Coagulation panel, uric acid levels; | **Notes:** Based on the results of a single controlled trial, a combination product (Rebixiao granule, RBXG) containing ash demonstrated no obvious toxic or adverse reactions.

ashwagandha *(Withania somnifera)* | **Uses:** Diabetes (type 2), diuretic, hypercholesterolemia, longevity/antiaging, osteoarthritis, Parkinson's disease; | **Preg:** Not recommended due to lack of sufficient evidence and historical use as an abortifacient; | **CIs:** Allergy/hypersensitivity, Pregnancy, Respiratory depression; | **ADRs:** abdominal pain, arrhythmias, ↓ blood pressure, dermatitis, diarrhea, ↓ FSH, immunosuppression, kidney lesions, mucous membrane irritation, nausea, ↑ platelet count, respiratory depression, sedation, ↑ T_4 levels, ↓ testosterone levels; | **Interactions:** Androgens (additive effects), anticoagulants/antiplatelets (↑ risk of bleeding), antidiabetic agents (↑ risk of hypoglycemia), antihypertensives (additive effects/↑ risk of hypotension), cholinesterase inhibitors (additive effects), CNS depressants (additive sedation), diuretics (additive effects/↑ risk of electrolyte imbalances), narcotics (↓ tolerance), paclitaxel (↑ effects), stimulants (antagonistic effects), thyroid hormones (altered effects); | **Dose:** 1–6 g of whole ashwagandha herb daily in capsule or tea form; 3–12 g of ashwagandha in combination with other herbs. Pediatric (8–12 years old): 2 g daily for 60 days; | **Monitor:** Blood glucose, blood pressure, coagulation panel, electrolytes, FSH, lipid profile, RBC count, testosterone, thyroid panel, WBC count; | **Notes:** Ashwagandha tablets may be standardized to 4.5 mg with anolides.

asparagus *(Asparagus officinalis)* | **Uses:** Dyspepsia, galactogogue; | **Preg:** Likely safe when consumed as a food; supplementation not recommended due to lack of sufficient evidence; | **CIs:** Hypersensitivity/allergy; | **ADRs:** primarily dermatological and pulmonary allergic reactions, including itchy conjunctivitis, runny nose, tightness of the throat and coughing during preparation of fresh asparagus; acute urticaria and contact dermatitis after ingestion of asparagus; chronic recurrent mechanical ileus of the small intestine has been caused by a high-fiber diet, including canned asparagus; | **Interactions:** Diuretics (additive effects); | **Dose:** Infusion: 45–60 g cut herb in 150 mL water daily, by mouth. Fluid extract (1:1 g/mL): 45–60 mL daily, PO. Alcoholic extract (1:5 g/mL): 225–300 mL

A

daily, PO; **Monitor:** Electrolytes; **Notes:** Volatile organic components are excreted in human urine after ingestion of asparagus. The detection of the excreted odor constitutes a genetic smell hypersensitivity.

aspartic acid **Uses:** Athletic performance enhancement, chronic fatigue syndrome; **Preg:** Mineral aspartates and supplemental aspartic acid are not recommended during pregnancy and lactation due to a lack of sufficient evidence; however, supplementation of pregnant women with magnesium aspartate decreased maternal hospitalizations, preterm delivery, and referral of the newborn to the neonatal intensive care unit; **CIs:** Allergy/hypersensitivity, Excessive intake; **ADRs:** large doses (> 10 g) associated with dehydration, diarrhea, gout, hepatotoxicity, kidney damage; **Interactions:** Antigout agents (↓ effects), antihypertensives (additive effects/↑ risk of hypotension), CNS depressants (antagonistic effects), hepatotoxic agents (↑ risk of liver damage), minerals (additive effects), nephrotoxic agents (↑ risk of kidney damage); **Dose:** General: 7–12 g over 24 hours. Exercise performance enhancement: 4–8 g of aspartic acid during the 24-hour period before an athletic event. Fatigue: 250 mg each potassium and magnesium aspartate daily; **Monitor:** Ammonia (plasma), arginine (plasma), blood glucose, blood pressure, hormone panel, LFTs, lipid profile, renal function tests; **Notes:** In mammals, aspartic acid is a nonessential amino acid, meaning that it can be synthesized in adequate quantities by the body. It is used to enhance absorption of mineral supplements.

astaxanthin **Uses:** Carpal tunnel syndrome, hyperlipidemia, male infertility, muscle strength, musculoskeletal injuries, rheumatoid arthritis; **Preg:** Not recommended due to lack of sufficient evidence; may alter reproductive hormones; **CIs:** Allergy/hypersensitivity; **ADRs:** aplastic anemia, ↓ blood pressure, gynecomastia, ↓ libido; **Interactions:** 5-alpha-reductase inhibitors (additive effects), androgens (additive effects), antihypertensive agents (additive effects/↑ risk of hypotension), calcium (↓ effects), carotenoids (↓ absorption of astaxanthin), CYP450 2B6 and 3A4 substrates (altered drug levels), estrogens (additive effects), rofecoxib (↓ effects); **Dose:** Up to 19.25 mg daily by mouth for up to 8 weeks; **Monitor:** Androgens, blood pressure, estrogens, calcium levels, immunoglobulins; lipid profile, PTH, WBC count; **Notes:** Astaxanthin has been used as a feed supplement and food coloring additive for salmon, crabs, shrimp, chickens, and egg production. A standard serving portion of four ounces of Atlantic salmon contains

A

from 0.5–1.1 mg of astaxanthin, whereas the same amount of sockeye salmon may contain 4.5 mg of astaxanthin.

astragalus *(Astragalus membranaceus)* | **Uses:** Aplastic anemia, athletic performance, burns, chemotherapy side effects, coronary artery disease, diabetes, heart failure, hepatitis, hepatoprotection, herpes, HIV, immune stimulation, menopausal symptoms, mental performance, myocarditis/endocarditis, renal failure, smoking cessation, tuberculosis, upper respiratory tract infection; | **Preg:** Not recommended due to insufficient evidence; related species may be fetotoxic or have abortifacient effects; | **CIs:** Allergy/hypersensitivity; Pregnancy; | **ADRs:** immunosuppression (high doses); | **Interactions:** Anticoagulants/antiplatelets (↑ risk of bleeding), antidiabetic agents (↑ risk of hypoglycemia), antihypertensives (↑/↓ effects), antilipemic agents (additive effects), antineoplastic agents (alter or interfere with effects), beta blockers (↓ effects), CNS stimulants (additive effects), cyclophosphamide (↓ cyclophosphamide-induced immunosuppression), diuretics (additive effects), immunosuppressants (alter or interfere with effects), propoxyphene (additive effects), steroidal agents (↑/↓ effects); | **Dose:** Extract: 20–500 mg of extract 3–4 times daily. Dried root: 1–60 g daily; 500–1,000 mg root capsules 3 times daily. Tinctures: 2–4 mL of a 1:1 water or alcohol whole root extract in 25% ethanol 3–4 times daily, and 3–5 mL of a tincture (1:5) in 30% ethanol 3 times daily; | **Monitor:** Blood pressure, blood glucose, chloride, coagulation panel, electrolytes, growth hormone, heart rate, lipid profile; | **Notes:** In theory, consumption of the tragacanth (gummy sap derived from astragalus) may reduce absorption of agents taken by mouth. Therefore, tragacanth and other agents should be taken at separate times.

autumn crocus *(Colchicum autumnale)* | **Uses:** Cancer (renal cell carcinoma), cirrhosis, constipation, gout, idiopathic thrombocytopenic purpura, low back pain, lymphedema (obstructive), psoriasis; | **Preg:** Not recommended due to insufficient evidence and possible hormonal effects. The constituent colchicine is known to induce birth defects; | **CIs:** Allergy/hypersensitivity, Concurrent use with colchicine, All parts of the plant are highly TOXIC (potential poisoning due to colchicine content), Pregnancy, Lactation; | **ADRs:** abdominal pain, burning mouth and throat, cardiac arrest, DEATH, diarrhea, hypovolemic shock, liver necrosis, multiorgan failure, nausea/vomiting, numbness, renal impairment; long-term use of colchicine is associated with agranulocytosis, aplastic anemia, DEATH, liver dysfunction, neuromuscular toxicity, peripheral neuritis, renal dysfunction; **Interactions:** May interact with agents with similar effects or related mechanisms of action (antineoplastic, antiarthritic, anti-inflammatory, immunomodulatory, laxative), colchicine (additive effects/↑ risk of toxicity), diuretics (↑ risk of electrolyte imbalances); **Dose:** PO: Up to 8 mg as a single dose (maximum 1 dose every 3 days); 1 mg daily for 2 days. Gout, oral: colchicine (active constituent) 1.2 mg followed by 0.6 mg at 1 hour (total 1.8 mg), corresponding to crocus seed 200 mg or corm (the root) 250 mg; **Monitor:** Immune parameters, LFTs, uric acid; **Notes:** The primary active ingredient of *Colchicum autumnale* is the alkaline substance colchicine. Colchicine has been used for centuries for the treatment of gout. In 2009, colchicine was FDA approved for this use, as well as familial Mediterranean fever. Colchicine may be poisonous when recommended doses are exceeded or if accidentally ingested. Colchicine intoxication may result in multiorgan failure and death.

avocado *(Persea americana)* **Uses:** Hypercholesterolemia, osteoarthritis, psoriasis; **Preg:** Likely safe when used as a food; supplemental amounts not recommended due to insufficient evidence; reduced milk production at doses greater than 20 g/kg in animals; **CIs:** Allergy/hypersensitivity to avocado, banana, chestnut, natural rubber latex; Monoamine oxidase inhibitors (MAOIs, ↑ risk of hypertensive crisis); **ADRs:** bronchial asthma, contact dermatitis, drowsiness, fever, gastrointestinal disorders, hepatotoxicity (from unrefined oil), migraine; **Interactions:** Anticoagulants (↑ metabolism or ↓ absorption), antilipemic agents (additive effects), MAOIs (↑ risk of hypertensive crisis); **Dose:** Fruit: Up to 1.5 avocados consumed daily for 2–4 weeks; 300 g avocado daily for 7 days; can decrease serum lipids. Avocado/soybean unsaponifiables (ASU): 300–600 mg daily for up to 2 years. Topical: Regividerm, containing avocado oil with 82.9 mg/kg vitamin E, applied twice daily for 12 months; **Monitor:** Lipid profile; **Notes:** Avocado oil is derived from the fruit pulp, which is a good source of potassium and vitamin D. Mexican avocado is reported to contain estragole and anethole, which have proven to be hepatotoxic in animals and structurally similar to safrole, a known carcinogen.

babassu *(Orbignya phalerata)* **Uses:** There are no scientific studies on the use of babassu for medical conditions; **Preg:** Not recommended due to insufficient evidence; **CIs:** Allergy/hypersensitivity; **ADRs:** likely safe when used in food amounts in people without underlying medical conditions; altered thyroid hormone levels, bleeding, chromoblastomycosis

B

(on contact) fungal infections; | **Interactions:** Anticoagulants/antiplatelets (↑ risk of bleeding), antithyroid agents (additive effects), thyroid hormones (antagonistic effects); | **Dose:** Insufficient evidence; | **Monitor:** Coagulation panel; thyroid hormones; | **Notes:** Babassu coconut (mesocarp) has been widely used as a source of food and for treatment of pain, fever, constipation, obesity, leukemia, rheumatism, ulcerations, tumors, wounds, and inflammation.

bacopa *(Bacopa monnieri)* | **Uses:** Anxiety, cognition, epilepsy, irritable bowel syndrome, memory; | **Preg:** Not recommended due to insufficient evidence; | **CIs:** Allergy/hypersensitivity; | **ADRs:** altered thyroid hormones, drowsiness, fatigue, nausea, palpitations, xerostomia; | **Interactions:** Calcium channel blockers (additive effects), CYP450 substrates (altered drug levels), phenytoin (↓ phenytoin-induced cognitive impairment), thyroid hormones (altered effects); | **Dose:** General: 50–150 mg PO 2 or 3 times daily. Anxiety: 30 mL bacopa syrup (12 g dry crude drug) PO daily in divided doses for 4 weeks. Cognitive function: 150 mg of Keenmind bacopa extract PO daily for 12 weeks. Epilepsy: 2 oz crude aqueous extract, or 2–4 mg/kg defatted alcoholic bacopa extract, PO daily for up to 5 months; | **Monitor:** Thyroid function panel; | **Notes:** Bacopa is used traditionally in India to anoint newborns to increase their intelligence. Caution is warranted in patients with thyroid disorder.

bael fruit *(Aegle marmelos)* | **Uses:** Dysentery (shigellosis); | **Preg:** Not recommended due to insufficient evidence and traditional use of bael leaf as an abortifacient; | **CIs:** Allergy/hypersensitivity, Pregnancy; Avoid large doses; | **ADRs:** owing to tannins, large quantities may result in digestive complaints and constipation; | **Interactions:** Antidiabetic agents (additive effects/↑ risk of hypoglycemia), thyroid hormones (altered effects); | **Dose:** Fruit powder: 2–12 g. Decoction: 28–56 mL. Infusion: 12–20 mL; | **Monitor:** Blood glucose; thyroid function panel; | **Notes:** Evidence suggests that bael is not effective for treating dysentery (shigellosis).

balas | **Uses:** Insufficient evidence; | **Preg:** Not recommended due to insufficient evidence; | **CIs:** Allergy/hypersensitivity; | **ADRs:** anxiety, arrhythmia (prolonged QT interval), bradycardia, ↑ glucose, hand tremor, headache, hyper-/hypotension, irritability, memory loss, nervousness, psychosis, seizures, tremor; | **Interactions:** Analgesics (additive effects), antidiabetic agents (antagonistic effects), bronchodilators (additive effects), CAFFEINE/METHYLXANTHINES (↑ risk of stimulatory adverse effects), CNS STIMULANTS (↑ risk of stimulatory adverse effects), dexamethasone (↓ effectiveness of dexamethasone), ergot derivatives (↑ risk of hypertension), MAO inhibitors (↑ risk of hypertensive crisis), QT PROLONGING AGENTS (↑ risk of QT prolongation), vasorelaxants (additive effects); | **Dose:** Capsules: 300 mg PO q a.m. Tincture (1:3 in 24% alcohol): 5–10 mL daily in divided doses. Tea: 10 g bala per cup water as tea steeped for at least 1 hr. Whole plant juice: pounded with some water given in doses of 1/4 seer (equal to 1/4 kg), used for the treatment of gonorrhea; | **Monitor:** Blood pressure, heart rate; | **Notes:** Bala, or *Sida cordifolia*, means young or strength in Sanskrit; it has been traditionally used in Ayurvedic medicine for inflammation, asthma, bronchitis, and nasal congestion. Ephedrine is a constituent of balas, which can increase heart rate and blood pressure.

bamboo *(Arundinaria japonica)* | **Uses:** There are no scientific studies on the use of bamboo for medical conditions; | **Preg:** Not recommended due to insufficient evidence; | **CIs:** Allergy/hypersensitivity; | **ADRs:** melanosis coli associated with ingestion of bamboo leaf; contact allergy; ↓ thyroid activity; | **Interactions:** Thyroid hormones (altered or interfere with effects); | **Dose:** Insufficient evidence; | **Monitor:** Thyroid function panel; | **Notes:** Preliminary studies suggest bamboo as an alternative bone substitute.

banaba *(Lagerstroemia speciosa)* | **Uses:** Diabetes; | **Preg:** Not recommended due to insufficient evidence; | **CIs:** Allergy/hypersensitivity; | **ADRs:** no adverse effects have been noted in the available research; | **Interactions:** Anticoagulants/antiplatelets (↑ risk of bleeding), antidiabetic agents (additive effects/↑ risk of hypoglycemia); xanthine oxidase inhibitors (↓ xanthine oxidase activity); | **Dose:** Diabetes: 32–48 mg daily for 2 weeks; | **Monitor:** Blood glucose, lipid profile; | **Notes:** Banaba is generally considered to be safe when taken orally for 15 days for the treatment of type 2 diabetes.

barberry (*Berberis* spp.) | **Uses:** There are no scientific studies on the use of barberry for medical conditions; | **Preg:** Not recommended due to insufficient evidence and traditional use as an abortifacient; ↑ risk for kernicterus in jaundiced newborns; | **CIs:** Allergy/hypersensitivity, Newborns, Pregnancy, Concurrent use with cyclosporine; | **ADRs:** bradycardia, DEATH (>500 mg berberine), dyspnea, eye irritation, giddiness, headache, hyperbilirubinemia, hyper-/hypotension, kidney

B

irritation (>500 mg berberine), lethargy, leucopenia, nausea, paresthesias, respiratory failure, respiratory spasms, vomiting; **Interactions:** Antiarrhythmic agents (↑ effects), anticholinergics (↓ effects), anticoagulants/antiplatelets (↑ risk of bleeding), antidiabetic agents (additive effects/↑ risk of hypoglycemia), anti-inflammatory agents (additive effects), antihistamines (additive effects), antihypertensives (additive effects/↑ risk of hypotension), carmustine (BCNU) (↑ effects), CNS depressants (additive effects/↑ risk of sedation), CYCLOSPORINE (↑ serum levels), CYP450 3A4 substrates (inhibits 3A4/may ↑ levels of drugs metabolized by CYP3A4), L-phenylephrine (↑ effects), tetracycline (↓ effects), yohimbine (↓ effects); **Dose:** Insufficient evidence; most herbal experts purport that barberry is generally well tolerated in recommended doses of 1.5–3 g daily; **Monitor:** Bilirubin, blood glucose, coagulation panel, interleukins, WBC count; **Notes:** The main constituent of barberry is berberine. See separate entry on berberine.

barley ***(Hordeum vulgare)*** **Uses:** Constipation, diabetes, hyperlipidemia, ulcerative colitis, weight loss; **Preg:** Likely safe in amounts found in food; excessive consumption of barley sprouts is not advised during pregnancy; **CIs:** Allergy/hypersensitivity, Celiac disease (due to gluten content); **ADRs:** abdominal fullness, ↑ alertness, asthma, eye, nose, or sinus irritation, increased heart rate, low blood sugar levels, low levels of iron in the blood (in infants), malnutrition (in infants), swollen skin, eyelids, arms or legs; **Interactions:** Antidiabetic agents (additive effects/↑ risk of hypoglycemia), antihypertensives (additive effects/↑ risk of hypotension), antilipemic agents (additive effects), oral agents (↓ effects/↓ absorption), sympathomimetics (additive effects); **Dose:** Germinated barley foodstuff (GBF): up to 30 g daily. Barley oil: 3 mL daily. Barley bran flour: 30 g daily. Barley beta-glucan extract: 3–5 g daily for 10 weeks; **Monitor:** Blood glucose, blood pressure, lipid profile, urine drug screens (hordenine constituent may result in false-positive opiate tests); **Notes:** Barley-containing foods (with at least 0.75 g soluble fiber per serving) are allowed by the FDA to bear labeling claims that they reduce the risk of coronary heart disease (CHD).

bay leaf ***(Laurus nobilis)*** **Uses:** There are no scientific studies on the use of bay leaf for medical conditions; **Preg:** Not recommended due to insufficient evidence and traditional use as an abortifacient; **CIs:** Allergy/hypersensitivity, Concurrent use of CNS depressants or narcotics; **ADRs:** contact dermatitis, occupational asthma, ingested whole leaves may become lodged in the gastrointestinal tract; | **Interactions:** ACE inhibitors (additive effects), alcohol (↓ absorption), drugs that lower seizure threshold (↑ risk of seizures); CNS depressants (additive sedation), narcotics (additive sedation); | **Dose:** Insufficient evidence; | **Monitor:** Insufficient evidence; | **Notes:** Bay leaf (*Laurus nobilis*) may be confused with California bay leaf (*Umbellularia californica*), also known as "California laurel" or "Oregon myrtle," or Indian bay leaf (*Cinnamoma tamala*).

bayberry (*Myrica* spp.) | **Uses:** Insufficient clinical evidence; | **Preg:** Not recommended due to insufficient evidence and warnings in secondary sources; | **CIs:** Allergy/hypersensitivity, Pregnancy, Lactation; | **ADRs:** gastrointestinal irritation, hepatotoxicity, vomiting; | **Interactions:** May interact with agents with related effects or mechanisms of action (analgesic, anxiolytic, antibiotic, anticoagulant, antifungal, antihypertensive, antilipemic, antiparasitic, antiviral, bronchodilator, cardiovascular, hormonal); | **Dose:** Insufficient evidence; | **Monitor:** Blood pressure, coagulation panel, hormone panel, lipid profile; | **Notes:** Evidence of bayberry safe consumption is currently lacking, although the bark, leaves, and fruits of several species of *Myrica* have been traditionally used and consumed without reports of adverse effects.

bean pod | **Uses:** Diabetes mellitus, obesity; | **Preg:** Not recommended due to insufficient evidence; | **CIs:** Allergy/hypersensitivity, Ingesting husks; | **ADRs:** abdominal pain, diarrhea, gastrointestinal upset, nausea/vomiting; | **Interactions:** Antidiabetic agents (↑ risk of hypoglycemia), diuretics (additive effects), laxatives (additive effects); | **Dose:** Tea: prepare with 2.5 g bean pods in 150 mL of boiling water for 10–15 minutes and then straining, 1 cup several times daily (do not exceed 5–15 g/day). Obesity: specific bean pod extract (Phase 2 dietary supplement): 445 mg/day PO or 1,500 mg PO bid; | **Monitor:** Blood glucose, electrolytes; | **Notes:** Bean pod may lower blood glucose levels.

bear's garlic *(Allium ursinum)* | **Uses:** There are no scientific studies on the use of bear's garlic for medical conditions; | **Preg:** Not recommended due to insufficient evidence; | **CIs:** Allergy/hypersensitivity; | **ADRs:** insufficient evidence; likely safe when consumed in food amounts; | **Interactions:** Anticoagulants/antiplatelets (↑ risk of bleeding), anti-inflammatory agents (additive effects), antihypertensive agents (additive effects/↑ risk of hypotension); | **Dose:** Insufficient evidence; | **Monitor:** Blood pressure, coagulation panel;

B

Notes: Although there are no known toxicities associated with bear's garlic consumption, there have been several reports of colchicine poisoning, resulting in gastroenterocolitis and sometimes fatal organ dysfunction, with ingestion of autumn crocus mistaken for bear's garlic.

bee pollen | **Uses:** Athletic performance enhancement, chemotherapy-induced adverse effects, memory, multiple sclerosis; | **Preg:** Not recommended due to insufficient evidence; | **CIs:** Allergy/hypersensitivity, Pollen allergy; | **ADRs:** abdominal cramps, anaphylaxis, anorexia, asthma, decreased memory, diarrhea, dyspnea, edema, erythema, gastrointestinal distress, hay fever, hepatitis (liver inflammation), hypereosinophilia, nausea, photosensitivity, pruritus, rash, vertigo, vomiting; | **Interactions:** Insufficient evidence; | **Dose:** 1–2 teaspoons, up to 3 times daily; | **Monitor:** LFTs, WBC count (eosinophil counts); | **Notes:** Bee pollen composition varies depending on plant source and geographic region.

beer | **Uses:** Anti-inflammatory, antioxidant, cardiovascular risk reduction, thrombosis; | **Preg:** Avoid use; | **CIs:** Allergy/hypersensitivity, CHF, Liver dysfunction, Pancreatitis; | **ADRs:** asthma, ↑ blood pressure, diarrhea, facial edema, hyperuricemia, hyponatremia, insomnia, liver damage, rash, ↑ risk of colorectal cancer, sedation, ↑ triglycerides, weight gain; | **Interactions:** Aspirin/NSAIDs (↑ risk of GI bleeding), barbiturates (↓ metabolism of barbiturates), benzodiazepines (↓ metabolism of benzodiazepines), cefamandole (disulfiram-like reaction), cefoperazone (disulfiram-like reaction), chlorpropamide (disulfiram-like reaction), cisapride (↑ blood alcohol levels), CNS DEPRESSANTS (additive sedation), DISULFIRAM (disulfiram reaction), ERYTHROMYCIN (↑ blood alcohol levels), griseofulvin (disulfiram-like reaction), H2-blockers (↑ blood alcohol levels), HEPATOTOXIC AGENTS (↑ risk of hepatotoxicity), metformin (↑ risk of lactic acidosis), narcotics (↓ metabolism of narcotics), niacin (↑ risk of flushing), sulfonamides (disulfiram-like reaction), tolbutamide (disulfiram-like reaction), WARFARIN (altered effects of warfarin); | **Dose:** Insufficient evidence; | **Monitor:** Folate levels, lipid profile (triglycerides), LFTs, MCV; | **Notes:** Drinking beer may not raise total mortality above the normal risk level providing imbibers do not exceed 168–280 g of alcohol a week for men and 84–140 g a week for women. Caution is warranted in patients with asthma, gout, hypertriglyceridemia, GERD/PUD, and psychiatric disorders.

beet ***(Beta vulgaris)*** | **Uses:** Diabetes, hypertension, hyperlipidemia, peritonitis; | **Preg:** Likely safe in amounts found in food; medicinal amounts not recommended due to insufficient evidence; **CIs:** Allergy/hypersensitivity; **ADRs:** occupational illness (including asthma, anaphylaxis, toxic poisoning, respiratory infections, and tularemia), allergic skin reactions, beeturia (red urine), likely safe when consumed in food amounts; **Interactions:** Antidiabetic agents (additive effects/ ↑ risk of hypoglycemia); antilipemic agents (additive effects/ ↑ HDL); oral agents (beet fiber may ↓ absorption); **Dose:** Up to 30 g beet fiber daily; **Monitor:** Blood glucose, lipid profile; **Notes:** The FDA has approved dehydrated beets and sugar beet extract flavor base as food additives or listed or affirmed them as Generally Regarded as Safe (GRAS).

belladonna *(Atropa belladonna)* **Uses:** Airway obstruction, headache, irritable bowel syndrome, menopausal symptoms, nervous system disturbances, otitis media, premenstrual syndrome (PMS), radiation therapy rash, sweating; **Preg:** Not recommended due to the potential for toxicity and adverse outcomes, including respiratory abnormalities, hypospadias (penile urethral anomalies in men), and eye/ear malformations; **CIs:** Allergy/hypersensitivity, Asthma, Glaucoma, Elderly, Gastrointestinal disorders, Obstructive uropathy, Pregnancy, Ulcerative colitis; ORAL USE in children; **ADRs:** acute psychosis, agitation, arrhythmias, birth defects, blisters, bloating, blurred vision, coma, confusion, constipation, convulsions, DEATH, difficulty breast feeding, dizziness, drowsiness, dry mouth/skin, dysarthria, dysuria, erythema, hallucinations, headache, hyperreflexia, hypertension, hyperthermia, leg cramps, lightheadedness, mental problems, muscle pain, muscle shakes/tremors, mydriasis, myocardial infarction, no muscle movement (especially not breathing), ↓ perspiration, photosensitivity, sedation, spasms, skin rash, stiff muscles, syncope, tachycardia, tachypnea, unsteadiness, urinary retention; **Interactions:** Anticholinergic agents (↑ anticholinergic effects and risk of adverse effects), CNS depressants (additive sedation), levodopa (↓ absorption); **Dose:** Leaf powder: maximum single dose 200 mg (0.6 mg total alkaloids, calculated as hyoscyamine), maximum daily dose 600 mg (equivalent to 1.8 mg total alkaloids). Root: maximum single dose 100 mg (0.5 mg total alkaloids), maximum daily dose 300 mg (equivalent to 1.5 mg total alkaloids). Belladonna extract: single dose 100 mg (0.5 mg total alkaloids), maximum daily dose 150 mg (equivalent to 2.2 mg total alkaloids); **Monitor:** Blood pressure, heart rate, urinalysis; **Notes:** There is extensive literature on the adverse effects and toxicity of belladonna, related principally to its known anticholinergic actions. Likely safe when taken in extremely dilute homeopathic preparations.

B

berberine | **Uses:** Heart failure, chloroquine-resistant malaria, diabetes (type 2), glaucoma, *Helicobacter pylori* infection, hypercholesterolemia, infectious diarrhea, parasitic infection (leishmania), thrombocytopenia, trachoma; | **Preg:** Not recommended due to insufficient evidence, traditional use as an abortifacient, and association with jaundice; | **CIs:** Allergy/hypersensitivity, Newborns, Pregnancy, Concurrent use with cyclosporine; | **ADRs:** abdominal discomfort, abdominal distention, abortion, alterations in gut flora, ↑ bilirubin, bleeding, bradycardia, DEATH, diarrhea, dyspnea, eczema, edema, eye irritation, facial flushing, faintness, flu-like symptoms, giddiness, headache, heart damage, hemolysis (in babies with glucose-6-phosphate dehydrogenase deficiency), hyperpigmentation (permanent), hyper-/hypotension, hypoglycemia, infertility, jaundice, kernicterus (bilirubin encephalopathy), kidney irritation, lethargy, liver damage, myocardial infarction, nausea, nephritis, nosebleed, osteoporosis, paresthesias, pruritus, respiratory failure, ventricular tachycardia, vomiting; | **Interactions:** Antiarrhythmic agents (altered effects), anticholinergics (↓ effects), anticoagulants/antiplatelets (↓ effects), antidiabetic agents (additive effects/↑ risk of hypoglycemia), anti-inflammatory agents (additive effects) antihistamines (additive effects), antihypertensives (additive effect/↑ risk of hypotension), carmustine (BCNU) (↑ effects), CNS depressants (additive effects/↑ risk of sedation), CYCLOSPORINE (↑ serum levels), CYP450 3A4 substrates (inhibits 3A4/may ↑ levels of drugs metabolized by CYP3A4), L-phenylephrine (↑ effects), tetracycline (↓ effects), yohimbine (↓ effects); | **Dose:** Hypercholesterolemia: 0.5 g PO bid for 3 months. Infectious diarrhea: berberine sulfate 400 mg as a single dose. Thrombocytopenia: Berberine bisulfate 5 mg 3 times daily (20 min before meals) for 15 days. Heart failure: 0.2 mg/kg per min IV for 30 min. Trachoma: 0.2% eyedrops for 8 weeks; | **Monitor:** Bilirubin, blood glucose, coagulation panel, interleukins, WBC count; | **Notes:** Berberine is found in many species, including barberry (*Berberis vulgaris*) and other *Berberis* spp., goldenseal (*Hydrastis canadensis*), and coptis or goldenthread (*Coptis* spp.).

bergamot ***(Citrus aurantium)*** | **Uses:** Anxiety, hypertension; | **Preg:** Not recommended due to lack of sufficient evidence; | **CIs:** Allergy/hypersensitivity, Oral use in large quantities (due to known toxicity); | **ADRs:** essential oils may be toxic if taken in large amounts; contact dermatitis, eye irritation (vapors), hepatotoxicity, photosensitivity, pigmentary changes (if applied topically); | **Interactions:** CYP450 substrates (inhibits enzyme/may alter drug levels/effects), photosensitizing agents (↑ risk of adverse effects), may interact with agents with similar effects or related mechanisms of action (antimicrobial, cardiovascular, prebiotic, neurological); | **Dose:** Insufficient evidence; | **Monitor:** LFTs; | **Notes:** The FDA and USDA list bergamot orange as Generally Recognized as Safe (GRAS) with oil used for flavoring. Not to be confused with bee balm (*Monarda* spp.), which is sometimes called bergamot.

B

beta-carotene | **Uses:** Asthma (prevention), carotenoid deficiency, cataract prevention, chemotherapy toxicity, chronic obstructive pulmonary disease (COPD), cognitive performance, cystic fibrosis, immune system enhancement, oral leukoplakia, osteoarthritis, pregnancy-related complication, sunburn prevention (erythema prevention); | **Preg:** Pregnancy category C (potential benefits may warrant use in pregnant women despite potential risks); | **CIs:** Allergy/hypersensitivity, Before and following angioplasty, Smoking; | **ADRs:** well tolerated in appropriate amounts; high amounts may ↑ risk of lung and prostate cancer, ↑ risk of cardiovascular disease; ↓ HDLs; | **Interactions:** Alcohol (↓ concentrations of beta-carotene, ↑ risk of liver toxicity), bile acid sequestrants (↓ absorption of beta-carotene), colchicine (↓ levels of beta-carotene), dietary fats (↑ beta-carotene absorption), HMG-CoA reductase inhibitors (↓ effects of HMG-CoA reductase inhibitors), neomycin (↓ beta-carotene absorption), niacin (↓ effects of niacin), olestra (interferes with beta-carotene), proton pump inhibitors (↓ beta-carotene absorption); | **Dose:** 15–180 mg supplemental beta-carotene by mouth has been studied for various indications; | **Monitor:** Lipid profile (HDL), serum carotenoid levels; | **Notes:** 1,800 mcg beta-carotene daily is sufficient to maintain adequate vitamin A levels.

beta-glucan | **Uses:** Antioxidant, breast cancer, burns, cancer, cardiovascular disease, diabetes, diagnostic procedure, heart protection during coronary artery bypass grafting (CABG), HIV/AIDS, hyperlipidemia, hypertension, infection, postoperative infection, weight loss; | **Preg:** Not recommended due to insufficient evidence; | **CIs:** Allergy/hypersensitivity; | **ADRs:** dizziness, flushing, headache, hyper-/hypotension, inflammatory airway disease, keratoderma, nausea, polyuria, urticaria, vomiting; | **Interactions:** Antidiabetic agents (additive effects/↑ risk of hypoglycemia), antihypertensive agents (additive effects/↑ risk of hypotension), antilipemic agents (additive effects), antineoplastic agents (additive effects), carmustine (↑ effects), cefazolin (synergistic effects), immunosuppressants (↓ additive effects of immunosuppressants), oral agents (↓ absorption due to soluble fiber content); | **Dose:** General (oral): 8–15 g. Burns: Applied to burns on the skin as a collagen

B

matrix for 24 hours, or injected. Cardiovascular disease: 0.75 g 4 times daily. Diabetes: 50–90 g carbohydrate portions of barley grain with meals for up to 12 weeks. Heart protection during CABG: up to 1,400 mg daily for 5 days before surgery. Hypertension: 5.52 g daily. Hyperlipidemia: 3–16 g daily. Immune stimulation (in patients with breast cancer): 1,3,/1,6-D-beta-glucan daily for 15 days; | **Monitor:** Blood glucose, blood pressure, lipid profile, WBC count; | **Notes:** Beta-glucan is derived from the cell walls of algae, bacteria, fungi, yeast, and plants. The beta-glucan found in yeast and mushrooms contains 1,3-glucan linkages and occasionally 1,6 linkages, whereas the beta-glucans from grains (i.e., oats and barley) contain 1,3 and 1,4 linkages. Yeast-derived beta-1,3/1,6-glucan purportedly has greater biological activity than the 1,3/1,4 counterparts.

betaine anhydrous | **Uses:** Cardiovascular disease (in homocysteinuric patients), hyperhomocysteinemia, hyperlipidemia, steatohepatitis (nonalcoholic), weight loss; | **Preg:** Not recommended due to insufficient evidence; | **CIs:** Allergy/hypersensitivity; | **ADRs:** bromhidrosis, diarrhea, ↑ cholesterol (when used with folic acid and vitamin B_6), mental changes, mild gastrointestinal adverse effects; | **Interactions:** Antilipemic agents (interfere with effects); | **Dose:** Adults: up to 15 g daily in divided doses. Children: 250 mg/kg for cystathionine beta-synthase deficiency; | **Monitor:** Lipid profile, liver function tests, plasma betaine levels; | **Notes:** Betaine anhydrous is not to be confused with betaine hydrochloride.

beta-sitosterol | **Uses:** Alopecia areata, benign prostatic hyperplasia (BPH), burns, HIV, hyperlipidemia, immune suppression, rheumatoid arthritis, tuberculosis (adjunct); | **Preg:** Not recommended due to insufficient evidence; | **CIs:** Allergy/hypersensitivity; Sitosterolemia; | **ADRs:** ↓ alpha and beta carotene levels, asthma, constipation, diarrhea, dyspnea, erectile dysfunction, hypoglycemia, ↓ libido, nausea, sitosterolemia; | **Interactions:** Acarbose (absorption ↑ by acarbose), acid-labile antibiotics (↑ absorption), activated charcoal (↓ by activated charcoal), anticoagulants/antiplatelets (↑ risk of bleeding), antidiabetic agents (↓ blood glucose), antilipemics (additive effects), bile acid sequestrants (↓ beta-sitosterol concentrations), carotene (↓ absorption and blood levels of alpha- and beta-carotene), COX inhibitors (additive effects), diosgenin (altered effects), ezetimibe (inhibits intestinal absorption of beta-sitosterol and reduces plasma concentrations); finasteride (synergistic effects), hormone therapies (altered effects); lifibrol (↓ beta-sterol), pravastatin/HMG-CoA reductase inhibitors (lower blood levels of beta-sitosterol); vitamin E (↓ absorption/blood levels of vitamin E); **Dose:** BPH: 60–130 mg in 2–3 divided doses; hyperlipidemia; 800 mg to 18 g in divided doses. However, daily doses of 6.6 g were found to be no more effective than doses of 1.6–3.2 g daily but may be associated with ↑ risk of side effects; **Monitor:** Blood glucose, coagulation panel, cortisol, DHEA, hormone levels, immune parameters, lipid profile, WBC count; **Notes:** Beta-sitosterol is one of the most common dietary phytosterols (plant sterols).

betel nut ***(Areca catechu)*** **Uses:** Anemia, dental cavities, schizophrenia, stimulant, stroke recovery, ulcerative colitis, xerostomia; **Preg:** Avoid use in pregnant or lactating women due to potential carcinogenic or fetotoxic effects; **CIs:** Allergy/hypersensitivity; Oral use (long-term or high doses), Pregnancy, Lactation, Asthma, Hepatitis (↑ risk of hepatocellular carcinoma); **ADRs:** abdominal cramps, anxiety (withdrawal symptom), arrhythmia, blurred vision, burning/dryness of the mouth, cancer, chest pain, confusion, diaphoresis, diarrhea, dyspnea, excitability, extreme moods, fever, gum and mouth problems, hallucinations, hepatotoxicity, hyper-/hypotension, hypoglycemia, immunosuppression, kidney disease, lacrimation, mania, memory problems, metabolic syndrome, movement retardation, mydriasis, myocardial infarction, nausea, problems with eye movement, pruritus, rash, red stained teeth/mouth/lips/stool, ↑ salivation, seizure, skin color changes, stiffness, tachypnea, thyroid problems, tremor, vomiting, urinary incontinence, wheezing. **Interactions:** Alcohol (↑ risk of oral cancer), anticholinergic agents (interfere with therapy), antidiabetic agents (additive effects/↑ risk of hypoglycemia), antihypertensive agents (↑ or ↓ blood pressure), anti-inflammatory agents (decreased effects), antilipemic agents (additive effects), antipsychotic agents (↑ extrapyramidal symptoms), cardiovascular agents (interfere with effects), chemotherapy (↑ risk of adverse effects), cholinergic agents (↑ risk of adverse effects), CNS stimulants (additive effects), glaucoma agents (↑ or ↓ effects), monoamine oxidase (MAO) inhibitors (↑ risk of hypertensive crisis); **Dose:** Ingestion of 8–30 g may be lethal; **Monitor:** Blood pressure, blood glucose, LFTs, lipid profile, serum calcitrol, serum copper, thyroid function panel, urinalysis; **Notes:** Betel nut is reportedly used by a substantial portion (approximately 10%) of the world's population as a recreational drug due to its CNS stimulant activity; it is the fourth most commonly used addictive substance in the world.

betony **(*Stachys* spp.)** **Uses:** There are no scientific studies on the use of betony for medical conditions; **Preg:** Not recommended due to insufficient evidence and traditional use as an abortifacient; | **Cls:** Allergy/hypersensitivity, Pregnancy; | **ADRs:** gastrointestinal irritation, hypoglycemia, hypotension; | **Interactions:** Antidiabetic agents (additive effects/↑ risk of hypoglycemia), antihypertensive agents (additive effects/↑ risk of hypotension), anxiolytic agents (↓ effects); | **Dose:** Tea: up to 4 g in 1 cup water, 3 times daily. Liquid extract: 1:1 in 25% ethanol, up to 4 mL 3 times daily. Tincture: 1:5 in 45% ethanol, up to 6 mL 4 times daily; | **Monitor:** Blood glucose; | **Notes:** Betony should not be confused with Canada lousewort (*Pedicularis canadensis*), which is commonly called wood betony.

bi yan pian | **Uses:** Insufficient evidence; | **Preg:** Not recommended due to insufficient evidence; | **Cls:** Allergy/hypersensitivity; | **ADRs:** bitter/stringent taste, excess dryness; | **Interactions:** Diuretics (↓ potassium levels), hormonal agents (altered effects), MAOIs (↑ risk of hypertensive crisis), potassium-depleting drugs (↓ potassium levels); | **Dose:** Oral, tablets: 3–4 tablets PO tid with warm water after meals; may increase to 5 tablets q3h, if needed. Tea (Breathe Easy, contains licorice root 300 mg, eucalyptus leaf 285 mg, bitter fennel fruit 255 mg, bi yan pian dry aqueous extract (8:1) 120 mg, along with a proprietary blend (540 mg) of peppermint leaf, calendula flower, pleurisy root, and ginger rhizome): to prepare tea, 8 oz of freshly boiled water should be poured over a tea bag in a ceramic cup, the cup should be covered and allowed to steep 10–15 minutes, then the tea bag should be gently squeezed to release the remaining extractive, 3 cups should be drunk daily or as needed; | **Monitor:** Potassium levels; | **Notes:** Bi yan pian, which literally translates from Chinese as "nasal inflammation tablets," is a combination formula of Chinese herbs that is used for rhinitis, sinusitis, and allergies. It contains *Xanthium sibiricum* fruit, *Magnolia denudata* flower, *Forsythia suspensa* fruit, *Ledebouriella divaricata* root, *Angelica dahurica* root, *Anemarrhena asphodeloides* rhizome, *Glycyrrhiza uralensis* root, *Schizonepeta tenuifolia* herb, *Chrysanthemum indicum* flower, *Schisandra chinensis* fruit, and *Platycodon grandiflorum* root. Use with extreme caution in patients with diabetes, hypertension, liver disorder, Parkinson's disease, kidney disease, hypokalemia, blood disorders, tuberculosis, thyroid disease, urinary incontinence, or peptic ulcers.

bilberry *(Vaccinium myrtillus)* | **Uses:** Artherosclerosis/peripheral vascular disease, cataracts, chronic venous insufficiency, diabetes mellitus, diarrhea, dysmenorrhea, fibrocystic breast disease, glaucoma, peptic ulcer disease, retinopathy; | **Preg:** Insufficient evidence; however, bilberry fruit is presumed to be safe on the basis of the use of bilberry as a food product in nonallergic individuals; **CIs:** Allergy/hypersensitivity; Leaves may be toxic; **ADRs:** bleeding, bruising, diarrhea, gastrointestinal upset, hypoglycemia, hypotension, poisoning (hydroquinone); **Interactions:** Anticoagulants/antiplatelets (↑ risk of bleeding), antidiabetic agents (additive effects/↑ risk of hypoglycemia), antihypertensives (additive effects/↑ risk of hypotension), estrogen (↓ estrogen absorption), hepatotoxic agents (↑ risk of liver damage, due to high tannin content); **Dose:** 80–480 mL of bilberry extract (25% anthocyanosides) daily by mouth in 2–3 divided doses; **Monitor:** Blood glucose, blood pressure, coagulation panel, LFTs; **Notes:** Bilberry is closely related to blueberry; its fruit extracts contain a number of biologically active components, including a class of compounds called anthocyanosides.

biminne **Uses:** There are no scientific studies on the use of biminne for medical conditions; **Preg:** Insufficient evidence; **CIs:** Allergy/hypersensitivity; **ADRs:** insufficient evidence; **Interactions:** Insufficient evidence; **Dose:** Insufficient evidence; **Monitor:** Insufficient evidence; **Notes:** Biminne is a Chinese herbal formula that consists of 11 different ingredients. Some of the active ingredients include extracts of Baikal skullcap (*Scutellaria baicalensis*), ginkgo (*Ginkgo biloba*), horny goat weed (*Epimedium sagittatum*), schisandra (*Schizandra chinensis*), Japanese apricot (*Prunus mume*), fang feng (*Ledebouriella divaricata*), and astragalus (*Astragalus membranaceus*).

bing gang tang **Uses:** Hepatitis C infection; **Preg:** Not recommended due to insufficient evidence; **CIs:** Allergy/hypersensitivity; **ADRs:** hepatotoxicity; **Interactions:** Hepatotoxic agents (↑ risk of liver damage); **Dose:** Insufficient evidence; **Monitor:** LFTs; **Notes:** Bing gan tang is a Chinese herbal formula that may have a possible role in improving chronic hepatitis when taken in combination with other agents.

biotin ***(vitamin H)*** **Uses:** Alopecia areata, biotin deficiency, biotin-responsive inborn errors of metabolism, cardiovascular disease risk (in diabetics), diabetes mellitus (type 2), hepatitis (in alcoholics), onychorrhexis (brittle fingernails), peripheral neuropathy, pregnancy supplementation, total parenteral nutrition (TPN); **Preg:** It has been suggested that biotin supplements should be considered for widespread use in pregnant women; **CIs:** Allergy/hypersensitivity; **ADRs:** toxicity with biotin intake has not been reported in the available literature; eosinophilic pleuropericardial effusion (high doses);

doses as high as 200 mL daily have been used in patients with inborn errors of metabolism without significant reported toxicity; | **Interactions:** Antibiotics (↓ biotin levels), antilipemic agents (additive effects), carbamazepine (↓ biotin levels), pantothenic acid (case of eosinophilic pleuropericardial effusion reported with concurrent use of biotin and pantothenic acid), phenobarbital (↓ biotin levels), primidone (↓ biotin levels), raw egg whites (↑ risk of biotin deficiency), smoking (↓ biotin levels); | **Dose:** Adults: The U.S. Recommended Dietary Allowance (RDA) for biotin is 300 mcg daily; adequate intake (AI) is 30 mcg daily. Infants (0–6 months): 5 mcg daily AI. Infants (7–12 months): 6 mcg daily AI. Children (1–3 years): 8 mcg daily AI. Children (4–8 years): 12 mcg daily AI. Children (9–13 years): 20 mcg daily AI. Adolescents (14–18 years): 25 mcg daily AI; | **Monitor:** Thyroid hormones (may give false-high free T_4 and false-low TSH); | **Notes:** Biotin deficiency is teratogenic in many animals.

birch (*Betula* spp.) | **Uses:** Actinic keratosis; | **Preg:** Not recommended due to insufficient evidence; | **CIs:** Allergy/hypersensitivity; | **ADRs:** allergic conjunctivitis (pinkeye), asthma, atopic dermatitis, atopic eczema, diuresis, eye redness, hepatotoxicity, itching, oropharyngeal itching, rhinoconjunctivitis, urticaria (hives), whealing, wheezing; | **Interactions:** Anticoagulants/antiplatelets (↑ risk of bleeding); diuretics (↑ diuretic effects), hepatotoxic agents (↑ risk of liver damage); | **Dose:** Homeopathic: One tablet PO of Betula 30C once a week for 4 weeks (no effects). Topical: Birch bark ointment; | **Monitor:** LFTs; | **Notes:** Birch bark contains a variety of potential apoptosis-inducing and anti-inflammatory substances such as betulinic acid, betulin, oleanolic acid, and lupeol.

bishop's weed (*Ammi majus*) | **Uses:** Psoriasis, tinea versicolor, vitiligo (leukoderma); | **Preg:** Not recommended due to insufficient evidence; | **CIs:** Allergy/hypersensitivity; | **ADRs:** contact dermatitis, headache, ↑ liver enzymes, nausea, photosensitivity, pigmentary retinopathy, rhinitis, urticaria, vomiting; | **Interactions:** Anticoagulants/antiplatelets (↑ risk of bleeding); CYP450 3A4 substrates (↑ levels of drugs metabolized by CYP450 3A4); hepatotoxic agents (↑ risk of liver damage), photosensitizing agents (additive effects/↑ risk of sun sensitivity); | **Dose:** 10-mg capsules of a preparation containing ultramicronized methoxypsoralen (8-MOP); therapeutic effective dose was found to be 0.25 mg/kg; | **Monitor:** Coagulation panel, LFTs; | **Notes:** The prescription drug methoxsalen was developed from bishop's weed.

B

bismuth | **Uses:** Duodenal ulcer, dyspepsia, gastritis, *Helicobacter pylori* infection and stomach ulcers, ileostomy odor control, pouchitis, renal cysts, tonsillitis; | **Preg:** Not recommended due to insufficient evidence. Bismuth salicylate should be avoided because salicylates are contraindicated in pregnancy; | **CIs:** Allergy/hypersensitivity, Pregnancy (high doses); | **ADRs:** bismuth-containing regimens are considered to be well tolerated; adverse effects are generally due to other components of bismuth-containing compounds. High doses may cause encephalopathy. Bismuth-containing regimens have been associated with alopecia, glandular atrophy, constipation, chronic gastritis, diarrhea, dysgeusia, nausea, vomiting, dark stools, blackening of the tongue, intestinal metaplasia, aplastic anemia, acute renal failure, facial paresthesia, pain, perirenal bleeding, fever, radio-opaque punctate opacities on the chest, and xerostomia; | **Interactions:** The salicylate component may have potential interactions with other anticoagulants, antidiabetic agents, hypouricemic agents, and other salicylates. Colloidal bismuth subcitrate may reduce aspirin-induced gastric microbleeding. Tripotassium dicitrato bismuthate may aid in nonsteroidal anti-inflammatory-induced ulcer. Most interactions are due to other components of bismuth-containing compounds. EDTA complexes with bismuth. Bismuth salicylate: acidifying agents (↑ salicylic acid levels), anticoagulants (↑ risk of bleeding), doxycycline (↓ effects), salicylates (↑ salicylic acid levels/toxicity), furazolidone (↑ effects); bismuth subnitrate: ↑ cisplatin, may ↓ acid production; bismuth biskalcitrate: ↓ by omeprazole; may interact with agents with similar effects or related mechanisms of action (antidiarrheal, antineoplastic, antiulcer, antiemetic, hepatotoxic); | **Dose:** Oral: Bismuth-containing compounds have been studied at doses up to 2,100 mg daily. Bismuth galliate: 200 mg bid for 1 week; | **Monitor:** Serum antibodies, magnesium levels, renal function panel; | **Notes:** Bismuth has been used for approximately 100 years for gastrointestinal symptoms, and it was the first drug shown to alter the natural history of peptic ulcer disease.

bitter almond *(Prunus amygdalus* var. *amara)* | **Uses:** Cancer; | **Preg:** Not recommended due to insufficient evidence and known toxicity; | **CIs:** Allergy/hypersensitivity; | **ADRs:** abdominal pain, bradypnea, coma, confusion, cyanide poisoning, DEATH, dizziness, drooping eyelids, drowsiness, headache, lethargy, muscle weakness, mydriasis, nausea, seizure, severe allergic reaction, skin color changes, slow brain function, tachypnea, vomiting, ↓ white blood cell count; | **Interactions:** Alcohol (↑ alcohol dehydrogenase), analgesics (additive effects), CNS depressants (additive sedation), immunosuppressants (additive effects), nephrotoxic agents (↑ risk of kidney damage); | **Dose:** Insufficient evidence, known toxicity; | **Monitor:** WBC count; | **Notes:** Bitter almond should not be confused with sweet almond. Sweet almond seeds do not contain amygdalin and can be eaten, whereas bitter almonds are toxic. Laetrile is an anticancer drug derived from amygdalin, which has not been found to be an effective chemotherapeutic agent. Multiple cases of cyanide poisoning, including deaths, have been associated with laetrile therapy.

bitter melon *(Momordica charantia)* **and MAP3O** | **Uses:** Cancer, diabetes, HIV; | **Preg:** Not recommended due to insufficient evidence and abortifacient/antifertility effects observed in animals; | **CIs:** Allergy/hypersensitivity; Glucose-6-phosphate dehydrogenase deficiency, Pregnancy, Lactation; | **ADRs:** abdominal pain, bleeding, bruising, ↑/↓ cholesterol levels, coma, convulsions, dyspnea, fever, headaches, hepatotoxicity, immunomodulation, infertility, hyper-/hypoglycemia, miscarriage, pruritus, rash; | **Interactions:** Antidiabetic agents (additive effects/↑ risk of hypoglycemia), antilipemic agents (additive effects), chemotherapeutic agents (reverse chemotherapy drug resistance), antiviral agents (additive effects), antiretroviral agents (additive effects), protease inhibitors (additive effects), P-glycoprotein-regulated agents (altered drug levels); | **Dose:** Juice: 100-mL doses. Dried fruit powder: 5 g 3 times daily for 3 weeks; | **Monitor:** Blood glucose, CD4 count, LFTs, lipid profile, sperm count, viral load; | **Notes:** The seeds and outer rind of bitter melon fruit contain a toxic lectin, which inhibits protein synthesis in the intestinal wall. The protein MAP30 has been the subject of viral and cancer research.

bitter orange *(Citrus aurantium)* | **Uses:** Aging, dementia, obesity, tinea corporis, tinea cruris, tinea pedis; | **Preg:** Not recommended due to insufficient evidence and known adverse effects; | **CIs:** Allergy/hypersensitivity; Cardiovascular conditions, Concurrent use with midazolam, Concurrent use with MAOI, Glaucoma, Pregnancy, Lactation; | **ADRs:** cardiovascular toxicity, cluster headache, difficulty in concentrating, dizziness, headache, hypertension, hyperthyroidism, lightheadedness, memory loss, migraine, myocardial infarction, photosensitivity (particularly in fair-skinned people), QT prolongation, seizure, stroke, syncope, tachyarrhythmia, tachycardia, unsteady gait, worsened narrow-angle glaucoma symptoms; | **Interactions:** Alpha-adrenergic agents (alter or interfere with effects), beta-adrenergic agents (alter or interfere with effects), caffeine (↑ blood pressure and heart rate), CNS stimulants (additive effects), CYP450 3A4 (↑ drug levels), dextromethorphan

(↑ dextromethorphan levels), MIDAZOLAM (↑ drug levels), MAO inhibitors (↑ risk of hypertensive crisis), QT prolonging agents (additive effects/↑ risk of arrhythmias); | **Dose:** Weight loss: 975 mg extract daily in combination with 900 mg St. John's wort and 528 mg caffeine. Fungal infections: 25% bitter orange oil emulsion 3 times daily, 20% bitter orange oil in alcohol 3 times daily, and 100% bitter orange oil once daily; | **Monitor:** Blood pressure, heart rate, LFTs, thyroid hormones; | **Notes:** Bitter orange contains synephrine, an alkaloid with similarities to the banned substance ephedrine. Caution is warranted in patients with headache, hypertension, long QT interval syndrome, and tachyarrhythmias.

black bryony *(Tamus communis,* syn. *Dioscorea communis)* | **Uses:** There are no scientific studies on the use of black bryony for medical conditions; | **Preg:** Not recommended due to insufficient evidence and known toxicity; | **CIs:** Allergy/hypersensitivity, ORAL USE; | **ADRs:** skin irritation and inflammation, poisoning, black bryony–associated toxidermia; | **Interactions:** Anti-inflammatory agents (additive effects); | **Dose:** Insufficient evidence; | **Monitor:** Cortisol levels, toxic symptoms; | **Notes:** Black bryony should not be confused with bryony species of the *Bryonia* genus. *Byronia* species, such as white bryony (*Bryonia alba*), are members of the Cucurbitaceae family and are unrelated to black bryony and other members of the Dioscoreaceae family.

black cohosh *(Actaea racemosa,* formerly *Cimicifuga racemosa)* | **Uses:** Breast cancer, infertility, menopausal symptoms, migraine (menstrual), osteoarthritis, rheumatoid arthritis; | **Preg:** Not recommended due to unclear evidence; traditionally used to stimulate labor; | **CIs:** Allergy/hypersensitivity; | **ADRs:** abdominal pain, bleeding, bradycardia, bruising, constipation, diaphoresis, dizziness, headache, "heaviness in the legs," ↑ risk of stroke and hormone-sensitive cancers, HEPATOTOXICITY, hypotension, muscle damage, nausea, osteoporosis, seizures, skin rash, vaginal bleeding, vision changes, vomiting, weight gain; | **Interactions:** Agents that lower seizure threshold (↑ risk of seizures), analgesics (additive effects), anesthetics (additive effects), anticoagulants/antiplatelets (↑ risk of bleeding), antidepressants, antihypertensives (additive effects/↑ risk of hypotension), anti-inflammatory agents (additive effects), cisplatin (↓ cytotoxic effects), CYP450 2D6 substrates (inhibits CYP2D6/altered drug levels), hepatotoxic agents (↑ risk of liver damage), HMG-CoA reductase inhibitors (↑ LFTs), hormonal agents (altered or interfere with effects), oral agents (↓ effects),

B

salicylates (additive effects), tamoxifen (↓ tamoxifen-induced hot flashes); | **Dose:** Recommended: 40–200 mg dried black cohosh rhizome daily in divided doses; 0.4–2 mL of a (1:10) 60% ethanol tincture of black cohosh daily. Traditional: Up to 1 g 3 times daily; | **Monitor:** Blood glucose, blood pressure, coagulation panel, LFTs; | **Notes:** Black cohosh (*Cimicifuga racemosa*) is not to be confused with blue cohosh (*Caulophyllum thalictroides*), which contains potentially cardiotoxic/vasoconstrictive chemicals. Black cohosh is also not to be confused with *Cimicifuga foetida*, bugbane, fairy candles, or sheng ma; these are species from the same family (Ranunculaceae) with different therapeutic effects.

black currant ***(Ribes nigrum)*** | **Uses:** Antioxidant, chronic venous insufficiency, hypertension, immunomodulation, muscle stiffness, night vision, phenylketonuria, rheumatoid arthritis, stress; | **Preg:** Based on traditional use, the fruit is likely safe in food amounts in pregnant or breastfeeding patients. Other uses (including black currant seed oil) are not recommended due to lack of sufficient evidence; | **CIs:** Allergy/hypersensitivity; | **ADRs:** diarrhea, mild gastrointestinal symptoms; | **Interactions:** Anticoagulants/antiplatelets (↑ risk of bleeding), antihypertensives (additive effects/↑ risk of hypotension), anti-inflammatory agents (additive effects), MAOIs (↑ risk of hypertensive crisis); | **Dose:** Oil: One capsule containing 500–1,000 mg black currant seed oil 3 times daily. Doses up to 6 g daily have been studied. Anthocyanins: Up to 17 mg daily for 2 weeks; | **Monitor:** Blood pressure, coagulation panel; | **Notes:** Black currant is composed of approximately 17% omega-6 gamma-linolenic acid (GLA) and 13% omega-3 alpha-linolenic acid (ALA).

black haw ***(Viburnum prunifolium)*** | **Uses:** There are no scientific studies on the use of black haw for medical conditions; | **Preg:** Contraindicated due to salicin content, despite its traditional use in preventing miscarriage and morning sickness; | **CIs:** Allergy/hypersensitivity (to aspirin or salicylates), History of nephrolithiasis (kidney stones), Pregnancy, Lactation, Pediatric use; | **ADRs:** bleeding, gastrointestinal upset, Reye's syndrome (when used in children), uterine spasms; | **Interactions:** Aspirin (↑ salicylate levels/toxicity), anticoagulants/antiplatelets (↑ risk of bleeding), minerals (↓ absorption of minerals); | **Dose:** Insufficient evidence; | **Monitor:** Coagulation panel; | **Notes:** Black haw (*Viburnum prunifolium*) should not be confused with *Sideroxylon lanuginosum* and *Viburnum lentago*, which may also commonly be known as black haw.

black hellebore *(Helleborus niger)* **Uses:** There are no scientific studies on the use of black hellebore for medical conditions; **Preg:** Avoid use due to abortifacient effects and historical use as a menstrual stimulant; **CIs:** Allergy/hypersensitivity, ORAL USE (due to cardiac glycoside toxicity); **ADRs:** arrhythmia, diarrhea, dizziness, dyspnea, gastrointestinal irritation, nausea, salivation, scratchy throat or mouth, skin irritation, suffocation, vomiting; **Interactions:** cardiac glycosides (additive effects/↑ risk of toxicity), diuretics (additive effects/↑ risk of electrolyte imbalances), macrolides (↑ risk of toxicity), narcotics (additive effects), quinine (↑ risk of toxicity), stimulant laxatives (↑ risk of toxicity), tetracycline (↑ risk of toxicity); **Dose:** Fluid extract: 2–10 drops. Solid extract: 1–2 grains. Powdered root: 10–20 grains as a drastic purge; 2–3 grains as an alterative. Decoction: 1 fluid oz once every 4 hours; **Monitor:** Cardiac function; **Notes:** Black hellebore contains cardiac glycosides and is POISONOUS even when taken in small-to-moderate doses. Black hellebore is not to be confused with *Veratrum* species, also known as false hellebores. Black hellebore is considered an obsolete and dangerous natural product.

black horehound *(Ballota nigra)* **Uses:** There are no scientific studies on the use of black horehound for medical conditions; **Preg:** Not recommended due to insufficient evidence; used traditionally to treat morning sickness; **CIs:** Allergy/hypersensitivity; **ADRs:** overdose may result in DEATH, ↓ absorption of iron and other minerals, neurosedative effects; **Interactions:** Antilipemic agents (additive effects), CNS depressants (additive sedation), dopamine agonists (additive effects), iron (↓ absorption); **Dose:** Dried herb: 2–4 g 3 times daily. Fluid extract: 1–3 g dried equivalent 3 times daily. Infusion: 2 oz fresh horehound leaves per 2.5 cups water. Syrup: 1 tsp syrup 3 times daily. Tincture: 0.1–0.2 g dried equivalent 3 times daily (1:10, 45% ethanol). **Monitor:** Iron levels, lipid profile; **Notes:** Black horehound should not be confused with white horehound (*Marrubium vulgare*) or water horehound (*Lycopus americanus*, also known as bugleweed). Black horehound may bind to dopamine (D2) receptors and adversely affect patients with Parkinson's disease or schizophrenia.

black mulberry *(Morus nigra)* **Uses:** There are no scientific studies on the use of black mulberry for medical conditions; **Preg:** Based on traditional use, black mulberry is likely safe in food amounts in pregnant or breastfeeding patients. Other uses are not recommended due to lack of sufficient evidence; | **CIs:** Allergy/hypersensitivity; | **ADRs:** insufficient evidence; | **Interactions:** Cytochrome P450 substrates (altered drug levels), antidiabetic agents (additive effects/↑ risk of hypoglycemia), CNS depressants (additive sedation), midazolam (↓ effects); | **Dose:** General: 2–4 mL of mulberry syrup or 4.5–15 g of powder or decoction; | **Monitor:** Blood glucose, LFTs; | **Notes:** Black mulberry is commonly used for its antioxidant properties. It is also popularly used in the preparation of flavored syrup used as a laxative.

black pepper *(Piper nigrum)* | **Uses:** Smoking cessation, stroke recovery (difficulty swallowing); | **Preg:** Not recommended due to insufficient evidence; | **CIs:** Allergy/hypersensitivity; | **ADRs:** airway irritation, DEATH (inhalation, case reports), dyspepsia, edema, esophageal cancer, gastric bleeding, gastrointestinal adverse effects, mucosal microbleeding, nasopharyngeal cancer, occupational rhinoconjunctivitis, respiratory arrest, respiratory irritation, *Salmonella oranienburg* infection, severe anoxia; | **Interactions:** Analgesics (additive effects), anti-inflammatory agents (additive effects), carbamazepine (↑ levels of carbamazepine), cholinesterase inhibitors (additive effects), CYP 450 3A4 (↑ levels of drugs metabolized by CYP3A4), digoxin (↓ effects), diuretics (additive effects), phenytoin (↑ levels of phenytoin), rifampin (↑ levels of rifampin), theophylline (↑ levels of theophylline); | **Dose:** Nasal inhalation of volatile black pepper oil for 1 minute for up to 1 month; | **Monitor:** Electrolytes, serum drug levels (carbamazepine, phenytoin, theophylline); | **Notes:** Black pepper, white pepper, green pepper, pink pepper, and red pepper are all differently preserved berries or seeds of the *Piper nigrum* plant.

black seed *(Nigella sativa)* | **Uses:** Allergies; | **Preg:** Not recommended due to insufficient evidence and possible ↓ effects on uterine contraction and contraceptive activity; | **CIs:** Allergy/hypersensitivity, Those attempting to conceive (↓ conception in animals); | **ADRs:** contraceptive activity, dermatitis, hepatotoxicity; | **Interactions:** Anti-inflammatories (additive effects), antilipemic agents (additive effects), buthionine sulfoximine (↑ toxicity of black seed), hepatotoxic agents (↑ risk of liver damage); | **Dose:** Oral: Up to 80 mg/kg daily (capsules), 1 tsp 3 times daily (oil). Topical: Up to 1 tsp applied to scalp. Otic: ½ tsp mixed 1:1 with olive oil and dripped in ear. Inhalation: vapor containing 1 tsp oil; | **Monitor:** Lipid profile, WBC count; | **Notes:** According to secondary sources, other names used for black seed are onion seed and black sesame (both of which are similar looking but unrelated).

Frequently, the seeds are referred to as black cumin; however, although this may refer to the seeds of *Nigella sativa*, this may also refer to the seeds of a different plant, *Bunium persicum*.

black tea ***(Camellia sinensis)*** | **Uses:** Asthma, cancer prevention, colorectal cancer, dental cavity prevention, diabetes, memory enhancement, metabolic enhancement, methicillin-resistant *Staphylococcus aureus* infection (MRSA), mouth cancer/oral leukoplakia, myocardial infarction prevention, obesity, osteoporosis prevention, stress; | **Preg:** Not recommended in high doses during pregnancy due to caffeine content. Caffeine may ↑ risk of miscarriage, intrauterine growth retardation, low birth weight, birth defects, ↑ risk of sudden infant death syndrome (SIDS); | **CIs:** Allergy/hypersensitivity; Pregnancy and lactation (in high doses); | **ADRs:** agitation, anxiety, arrhythmia, cancer, dizziness, dyspepsia, excitement, hyperglycemia, hypertension, hypokalemia, hyponatremia, incontinence, insomnia, iron deficiency, microcytic anemia, muscle spasm, polyuria, psychosis, restlessness, rhabdomyolysis, seizure, skin rashes, stained teeth, tachycardia, thrombosis, tremor; | **Interactions:** Adenosine (caffeine is competitive inhibitor of adenosine), alcohol (↑ caffeine concentrations), anticoagulants/antiplatelets (↑ risk of bleeding), antidiabetic effects (altered or interfere with effects), bitter orange (additive stimulant effects/↑ of adverse cardiovascular effects), calcium (↑ calcium excretion), cimetidine (↓ caffeine clearance), clozapine (↑ risk of toxicity of clozapine), contraceptives (↑ caffeine concentrations), CNS depressants (antagonistic effects), CNS stimulants (additive stimulant effects), creatine (↑ risk of adverse cardiovascular effects), CYP450 substrates (altered drug levels), dipyridamole (↓ vasodilation), disulfiram (↓ clearance/↑ half-life of caffeine), echinacea (↑ effects), ephedrine (additive stimulant effects), estrogens (↑ caffeine concentrations), fluconazole (↑ caffeine effects), iron (↓ iron absorption), grapefruit (↑ caffeine concentrations), lithium (↑ lithium levels), magnesium (↑ excretion of magnesium), MAO inhibitors (↑ risk of hypertensive crisis), mexiletine (↑ caffeine effects), milk (↓ effects of black tea), pentobarbital (antagonistic effects), phenothiazines (precipitation of fluphenazine solutions), phenylpropanolamine (↑ blood pressure/stimulant effects), quinolones (↑ caffeine effects), terbinafine (↑ caffeine effects), theophylline (↑ theophylline levels), TCAs (precipitation of TCA solutions), verapamil (↑ caffeine concentrations), warfarin (↓ effects of warfarin), yohimbine (↑ risk of hypertensive crisis); | **Dose:** Heart disease prevention: 250–900 mL of tea, taken by mouth daily for up to 4 weeks. Mental performance: 400 mL taken 3 times daily. Dental cavity prevention: 20 mL of black tea gargled for 60 seconds daily; | **Monitor:** Blood pressure, blood glucose, ferritin, heart rate, plasma homocysteine, LFTs, renal function tests, theophylline levels, uric acid levels; | **Notes:** Green tea, black tea, and oolong tea come from the same plant. Much of the interactions of black tea are related to caffeine content.

black walnut *(Juglans nigra)* | **Uses:** There are no scientific studies on the use of black walnut for medical conditions; | **Preg:** Not recommended due to insufficient evidence on oral use and anecdotal evidence that topical black walnut may be unsafe to use by pregnant or lactating women; | **CIs:** Allergy/hypersensitivity; | **ADRs:** abdominal upset, dermatitis (when used topically), diarrhea, esophageal cancer, mouth cancer, ↑ risk of hepatotoxicity and nephrotoxicity (due to tannins), hypertension, lip leukoplakia, nasal cancer, stomach cancer; | **Interactions:** Antihypertensives (antagonistic effects), anti-inflammatory agents (additive effects), hepatotoxic agents (↑ risk of liver damage), laxatives (additive effects), nephrotoxic agents (↑ risk of renal damage), oral agents (precipitation of some oral drugs by tannins); | **Dose:** Oral: Powdered black walnut capsules (500 mg and 1,000 mg), 3 times daily for a maximum of 6 weeks. Topical: Black walnut topically twice daily; | **Monitor:** Blood pressure, LFTs, renal function panel; | **Notes:** The U.S. Food and Drug Administration (FDA) issued a press release on July 14, 2003, announcing the availability of a qualified health claim stating that eating 1.5 oz per day of walnuts as part of a diet low in saturated fat and cholesterol may reduce the risk of heart disease, due to the essential fatty acids contained in walnuts, which have been shown to protect against heart disease. Black walnuts contain a high amount of tannins (approximately 455) and may increase the risk of various cancers.

blackberry *(Rubus fructicosus)* | **Uses:** Antioxidant; | **Preg:** Based on traditional use, blackberry is likely safe in food amounts in pregnant or breastfeeding patients. Other uses are not recommended due to lack of sufficient evidence; | **CIs:** Allergy/hypersensitivity; | **ADRs:** sporotrichosis possibly due to picking blackberries; | **Interactions:** Antineoplastic agents (additive effects, due to antioxidant effects); | **Dose:** Insufficient evidence; | **Monitor:** Insufficient evidence; | **Notes:** May be prone to mold growth.

blessed thistle *(Cnicus benedictus)* | **Uses:** Abortifacient, dyspepsia/indigestion/flatulence, viral infections; | **Preg:** Avoid during pregnancy due to traditional use as an abortifacient; not recommended during lactation due to insufficient evidence; | **CIs:** Allergy/hypersensitivity (to Asteraceae/Compositae family, including ragweed, chrysanthemums, marigolds, daisies, etc.), Infectious/inflammatory bowel disease, Pregnancy, Lactation; | **ADRs:** abdominal discomfort, birth defects, bleeding, bruising, dyspepsia, dyspnea, gastric ulcer, hepatotoxicity, nasopharyngeal cancer, nephrotoxicity, pruritus, urticaria, vomiting; | **Interactions:** Antacids (↓ effectiveness), anticoagulants/antiplatelets (↑ risk of bleeding), anti-inflammatory agents (additive effects); | **Dose:** Tincture: 7.5–10 mL (1.5 g/L blessed thistle) 3 times daily. Liquid extract (1:1 g/mL in 25% alcohol): 1.5–3.0 mL 3 times daily. Infusion: 1.5–2 g of blessed thistle in 150 mL water, 3 times daily. Tea: 1.5–3 g of dried blessed thistle flowering tops steeped in boiling water 3 times daily; | **Monitor:** Coagulation panel; | **Notes:** Blessed thistle should not be mistaken for milk thistle (*Silybum marianus*) or other members of the thistle family.

bloodroot ***(Sanguinaria canadensis)*** | **Uses:** Plaque/gingivitis, periodontal disease; | **Preg:** Not recommended due to insufficient evidence and traditional use as an emmenagogue; | **CIs:** Allergy/hypersensitivity; Glaucoma (high doses), Infectious/inflammatory bowel conditions, Oral lesions, Pregnancy, Lactation; | **ADRs:** abdominal cramping, CNS depression, cognitive impairment, contact dermatitis, diarrhea, disfiguration of skin and tissue, drowsiness, dysgeusia, dysplastic lesions of the lip and mucosa, formation of an eschar, glaucoma, increased response time, irritation, lead poisoning, leukoplakia, myasthenia, obscured visual perception, polydipsia, staining of the tongue, teeth and fillings, syncope, ulceration, vertigo, vomiting; | **Interactions:** Antihypertensives (additive effects/↑ risk of hypotension), CNS depressants (additive sedation), cytochrome P450 substrates (altered drug levels), hormonal agents (altered effects); | **Dose:** Oral rinse: 300 mcg/mL sanguinaria extract twice daily for up to 6 months, oral rinses containing 0.01% sanguinarine daily for up to 6 weeks; | **Monitor:** Blood pressure, pregnancy hormones, WBC count; | **Notes:** The active constituent of bloodroot is thought to be sanguinarine, which may have antimicrobial and antiplaque activity.

blue cohosh ***(Caulophyllum thalictroides)*** | **Uses:** There are no scientific studies on the use of blue cohosh for medical conditions; | **Preg:** Not recommended due to known maternal and fetal toxicity and traditional use as an abortifacient or for labor induction; | **CIs:** Allergy/hypersensitivity; PREGNANCY, Lactation; | **ADRs:** abdominal pain, angina,

B

aplastic anemia, ataxia, cardiotoxic effects, coma, congestive heart failure, cramping, diarrhea, fasciculations, headache, hyperglycemia, hypertension, hyperthermia, hyperventilation, hypotension, irregular pulse, myasthenia, mydriasis, myocardial infarction, nausea, nystagmus, polydipsia, seizures, shock, stroke, tachycardia, uterine contractions, vomiting; | **Interactions:** Antidiabetic agents (↓ effectiveness), antihypertensive agents (↓ effectiveness), antispasmodic agents (↑ effectiveness), cocaine (additive effects, possible contamination), nicotine (↓/↑ effects), oxytocin (additive effects); | **Dose:** Decoction: 4 g twice daily or 1–3 g every 3 to 4 hours. Fluid extract: 0.5–1.0 mL (1:1 in 70% alcohol) 3 times daily. Infusion: 2–4 fluid ounces (1 oz root to 1 pint boiling water) 3 or 4 times daily. Tea: 1 tsp dried root in 1 cup water, taken twice daily. Tincture: 30 drops in 2 cups of water, or 15 drops in a cup of warm water every half hour. Whole herb: 300–1,000 mg of dried herb up to 3 times daily. | **Monitor:** Blood glucose, blood pressure, pregnancy; | **Notes:** Blue cohosh (*Caulophyllum thalictroides*) should not be confused with black cohosh (*Cimicifuga racemosa*), an over-the-counter herbal supplement sold as a menopause and menstrual remedy.

blue flag ***(Iris versicolor)*** | **Uses:** There are no scientific studies on the use of blue flag for medical conditions; | **Preg:** Not recommended due to insufficient evidence and known toxicity; | **CIs:** Allergy/hypersensitivity, ORAL USE, Pregnancy, Lactation; | **ADRs:** abdominal pain and cramping (persistent), dermatitis, emesis, gastroenteritis (resulting in DEATH), mucosal irritation, nausea, neuralgic pain, poisoning, skin eruptions, vomiting; | **Interactions:** Anti-inflammatory agents (additive effects), diuretics (additive effects), emetics (additive effects), oral agents (↓ effectiveness, due to purgative effects); | **Dose:** Decoction: 1 tsp of dried herb simmered in water 3 times daily. For poisonous stings and bites, 1 oz of the powdered root boiled in 1 pint of water. Dried rhizome: 0.6–2 g. Fluid extract: 0.5–1 drachm, or 1–2 mL 3 times daily. Powdered root: 20 grains. Solid extract: 10–15 grains. Tincture: 1–5 mL 3 times daily, or 1–3 drachms; | **Monitor:** Toxic symptoms (oral use); | **Notes:** According to expert opinion, fresh rhizome should only be applied topically and never taken internally because it may irritate the mouth and is much more likely to cause nausea and diarrhea.

boldo ***(Peumus boldus)*** | **Uses:** There are no scientific studies on the use of boldo for medical conditions; | **Preg:** Not recommended due to insufficient evidence and possible fetal alterations. The German Commission E notes no contraindications to the use of ascaridole-free boldo preparations in pregnancy and lactation. **CIs:** Allergy/hypersensitivity; Alcoholism, Bile duct obstruction, Liver disease, Pregnancy; **ADRs:** HEPATOTOXICITY (due to ascaridole content), skin irritation; **Interactions:** Anticoagulants/antiplatelets (↑ risk of bleeding), anti-inflammatory agents (additive effects), diuretic agents (additive effects), hepatotoxic agents (↑ risk of liver damage); **Dose:** Liquid extract: 1:1 in 45% alcohol, 0.1–0.3 mL 3 times daily. Tea/infusion: 60–200 mg dried leaf 3 times daily as a tea. Tincture: 1:10 in 60% alcohol, 0.5–2 mL 3 times daily; **Monitor:** Coagulation panel, LFTs; **Notes:** Boldo has Generally Recognized as Safe (GRAS) status for use in foods in the United States.

boneset ***(Eupatorium perfoliatum)*** **Uses:** Colds/flu; **Preg:** Not recommended due to insufficient evidence and toxic pyrrolizidine alkaloids; **CIs:** Allergy/hypersensitivity (to Asteraceae/Compositae family, including ragweed, chrysanthemums, marigolds, daisies, etc.), Alcoholism, Kidney conditions, Liver disease; **ADRs:** arrhythmia, coma, contact dermatitis, DEATH, diaphoresis, diarrhea (severe), diuresis, HEPATOTOXICITY, myasthenia, nausea, vomiting; **Interactions:** Anti-inflammatory agents (additive effects), diuretic agents (additive effects), hepatotoxic agents (↑ risk of liver damage); **Dose:** Tea: 1–2 g or 1–3 tsp herb per cup, up to 6 cups daily for 2 days. Liquid extract (1:1 in 25% alcohol): 1–2 mL 3 times daily, 0.5–1 drachm, or 1–3 grains. Powder: 12–20 grains. Tincture (1:5 in 45% alcohol): 1–4 mL 3 times daily; **Monitor:** Electrolytes, LFTs, renal function panel; **Notes:** Avoid confusion with gravel root (*Eupatorium purpureum*), which is also known as boneset. Snakeroot is a common name used for poisonous Eupatorium species, but boneset should not be confused with *Ageratina* spp., which are more commonly known as snakeroot. Boneset contains hepatotoxic pyrrolizidine alkaloids.

borage ***(Borago officinalis)*** **Uses:** Acute respiratory distress syndrome; periodontitis/gingivitis; rheumatoid arthritis; alcohol-induced hangover; asthma; atopic dermatitis; cystic fibrosis; hyperlipidemia; infant development/neonatal care (in preterm infants); malnutrition (inflammation complex syndrome); seborrheic dermatitis (infantile); stress; supplementation in preterm and very low birth weight infants (fatty acids); **Preg:** May be contraindicated in pregnancy due to teratogenic and labor-inducing effects of prostaglandin E agonists; **CIs:** Allergy/hypersensitivity; Immunocompromised, Liver disease, Pregnancy, Seizure disorders; **ADRs:** flatulence, HEPATOTOXICITY (due to pyrrolizidine alkaloid content), hyperglycemia, ↓ seizure threshold; | **Interactions:** Anticoagulants (↑ risk of bleeding), anticonvulsants (altered or interferes with effects), antilipemic agents (additive effects), drugs that lower seizure threshold (↑ risk of seizures), hepatotoxic agents (↑ risk of liver damage), NSAIDs (↓ effects of borage); | **Dose:** Up to 3 g daily; | **Monitor:** Blood glucose, coagulation panel, immune parameters, LFTs, lipid profile; | **Notes:** Although one meta-analysis has identified borage as unsafe, borage did not cause any adverse effects in two clinical trials. Some products contain hepatotoxic pyrrolizidine alkaloids.

boron | **Uses:** Boron deficiency, cognitive function; hormone regulation; osteoarthritis; osteoporosis; vaginitis; | **Preg:** Not recommended due to insufficient evidence; | **CIs:** Allergy/hypersensitivity; Children/infants (high doses), Hormone-sensitive conditions, Pregnancy (high doses), Renal failure; | **ADRs:** abdominal pain, agitation, alopecia, anemia, cough with mucus discharge, dehydration, depression, diarrhea, dryness of the mouth or nose, excitability, eye irritation, fever, headache, hepatotoxicity, hyper-/hypoglycemia, hypertension, hyperthermia, infant death, infertility, irritability, lethargy, nausea, nephrotoxicity, seizure, skin rash/redness/peeling, sore throat, ↑ steroid hormone levels, testicular toxicity, toxicity, tremors, weakness, vomiting (blue-green in color). Boron may also affect the blood levels of calcitonin, insulin, phosphorus, vitamin D_2, calcium, copper, magnesium, or thyroxine; | **Interactions:** Analgesics (additive effects), androgens (additive effects), anti-inflammatory agents (additive effects), antilipemic agents (additive effects), dopaminergic agents (altered effects), estrogens (↑ estrogen levels/effects), hepatotoxic agents (↑ risk of liver damage), nephrotoxic agents (↑ risk of kidney damage), osteoporosis agents (additive effects); | **Dose:** General: acute bolus of 11.6 mg boron (given as 102.6 mg sodium tetraborate decahydrate). Bodybuilding aid: 2.5 mg daily for 7 weeks. Dietary intake: The average reported boron intake in the American diet is 1.17 mg/day for men, 0.96 mg/day for women, and 1.29–1.47 mg/day for vegetarians. Improvement of cognitive function: 3 mg of elemental boron PO daily. Menopausal symptoms: 2.5–3 mg of elemental boron daily. Osteoarthritis: 3–6 mg of elemental boron (as sodium tetraborate decahydrate) daily for up to 8 weeks. Osteoporosis: 3 mg daily for 1 year. Psoriasis: A combination formula of 1.5% boric acid with 3% zinc oxide applied to the skin as needed. Vaginitis: Boric acid powder capsules administered vaginally daily; | **Monitor:** BMI, calcium levels, estrogen levels, lipid profile, LFTs, magnesium levels, renal function test, thyroid function panel, vitamin D levels; | **Notes:** Boron is a micronutrient found in plants and is thought to be essential for animal growth and development.

boswellia *(Boswellia serrata)* | **Uses:** Asthma, arthritis, Crohn's disease, ulcerative colitis; | **Preg:** Not recommended due to insufficient evidence and traditional use as an abortifacient; | **CIs:** Allergy/hypersensitivity; Pregnancy; | **ADRs:** abdominal pain and fullness, diarrhea, dyspepsia, gastrointestinal upset, menorrhagia, miscarriage, nausea, rash, skin rash; | **Interactions:** Analgesics (additive effects), anti-inflammatory agents (additive effects), antilipemics (additive effects), antineoplastic agents (additive effects), CNS depressants (additive sedation), CYP450 substrates (altered drug levels); | **Dose:** 200- to 1,200-mg capsules 3 times daily for up to 8 months. | **Monitor:** LFTs, lipid profile; | **Notes:** Boswellia has traditionally been used for topical conditions, including acne, bacterial infections, fungal infections, boils, wound healing, scars, wrinkles, and varicose veins.

bovine cartilage | **Uses:** Acne, anal fissures, anal pruritus, cancer, hemorrhoids, mandibular alveolitis, osteoarthritis, poison oak, psoriasis, rheumatoid arthritis, skin care (laser resurfacing adjunct); | **Preg:** Not recommended due to insufficient evidence; | **CIs:** Allergy/hypersensitivity; | **ADRs:** oral: bloating, diarrhea, fatigue, gastrointestinal upset, nausea, nephrotic syndrome, scrotal swelling; subcutaneous: edema, local redness, pruritus, urticaria; | **Interactions:** Antiangiogenic agents (additive effects), antiarthritic agents (additive effects), antineoplastics (additive effects), immunosuppressants (altered effects); | **Dose:** Oral: capsules (3 g) 3 times daily. Topical: ointment (10% powdered bovine cartilage) applied every 2–4 hours for 8 days; 5% bovine cartilage 2 or more times daily; paste (powdered bovine cartilage and saline) packed into tooth socket. Parenteral subcutaneous: weekly or biweekly 5–25 g for most indications; experimental doses have been up to 300 g. Rectal: 2.2 g bovine cartilage, as a 2% suppository, 3 or more times a day; | **Monitor:** Tuberculosis tests; | **Notes:** Bovine cartilage, as a dietary supplement, typically is a preparation of bovine tracheal cartilage.

bovine colostrum | **Uses:** Colitis, cryptosporidiosis, diarrhea, exercise performance enhancement, immune function, *Helicobacter pylori* infection, multiple sclerosis, oral hygiene, postoperative recovery, rotavirus, sore throat, upper respiratory tract infection; | **Preg:** Not recommended due to insufficient evidence and recommendations from secondary sources;

B

Cls: Allergy/hypersensitivity; Pregnancy, Lactation, Cancer or ↑ cancer risk (due to growth factors found in colostrum); **ADRs:** atherosclerosis, bloating, diarrhea, digestive problems, nausea/vomiting, rashes, ↑ risk of cancers (including prostate, colorectal, breast, and lung), skin eruptions; **Interactions:** Antidiabetic agents (additive effects/↑ risk of hypoglycemia), antidiarrheals (additive effects), antineoplastic agents (↓ effects), NSAIDs (↓ effects); **Dose:** Adults: 400–5,000 mg 1–3 times daily in tablet, powder, or solution. Children: 7–20 g 3 times daily for up to 14 days; **Monitor:** GI effects, lipids, immune parameters; **Notes:** Bovine colostrum is the premilk fluid produced from cow mammary glands during the first 2–4 days after birth. Bovine colostrum confers growth, nutrient, and immune factors to the offspring.

boxwood *(Buxus sempervirens)* **Uses:** HIV/AIDS; **Preg:** Not recommended due to insufficient evidence; **Cls:** Allergy/hypersensitivity; **ADRs:** blood pressure ↑/then blood pressure ↓, contact dermatitis; **Interactions:** Antihypertensive agents (altered effects), antiretroviral agents (may ↑ CD4 and CD8 counts, ↓ viral load), cholinergic agents (altered effects), steroids (additive effects); **Dose:** Insufficient evidence; **Monitor:** Blood pressure, CD4 counts, CD8 counts, viral load; **Notes:** An extract of boxwood, SPV-30 (Arkopharma, France), has been studied for its potential effects in HIV and AIDS; however, claims for SPV-30 have been controversial.

branched-chain amino acids (BCAAs) **Uses:** Alcoholic hepatitis, athletic performance enhancement, hepatic encephalopathy, hepatocellular carcinoma, hormone regulation (male), immunomodulation, liver cirrhosis, muscle atrophy, phenylketonuria, spinocerebellar degeneration, tardive dyskinesia, total parenteral nutrition (TPN); **Preg:** Not recommended due to insufficient evidence; **Cls:** Allergy/hypersensitivity; **ADRs:** ↑ ammonia levels, fatigue, hepatotoxicity, ↑ hormone production; **Interactions:** Anesthesia (↑ BCAA effects), antidiabetic agents (additive effects/↑ risk of hypoglycemia), antineoplastics (additive effects), corticosteroids (↓ metabolism of BCAAs), diazoxide (↓ BCAA effects), epinephrine (↓ BCAA levels), erythropoietin (normalizing erythropoietin normalizes BCAA levels), levodopa (↓ effectiveness of levodopa), thyroid hormones (↓ metabolism of BCAAs); **Dose:** Oral: 68–240 mg/kg/day; 60–80 g total amino acids (51% BCAAs); Aminoleban EN 100 g daily for 1 year; **Monitor:** Amino acid levels, renal function tests, urine tests; **Notes:** The three BCAAs are leucine, isoleucine and valine; they are called branched-chain amino acids because they are aliphatic, meaning that they are nonlinear and have side chains.

breadfruit | **Uses:** Insufficient evidence; | **Preg:** Not recommended due to insufficient evidence; | **CIs:** Allergy/hypersensitivity; | **ADRs:** unpleasant taste, urticaria; | **Interactions:** 5-alpha reductase inhibitors (synergistic effects), anthelmintics (additive effects), anticoagulants/antiplatelets (↑ risk of bleeding), antineoplastic effects (additive effects), inotropes (antagonize effects); | **Dose:** Insufficient evidence; | **Monitor:** Coagulation panel; | **Notes:** Breadfruit tree preparation is believed to lower hypertension, and it has also been studied to treat taeniasis (a digestive tract infection caused by tapeworms).

brewer's yeast | **Uses:** *Clostridium difficile* colitis, diabetes, hyperlipidemia, mood enhancement, PMS, upper respiratory tract infection; | **Preg:** Not recommended due to insufficient evidence; | **CIs:** Allergy/hypersensitivity; | **ADRs:** allergic reactions, flatulence, fungemia, gastrointestinal upset, local exanthemas, migraine headache, pruritus, Quincke's edema; | **Interactions:** Antidiabetic agents (↑ risk of hypoglycemia), antifungals (↓ effectiveness of brewer's yeast), antilipemic agents (additive effects), antineoplastic agents (additive effects), chromium (↑ risk of chromium toxicity), immunosuppressants (antagonize effects), MAOIs (↑ risk of hypertensive crisis), vitamin D (brewer's yeast is a source of vitamin D/ ↑ levels of vitamin D) | **Dose:** 500 mg–6 g PO qd; | **Monitor:** Blood glucose, lipid profile; | **Notes:** Brewer's yeast contains tyramine and chromium.

bromelain | **Uses:** Burns, cancer, COPD, digestion, inflammation, knee pain, muscle soreness, nutritional supplement, osteoarthritis (knee), rash, rheumatoid arthritis, sinusitis, steatorrhea, urinary tract infection (UTI); | **Preg:** Not recommended due to insufficient evidence and purported ↑ in menstrual bleeding; | **CIs:** Allergy/hypersensitivity to pineapples, tree or grass pollen, carrots, celery, fennel, bees, latex, or flour; Liver/kidney disease (↓ bromelain elimination), Bleeding disorders; | **ADRs:** bleeding, diarrhea, drowsiness, dyspnea, gastrointestinal upset, irritation of mucus membranes, menstrual irregularities, nausea, throat swelling, sedation, tachycardia, vomiting; | **Interactions:** Amoxicillin (↑ levels of amoxicillin), analgesics (additive effects), anti-inflammatory agents (additive effects), anticoagulants/antiplatelets (↑ risk of bleeding), antihypertensives (additive effects/↑ risk of hypotension), antineoplastic agents (additive effects), CNS depressants (additive sedation),

B

immunosuppressants (altered effects), magnesium (may ↑ bromelain), tetracycline antibiotics (↑ absorption/levels of tetracyclines), zinc (↓ bromelain effects); | **Dose:** Tablets: 80- to 1,000-mg tablets up to 3 times daily. Cream: 35% bromelain in an oil base; | **Monitor:** Coagulation panel, CBC, electrolytes, heart rate; | **Notes:** Bromelain is a sulfur-containing proteolytic digestive enzyme that is extracted from the stem and the fruit of the pineapple plant (*Ananas comosus* family).

broom corn | **Uses:** Insufficient evidence; | **Preg:** Not recommended due to insufficient evidence; | **CIs:** Allergy/hypersensitivity; | **ADRs:** insufficient evidence; | **Interactions:** Insufficient evidence; | **Dose:** Decoction: 2 oz of seeds to 1 quart of water, boil to 1 pint; | **Monitor:** N/A; | **Notes:** Broom contains large amounts of starch as well as protein, fatty oil, thiamine, riboflavin, and dhurrin (a cyanogenic glycoside). It has been used as a diuretic and demulcent.

bryonia | **Uses:** Insufficient evidence; | **Preg:** Avoid use due to abortifacient effects; | **CIs:** Allergy/hypersensitivity, Infectious/inflammatory GI conditions, ingestion of berries and root; | **ADRs:** oral: colic, convulsions, diaphoresis, diarrhea, dizziness, hypoglycemia, mydriasis, nausea/VOMITING, nephrotoxicity, nervousness, ↓ temperature, vertigo; topical: blisters, irritation; | **Interactions:** Antidiabetic agents (↑ risk of hypoglycemia), immunosuppressants (altered effects), nephrotoxic agents (↑ risk of kidney damage); | **Dose:** Insufficient evidence; | **Monitor:** Blood glucose, renal function tests; | **Notes:** Historically, bryonia was used as an emetic or laxative; however, oral ingestion of bryonia is unsafe and may be fatal.

buchu ***(Agathosma betulina)*** | **Uses:** There are no scientific studies on the use of buchu for medical conditions; | **Preg:** Not recommended due to insufficient evidence and traditional use as an abortifacient; | **CIs:** Allergy/hypersensitivity; Urinary tract inflammation; | **ADRs:** bleeding, diarrhea, gastrointestinal upset, hepatotoxicity, menorrhagia; | **Interactions:** Anticoagulants/antiplatelets (↑ risk of bleeding), cardiac glycosides (↑ risk of adverse effects), diuretic agents (↑ additive effects); | **Dose:** Insufficient evidence; | **Monitor:** Coagulation panel, electrolytes, LFTs; | **Notes:** Not to be confused with Indian buchu (*Myrtus communi*), which is an unrelated plant.

buckhorn plantain ***(Plantago coronopus)*** | **Uses:** There are no scientific studies on the use of buckhorn plaintain for medical conditions; | **Preg:** Not recommended due to insufficient evidence; | **Cls:** Allergy/hypersensitivity; | **ADRs:** insufficient evidence; | **Interactions:** Insufficient evidence; | **Dose:** Insufficient evidence; | **Monitor:** Insufficient evidence; | **Notes:** In the Canary Islands, buckhorn plantain is used for the treatment of kidney and urinary diseases.

buckwheat | **Uses:** Chronic venous insufficiency, diabetes, diabetic retinopathy, hyperlipidemia; | **Preg:** Not recommended due to insufficient evidence; | **Cls:** Allergy/hypersensitivity; | **ADRs:** anaphylaxis, asthma, conjunctivitis, diarrhea, edema, gastrointestinal upset, hypotension, nausea/vomiting, photosensitization, pruritus, shock, urticaria; | **Interactions:** Antidiabetic agents (↑ risk of hypolglycemia), antihypertensives (↑ risk of hypotension), antilipemic agents (additive effects), antineoplastic agents (additive effects), diuretics (altered effects), laxatives (additive effects), photosensitizers (↑ risk of photosensitivity); | **Dose:** Chronic venous insufficiency: buckwheat (100% *Fagopyrum esculentum*, standardized to a total flavonoid content of 5% yielding a daily dosage of 270 mg of rutin) tea PO × 3 mo. Diabetes: 70–100 g flour or grain PO qd. Diabetic retinopathy: 2 tablets (containing 0.5 g buckwheat herb and 0.03 g troxerutin) of pressed buckwheat herb PO 3 times/day × 3 mo. Hyperlipidemia (raise HDL): 100 g sifted buckwheat flour PO qd × 4 wk; | **Monitor:** Blood glucose, blood pressure, lipid profile; | **Notes:** Caution is warranted in patients with celiac disease.

bugleweed (*Lycopus* spp.) | **Uses:** There are no scientific studies on the use of bugleweed for medical conditions; | **Preg:** Not recommended due to insufficient evidence and possible hormonal effects; | **Cls:** Allergy/hypersensitivity; Pregnancy, Lactation; | **ADRs:** goiter, hyperprolactinemia, hypoglycemia; | **Interactions:** Antidiabetic agents (additive effects/↑ risk of hypoglycemia), CNS depressants (additive sedation), antihypertensive agents (additive effects/↑ risk of hypotension), hormonal agents (altered effects), thyroid hormones (↓ effects of thyroid hormones); | **Dose:** General: up to 2 g above-ground plant or root. Fluid extract: 10–30 drops. Infusion: 1 oz herb per cup. Dry extract: 1–4 grains. Tea: 1–2 g herb; | **Monitor:** Blood pressure, blood glucose, thyroid function tests; | **Notes:** Not to be confused with *Ajuga reptans*, also called bugleweed in the scientific literature.

bulbous buttercup ***(Ranunculus bulbosus)*** | **Uses:** There are no scientific studies on the use of bulbous buttercup for medical conditions; | **Preg:** Not recommended due to insufficient evidence; | **CIs:** Allergy/hypersensitivity; | **ADRs:** blisters and swelling (topical); ingestion causes abdominal pain, mouth blisters, diarrhea, hepatotoxicity, respiratory failure (due to protoanemonin), ventricular arrhythmia; | **Interactions:** Antiarrhythmic agents (altered effects), hepatotoxic agents (↑ risk of liver damage); | **Dose:** 6–8 drops of tincture for shingles; | **Monitor:** Heart rate, liver function tests; | **Notes:** All parts of the bulbous buttercup are now known to be poisonous. The active properties of bulbous buttercup are thought to be destroyed upon heating or drying.

bupleurum *(Bupleurum chinense)* | **Uses:** Brain damage (minimal, in children), fever, hepatitis, hepatocellular carcinoma, thrombocytopenic purpura; | **Preg:** Not recommended due to insufficient evidence; | **CIs:** Allergy/hypersensitivity; | **ADRs:** abdominal bloating, anorexia, bleeding, ↑ bowel movements, bruising, drowsiness, dyspepsia, flatulence, hepatotoxicity, hyper-/hypoglycemia, hyper-/hypotension, lethargy, nausea, pneumonitis, pruritus, pulmonary edema, sedation, tachycardia, urticaria, wound healing; | **Interactions:** Anticoagulants/antiplatelets (↑ risk of bleeding), antidiabetic agents (altered effects/↑ risk of hypoglycemia), antihypertensives (additive effects/↑ risk of hypotension), antilipemic agents (additive effects), antineoplastic agents (additive effects), cholinesterase inhibitors (additive effects), corticosteroids (additive effects), CNS depressants (additive sedation), diuretics (additive effects), hepatotoxic agents (↑ risk of liver damage), immunosuppressants (interfere with effects), lamivudine (↑ effects), tolbutamide (↓ absorption); | **Dose:** Insufficient evidence; | **Monitor:** ACTH levels, blood glucose, coagulation panel, LFTs, lipid profile; | **Notes:** The effects of *Bupleurum* species are unclear.

burdock *(Arctium lappa)* | **Uses:** Diabetes, cancer (quality of life); | **Preg:** Not recommended due to insufficient evidence, toxic anthraquinone glycosides in burdock root and oxytocic and uterine stimulant activities observed in animals; | **CIs:** Allergy/hypersensitivity; | **ADRs:** allergic dermatitis, anticholinergic reactions (mydriasis, tachycardia, urinary retention, xerostomia), bradycardia, contact dermatitis, diuresis, erythema, estrogenic effects, exudative reactions, eye trauma, hyper-/hypoglycemia, ophthalmia, pruritus; | **Interactions:** Anticoagulants/antiplatelets (↑ risk of bleeding), antidiabetic agents (additive effects/↑ risk of hypoglycemia), anti-inflammatory agents (additive effects), antiretroviral agents (additive effects), diuretics (additive effects), estrogens (additive effects); | **Dose:** Insufficient evidence; | **Monitor:** Coagulation panel, blood glucose, electrolytes; **Notes:** Burdock has historically been used to treat a wide variety of ailments, including arthritis, diabetes, and hair loss. It is a principal herbal ingredient in the popular cancer remedies Essiac and Hoxsey formula.

burnet **Uses:** Insufficient evidence; **Preg:** Not recommended due to insufficient evidence; **CIs:** Allergy/hypersensitivity; **ADRs:** Insufficient evidence; **Interactions:** Anticoagulants/antiplatelets (counteract effects), diuretics (additive effects); **Dose:** Decoction: 4.5–15 g PO qd; **Monitor:** Coagulation panel; **Notes:** Burnet leaves and roots contain tannins and triterpenoids, which have been isolated and studied for potential anticancer activity.

butanediol **Uses:** Narcolepsy; **Preg:** Not recommended due to insufficient evidence; **CIs:** Allergy/hypersensitivity, Oral use; **ADRs:** acute respiratory acidosis, addiction, aggression, agitation, amnesia (short-term), anxiety, apnea, ataxia, bradycardia, cognitive impairment, coma, combativeness, confusion, DEATH, delusions, depression, diaphoresis, dizziness, drowsiness, euphoria, fasciculation, flailing, hallucinations, hepatotoxicity, hyperglycemia, hypersalivation, hypertension, hypothermia, insomnia, lethargy, lightheadedness, miosis, nephorotoxicity, nystagmus, psychosis, pulmonary edema, sedation, seizures, unconsciousness, unresponsiveness to pain, urinary incontinence, vertigo, visual disturbances, vomiting; **Interactions:** AMPHETAMINES (severe adverse effects), anticonvulsants (antagonistic effects), ANTIPSYCHOTIC AGENTS (potentiate the effects of gamma hydroxybutyrate [GHB]/metabolite of butanediol), BENZODIAZEPINES (additive sedation), CNS DEPRESSANTS (additive sedation), CNS STIMULANTS (antagonistic effects), methamphetamine (↑ risk of seizures), muscle relaxants (additive effects/severe adverse effects), opiate antagonists (synergistic effects), protease inhibitors (fatal reaction); **Dose:** Oral: Up to 3 g twice daily at bedtime, 4 hours apart (unclear evidence of benefit); **Monitor:** Blood pressure, body temperature, butanediol/GHB levels, heart rate, LFTs, renal function tests; **Notes:** Butanediol is metabolized to GHB, commonly known as the "date rape" drug. Although available as a prescription for sleep disorders in some other countries, GHB was banned in the United States by the FDA in 1990 because of the dangers associated with its use. It has since been approved only for the treatment of a rare form of narcolepsy. In Europe, GHB has been used as an anesthetic and experimentally to treat alcohol withdrawal.

B

butcher's broom *(Ruscus aculeatus)* | **Uses:** Chronic venous insufficiency, diabetic retinopathy, edema (calcium antagonist–induced), hemorrhoids, lymphedema, premenstrual syndrome, soft tissue injuries, varicose veins; | **Preg:** Not recommended due to insufficient evidence, although when taken by pregnant women for venous insufficiency, embryotoxic or adverse effects were not noted; | **CIs:** Allergy/hypersensitivity; | **ADRs:** generally well tolerated in clinical trials, with few adverse events reported, including contact dermatitis, gastrointestinal and epigastric discomfort, and vasoconstriction; | **Interactions:** Alpha-adrenergic agents (alter or interfere with effects), antibacterial agents (additive effects), antifungal agents (additive effects), MAOIs (↑ risk of hypertensive crisis due to tyramine content), antihypertensive agents (↓ effects), may interact with agents with similar effects or related mechanisms of action (anti-inflammatory, vasoconstrictive, diuretic); | **Dose:** Oral: Up to three 150-mg capsules (containing 33 mg total extract of ruscogenin and neoruscogenin per capsule) up to 3 times daily. Topical: 4–6 g cream containing 64–96 mg of *Ruscus* extract has been applied 2 to 3 times daily on both legs for 3 weeks; | **Monitor:** Blood pressure, electrolytes; | **Notes:** Not to be confused with Scotch broom flower, scotch broom herb, Spanish broom

butterbur *(Petasites hybridus)* | **Uses:** Allergic rhinitis prevention, migraine prevention, allergic skin disease, asthma; | **Preg:** Not recommended due to insufficient evidence; | **CIs:** Allergy/hypersensitivity; | **ADRs:** abdominal upset, constipation, diarrhea, discolored stool, drowsiness, dysphagia, dyspnea, eye discoloration, fatigue, headache, hepatotoxicity/↑ LFTs, itchy eyes, pruritus, severe nausea, skin discoloration, vomiting; | **Interactions:** Anticholinergic agents (additive effects), hepatotoxic agents (↑ risk of liver damage); | **Dose:** Allergic rhinitis: Tablets (standardized to 7.5 mg petasin (Tesalin) and isopetasin per 50-mg tablet) twice daily. Tesalin tablets containing 8 mg total petasin up to 4 times daily. Asthma: 50–150 mg butterbur (Petaforce) in 2–3 divided daily doses. Migraine prevention: 50–75 mg Petadolex twice daily for up to 4 months. Other/General: tea (1 tsp per cup) 3 times daily. Tincture: 1–2 mL 3 times daily; | **Monitor:** LFTs; | **Notes:** Raw, unprocessed butterbur plant should not be ingested due to hepatotoxic and carcinogenic pyrrolizidine alkaloids.

cabbage, broccoli, cauliflower, collard, kale, Brussels sprouts, kohlrabi *(Brassica oleracea)* | **Uses:** Breast engorgement in lactating women, cancer (bladder, colorectal, gastric, lung), fibromyalgia, hyperlipidemia, *Helicobacter pylori* infection; | **Preg:** Likely safe in food amounts in pregnant or breastfeeding patients based on traditional use; recommended as a good source of folic acid. Other uses are not recommended due to lack of sufficient evidence; | **CIs:** Allergy/hypersensitivity, Thyroid conditions; | **ADRs:** in general, *Brassica* vegetables are considered safe and well tolerated when consumed in dietary amounts; may cause flatulence, flushing, pruritus, ↓ iodine uptake; | **Interactions:** Acetaminophen (↑ elimination, ↓ levels of acetaminophen), CYP450 1A2 (↓ effectiveness), glucuronidated drugs (↓ drug levels), warfarin (↓ effects of warfarin/due to vitamin K content), thyroid hormones (altered effects); may interact with agents with similar effects or related mechanisms of action (antidiabetic, antilipemic, antineoplastic, hormonal); | **Dose:** Oral: up to 1 L cabbage juice daily; up to 160 g vegetable daily; 500 mg of a blend containing 100 mg ascorbigen and 400 mg broccoli powder daily for 1 month. Topical: Extract-containing cream applied to engorged breasts between feedings in lactating women; | **Monitor:** Blood glucose, coagulation panel, lipid profile, TSH test; | **Notes:** Cabbage, broccoli, cauliflower, collard, kale, Brussels sprouts, and kohlrabi are all cultivars (varieties) of *Brassica oleracea*; the wild form is called colewort or cole plant.

caffeine | **Uses:** Alertness, asthma, athletic performance, cirrhosis, cognitive enhancement, diabetes, headache, ischemic stroke, kwashiorkor, menstruation, migraine, pain, Parkinson's disease, respiratory disorders, weight loss; | **Preg:** Not recommended. Caffeine may ↑ risk of delayed conception (> 301 mg caffeine daily maternal intake), SIDS (> 400 mg daily), low birth weight infants (> 150 mg daily), miscarriage (> 100 mg daily), tremors in infants (> 500 mg daily), ↓ hematocrit and hemoglobin (> 450 mL coffee daily), birth defects (> 1,100 mg daily); | **CIs:** Allergy/hypersensitivity, Hypertension, Liver dysfunction, Arrhythmias, Breast disease, Concomitant CNS stimulants and other agents that may interact adversely with caffeine; | **ADRs:** acid reflux, agitation, angina, anxiety, arrhythmia, bone loss, cancer, convulsions, delirium, diarrhea, dizziness, dyspepsia, dysphagia, excitement, gastric irritation, hyperglycemia, hypernatremia, hypertension, hypokalemia, incontinence, increased intraocular pressure, insomnia, iron deficiency, metabolic acidosis, microcytic anemia, multiple sclerosis, muscle spasm, nausea, nervousness, polyuria, psychosis, respiratory alkalosis, restlessness, rhabdomyolysis, seizure, skin rashes, tachycardia, tachypnea, thrombosis, tremor; | **Interactions:** Adenosine (caffeine is competitive inhibitor of adenosine), alcohol

(↑ caffeine concentrations), analgesics (accelerates absorption, enhances analgesic effects), antibiotics (altered effects), anticoagulants/antiplatelets (↑ risk of bleeding), antidiabetic agents (altered or interfere with effects), antihypertensives (antagonistic effects), antineoplastics (enhance the cytotoxicity), beta blockers (antagonistic effects), bitter orange (additive stimulant effects/↑ of adverse cardiovascular effects), calcium (↑ calcium excretion), cimetidine (↓ caffeine clearance), clozapine (↑ risk of toxicity of clozapine), contraceptives (↑ caffeine concentrations), CNS depressants (antagonistic effects), CNS stimulants (additive stimulant effects), creatine (↑ risk of adverse cardiovascular effects), CYP450 substrates (altered drug levels), dipyridamole (↓ vasodilation), disulfiram (↓ clearance/↑ half-life of caffeine), dopaminergic drugs (additive effects), echinacea (↑ effects), ephedrine (additive stimulant effects), estrogens (↑ caffeine concentrations), fluconazole (↑ caffeine effects), fluvoxamine (↑ levels of caffeine), furafylline (↑ levels of caffeine), haloperidol (reduced haloperidol-induced catalepsy), hydrocortisone (added beneficial effects), iron (↓ iron absorption), grapefruit (↑ caffeine concentrations), lithium (↑ lithium levels), magnesium (↑ excretion of magnesium), MAOIs (↑ risk of hypertensive crisis), methoxsalesen (inhibitor of caffeine metabolism), mexiletine (↑ caffeine effects), nicotine (altered effects), opiates (potentiate analgesic effects), pentobarbital (antagonistic effects), phenothiazines (precipitation of fluphenazine solutions), phenylpropanolamine (↑ blood pressure/stimulant effects), phenytoin (↑ caffeine clearance), quinolones (↑ caffeine levels), terbinafine (↑ caffeine effects), theophylline (↑ theophylline levels), TCAs (precipitation of TCA solutions), verapamil (↑ caffeine concentrations), warfarin (↓ effects of warfarin), yohimbine (↑ risk of hypertensive crisis); | **Dose:** Light intake: < 150 mg daily. Heavy intake: > 400 mg daily. Excessive: >1,100 mg daily; | **Monitor:** Blood pressure, blood glucose, ferritin, heart rate, plasma homocysteine, LFTs, renal function tests, theophylline levels, uric acid level; | **Notes:** Caffeine naturally occurs in a number of plants, including coffee (*Coffea* spp.), tea (*Camellia sinensis*), and guarana (*Paullinia cupana*).

cajeput *(Melaleuca quinquenervia,* syn. *Melaleuca leucadendron)* | **Uses:** Insufficient clinical evidence; | **Preg:** Not recommended due to insufficient evidence; | **CIs:** Allergy/hypersensitivity; | **ADRs:** atopic dermatitis, ↓ blood glucose, carcinogenicity; | **Interactions:** Cocaine (↑ anesthetic effects), antidiabetic agents (additive effects/↑ risk of hypoglycemia), antihypertensives (additive effects/↑ risk of hypotension), CYP450 substrates (inhibits enzyme activity);

Dose: Insufficient evidence; Monitor: Blood glucose, blood urea nitrogen (BUN), Notes: Cajeput oil should not be confused with tea tree oil, although the plants are part of the same genus.

calamus *(Acorus calamus)* **Uses:** Insufficient clinical evidence; **Preg:** Not recommended due to insufficient evidence and potential antifertility effects; **CIs:** Allergy/hypersensitivity; ORAL USE (toxic); pediatric use (possible death due to dynamic ileus); **ADRs:** adynamic ileus (intestinal obstruction), contact dermatitis, DEATH, gastrointestinal disturbance, gastrointestinal toxicity, nephrotoxicity; **Interactions:** Amphetamines (↓ effects), antibacterial agents (additive effects), anticholinergic agents (additive effects), anticonvulsants (additive effects), antifungal agents (additive effects), antilipemic agents (additive effects), anti-inflammatory agents (additive effects), antispasmodics (altered effects), CNS depressants (additive sedation), calcium channel blockers (additive effects); **Dose:** Insufficient evidence; **Monitor:** Lipid profile, renal function tests; **Notes:** Traditional medicine includes use of the rhizome, and the herb's main traditional uses include therapy for colic, dyspepsia, and flatulence.

calcium **Uses:** Antacid, black widow spider bite, bone stress injury prevention, calcium deficiency, cancer, cardiopulmonary resuscitation (CPR), colorectal cancer, growth (low birth weight infants), hyperkalemia, hyperparathyroidism, HTN, lead toxicity (acute symptom management), magnesium toxicity, obesity, osteomalacia/rickets, osteoporosis, PMS, preeclampsia, vaginal disorders; **Preg:** The National Academy of Sciences recommends that women who are pregnant or breastfeeding consume calcium daily. Calcium supplementation may be recommended during pregnancy to prevent bone density loss; **CIs:** Allergy/hypersensitivity, History of ventricular fibrillation, Hypercalcemia, Hypophosphatemia, Renal stones, Sarcoidosis; **ADRs:** abdominal pain, arrhythmias, calcium deposits (in heart and kidney), chalky taste, coma, confusion, constipation, gastrointestinal irritation, headache, irritability, myocardial infarction, nausea/vomiting, nephrotoxicity, polydipsia, polyuria, renal calculi, skin reactions, urinary incontinence; **Interactions:** Alcohol (↓ calcium absorption), aluminum-containing compounds (↓ calcium levels), anticonvulsants (↓ calcium levels), bile acid sequestrants (↓ calcium levels), bisphosphonates (↓ absorption of bisphosphonates), caffeine (↓ calcium levels), calcium channel blockers (↓ effects of calcium channel blockers), cardiac glycoside (↑ risk of arrhythmias), CEFTRIAXONE (calcium salts in lungs and kidneys, in

C

neonates), corticosteroids (↓ calcium levels, ↑ risk of bone loss), diuretics (↓ calcium levels/↑ risk of milk-alkali syndrome in patients using thiazide diuretics), estrogen (↑ calcium absorption), fiber (↓ calcium levels), fluoroquinolone antibiotics (forms precipitates with quinolones/↓ calcium and fluoroquinolone levels), H2 blockers (↓ calcium levels), levothyroxine (↓ effectiveness of levothyroxine/↓ calcium levels), magnesium (↓ calcium levels), mineral oil (↓ calcium levels), orlistat (↓ calcium absorption), phosphorus (may ↓ absorption), potassium (↓ calcium excretion), proton pump inhibitors (↓ calcium levels), sodium (↓ calcium levels), sotalol (forms precipitates), stimulant laxatives (↓ calcium levels), tetracyclines (↓ calcium and tetracyclines), vitamin D (↑ calcium absorption); **Dose:** Doses ranging from 400–3,000 mL daily of a calcium supplement have been taken PO in several studies. Recommended doses may vary depending on specific indication; **Monitor:** Bone mineral density, calcium levels, renal function tests; **Notes:** Adequate intake (AI) recommendations for calcium are 1,000 mL for men and women ages 19–50 and 1,200 mL for individuals older than age 50.

calendula *(Calendula officinalis)* **Uses:** Otitis media, radiation skin protection, skin inflammation, venous leg ulcers, wound and burn healing; **Preg:** Not recommended due to insufficient evidence and possible abortifacient effects; **CIs:** Allergy/hypersensitivity, Pregnancy, Lactation, Chronic use; **ADRs:** allergic reactions, ↑ or ↓ blood sugar levels, drowsiness, hepatotoxicity, hypotension, nephrotoxicity, skin and eye irritation; **Interactions:** Antidiabetic agents (additive effects/ ↑ risk of hypoglycemia), antihypertensive agents (additive effects/↑ risk of hypotension), antilipidemic agents (additive effects), antineoplastic agents (additive effects), CNS depressants (additive sedation), hepatotoxic agents (↑ risk of liver damage), nephrotoxic agents (↑ risk of kidney damage); **Dose:** Topical: ointments (2%–5%) applied 3–4 times daily as needed, or 1:1 tincture in 40% alcohol or 1:5 in 90% alcohol diluted at least 1:3 with water for compresses; **Monitor:** Blood glucose, LFTS, lipid profile, renal function tests; **Notes:** Not to be confused with the common garden or French marigold (*Tagetes spp.*), African marigold (*T. erecta*), or Inca marigold (*T. minuta*).

California jimson weed *(Datura wrightii)* **Uses:** Insufficient clinical evidence; **Preg:** Not recommended due to insufficient evidence and potential adverse effects; **CIs:** Allergy/hypersensitivity; Oral use (TOXIC); **ADRs:** toxic symptoms: aggressive behavior, ataxia, blurred vision, coma, confusion, DEATH, dyspnea, euphoria, fatigue, hallucinations, headache, hypohydrosis, insomnia, panic, polydipsia,

RESPIRATORY DEPRESSION, seizures, speech disorders, tachycardia, xerosis, xerostomia; | **Interactions:** Anesthesia (↑ risk of respiratory depression), anticholinergic agents (additive effects), anticoagulants/antiplatelets (↑ risk of bleeding), antidepressants (↑ risk of adverse effects), antihypertensive agents (additive effects/↑ risk of hypotension), phenothiazines (↑ risk of adverse effects); | **Dose:** General: 0.125–0.25mg L-hyoscyamine 3–4 times daily, 0.4–0.6 mg of atropine (4–6 seeds) or 0.4–0.8 mg (8–16 seeds) of scopolamine. Ophthalmic: Atropine and scopolamine may be applied to the eye; however, the plant itself should not be applied to the eye; | **Monitor:** Blood pressure, coagulation panel, toxic effects; | **Notes:** *Datura wrightii* is a POISONOUS plant. Use of this plant may cause respiratory depression and death. *Datura* species contain atropine and scopolamine, which may induce visual and auditory hallucinations, confusion, panic, and other conditions.

C

California poppy *(Eschscholzia californica)* | **Uses:** Insufficient clinical evidence; | **Preg:** Not recommended due to insufficient evidence; | **CIs:** Allergy/hypersensitivity; | **ADRs:** fatigue ("morning sluggishness"), ↓ motor skills, muscular stiffness, nausea; | **Interactions:** Analgesics (additive effects), antidepressant agents (additive effects), antihypertensive agents (additive effects/↑ risk of hypotension), CNS depressants (additive sedation); | **Dose:** Insufficient evidence; | **Monitor:** Blood pressure; | **Notes:** In the same family (Papaverceae) as the opium poppy (*Papaver somniferum*).

camphor | **Uses:** Cough, functional cardiovascular disorders, onychomycosis, orthostatic hypotension, osteoarthritis, pain, pruritus; | **Preg:** Not recommended due to insufficient evidence and traditional use as an abortifacient; | **CIs:** Allergy/hypersensitivity, Infectious or inflammatory gastrointestinal conditions, Injured or broken skin, Intermittent acute porphyria, Nasal application on infants and children, Pregnancy; | **ADRs:** eczema; toxic effects with oral use: agitation, apnea, blurry vision, HEPATOTOXICITY (large quantities), nausea/vomiting, nephrotoxicity, neuromuscular hyperactivity, respiratory depression, rigidity, SEIZURES (large quantities), shock, spasticity, tachycardia, tremulousness; | **Interactions:** Drugs that lower seizure threshold (↑ risk of seizures); hepatotoxic agents (↑ risk of liver damage); nephrotoxic agents (↑ risk of kidney damage); | **Dose:** Topical: 10%–20% in semisolid preparations of camphor, or 1%–10% in camphor spirits, apply 3%–11% ointment 3–4 times per day to areas that hurt; | **Monitor:** LFTs; | **Notes:** Camphor and camphor containing products are generally applied as topical formulations. Ingestion of such preparations is not recommended because they are potentially poisonous and may induce a number of adverse and potentially fatal side effects.

C

Canada balsam *(Abies balsamea)* | **Uses:** Insufficient clinical evidence; | **Preg:** Not recommended due to insufficient evidence and traditional use as an abortifacient; | **CIs:** Allergy/hypersensitivity; | **ADRs:** contact dermatitis, diarrhea, nausea; | **Interactions:** Antineoplastics (additive effects); | **Dose:** Insufficient evidence; | **Monitor:** Insufficient evidence; | **Notes:** Canada balsam is sometimes mistaken for balm of Gilead, a tree in the *Populus* genus.

canthaxanthin ($C_{40}H_{52}O_2$) | **Uses:** Cancer, erythropoietic protoporphyria, photodermatoses/pigmentation disorders, photosensitivity, polymorphous light eruptions, psoriasis, vitiligo; | **Preg:** Not recommended due to insufficient evidence; | **CIs:** Allergy/hypersensitivity, Hypersensitivity to vitamin A; | **ADRs:** abdominal cramps, aplastic anemia, diarrhea, discolored palms, soles, and stools (orange color), nausea, pruritus, retinal granules (reversible), urticaria; serious side effects are rare; | **Interactions:** Bleomycin (protective effects), beta-carotene (↓ bioavailability of the canthaxanthin), may interact with agents with similar effects or related mechanisms of action (antiallergenic, antineoplastic, antioxidant, hypolipidemic, carotenoid); | **Dose:** Oral: up to 250 mg daily; | **Monitor:** Lipid profile, immune parameters, retinograms; | **Notes:** Canthaxanthins are carotenoids present in variable levels in the human population; it is derived entirely from the diet because humans do not produce canthaxanthin.

caper *(Capparis spinosa)* | **Uses:** Cirrhosis; | **Preg:** Not recommended due to insufficient evidence; | **CIs:** Allergy/hypersensitivity; | **ADRs:** hypoglycemia, hypotension, iron overload, photosensitivity; | **Interactions:** Antidiabetic agents (additive effects/↑ risk of hypoglycemia), antihypertensive agents (additive effects/↑ risk of hypotension), anti-inflammatory agents (additive effects), diuretics (additive effects), iron (↑ iron levels), photosensitizers (↑ risk of phototoxicity); | **Dose:** Three tablets Liv-52 (a combination product from Himalayan Co. India) daily for 6 months; | **Monitor:** Blood glucose, blood pressure, iron levels; | **Notes:** Caper is used traditionally to relieve rheumatism, reduce flatulence, and improve liver function.

caprylic acid (octanoic acid) | **Uses:** Epilepsy (pediatric); diagnostic tests; | **Preg:** Not recommended due to insufficient evidence; **CIs:** Allergy/hypersensitivity; Medium-chain acyl-CoA dehydrogenase (MCAD) deficiency, Renal calculi; **ADRs:** abdominal bloating and pain, ↓ calcium, diarrhea, drowsiness, dyspepsia, GERD, ↓ immune function, lethargy, nausea/vomiting, renal calculi; **Interactions:** Indomethacin (↓ effects of caprylic acid), nimodipine (additive effects), warfarin (↓ effects); **Dose:** General: 300–1,200 mg daily, preferably 30 minutes before meals. 13 C octanoic acid breath test: 100 mg 1–(13) C octanoic acid added to 40 g of oil (10) or a solid meal (11) for a labeled octanoic acid breath test to evaluate gastric emptying; **Monitor:** Coagulation panel; **Notes:** Nutritionists recommend caprylic acid for use in treating candidiasis and bacterial infections.

C

capsicum (*Capsicum annuum, Capsicum frutescens, Capsicum* spp.) **Uses:** Clotting disorders, diarrhea, digestion problems, fibromyalgia (topical), heart disease (prevention), migraine headache, neuralgias (topical), neuropathies (topical), peptic ulcers, perennial rhinitis, pain (topical, low back pain, postoperative), prurigo nodularis (topical), rhinitis, weight loss; **Preg:** Not recommended due to insufficient evidence; **CIs:** Allergy/hypersensitivity, Damaged skin/open wounds (topical), Infectious and inflammatory GI conditions (oral); **ADRs:** bleeding, burning (topical), contact dermatitis (topical), cough, flushing, gastroenteritis, GI irritation, hepatotoxicity, lacrimation, mucous membrane irritation, nephrotoxocity, ocular irritation, redness (topical), rhinorrhea, sweating, tachyphylaxis, urticaria (topical); **Interactions:** ACE inhibitors (added cough), anticoagulants/antiplatelets (↑ risk of bleeding), cocaine (↑ cocaine effects), CNS depressants (additive effects), theophylline (enhanced theophylline absorption); **Dose:** Intranasal, for rhinitis: 4 mcg per puff, one puff in each nostril, 3 times daily, with each puff separated by 30 minutes, for 3 consecutive days. Oral: fruit: 30–120 mg PO tid; tincture: 0.6–2 mL/dose PO; oleoresin: 0.6–2 mg/dose PO. Oral, general: 30–400 mg, 1–4 capsules, 10–15 drops in water 4 times per day have also been used. Topical, creams contain 0.025%–0.075% capsaicin, apply topically tid-qid; **Monitor:** LFTs (oral), kidney function (oral); **Notes:** Capsicum (or cayenne) alters temperature regulation and stimulates circulation.

caraway *(Carum carvi)* **Uses:** Dyspepsia; **Preg:** Likely safe in food; possibly unsafe in medicinal amount based on reports that caraway may stimulate menstruation; **CIs:** Allergy/hypersensitivity; **ADRs:** contact dermatitis, eructation, flatulence, nausea, seizures, substernal burning sensation, syncope; | **Interactions:** Antidiabetic agents (↑ risk of hypoglycemia), antilipemic agents (additive effects); | **Dose:** Dyspepsia: 50–100 mg PO qd with peppermint oil; dried fruit: 1–6 g PO qd; tea: 1–2 tsp of dried seeds submersed in 150 mL boiling water for 5–10 minutes and then strained; | **Monitor:** Blood glucose, lipid profile; | **Notes:** Caraway oil is often marketed as a combination product with peppermint oil.

cardamom *(Elettaria cardamomum)* | **Uses:** Insufficient clinical evidence; | **Preg:** Based on traditional use, likely safe in food amounts in pregnant or breastfeeding patients. Other uses are not recommended due to lack of sufficient evidence; | **CIs:** Allergy/hypersensitivity, Gallstones; | **ADRs:** allergic contact dermatitis, gallstone colic (spasmodic pain); | **Interactions:** Anticoagulant agents (↑ risk of bleeding), CYP450 substrates (altered drug levels), indomethacin (additive effects), muscarinic agents (↓ effects); | **Dose:** General: 1.5 g ground seeds daily. Infusion: 1 tsp crushed seeds in tea. Tincture: 1–2 g herb; | **Monitor:** Coagulation panel; | **Notes:** The spice known as cardamom is the fruit of several plants of the *Elettaria, Aframomum* and *Amomum* genera in Zingiberaceae, or ginger family. In general, *Aframomum* is used as a spice. *Elettaria* is used both as a spice and as medicine, and *Amomum* is used as an ingredient in traditional medicine.

carnosine (beta-alanyl-L-histidine) | **Uses:** Autism, cataracts, exercise performance, eye disorder; | **Preg:** Not recommended due to insufficient evidence; | **CIs:** Allergy/hypersensitivity; | **ADRs:** eyedrops: blurred vision, burning, ocular discomfort, ocular dryness, stinging; oral: insomnia, irritability; | **Interactions:** antihypertensives (↑ risk of hypotension); | **Dose:** Eyedrops, 1%–5%: instill 1–2 drops in each eye 3–4 times/day; oral: 100–600 mg/day; | **Monitor:** Blood pressure; | **Notes:** Carnosine supplements have been popular among body builders and athletes for improving muscular fatigue. Carnosine has been called a "longevity nutrient" and the "antiaging and antioxidant dipeptide."

carob *(Ceratonia siliqua)* | **Uses:** Diarrhea (in children), GERD (in infants), hypercholesterolemia; | **Preg:** Not recommended due to insufficient evidence; | **CIs:** Allergy/hypersensitivity, Metabolic disorders, Mineral deficiencies, Underweight infants, Renal disorders, Acute diarrhea; | **ADRs:** abdominal fullness, asthma, diarrhea, hypotension, ↓ mineral absorption, necrotizing enterocolitis (an inflammation of nerve cells in the intestine) in low birth weight infants, rash, rhinitis, urticaria (hives), ↓ urea, creatinine and phosphorus, vomiting; | **Interactions:** antidiabetic agents (additive effects/↑ risk of hypoglycemia), antihypertensive agents (additive effects/↑ risk of hypotension), laxatives (additive effects), oral agents (↓ absorption); | **Dose:** Adult: 20–30 g daily with liquid. Children: 15 g daily mixed with food or liquid. Hyperlipidemia: 50–100 mg PO tid; | **Monitor:** blood glucose, lipid profile, mineral levels, uric acid; | **Notes:** Carob bean gum (also known as locust bean gum) is commonly used as a food thickener.

carqueja (*Baccharis* spp.) | **Uses:** Insufficient clinical evidence; | **Preg:** Not recommended due to insufficient evidence; | **CIs:** Allergy/hypersensitivity; | **ADRs:** insufficient evidence; | **Interactions:** Antidiabetic agents (additive effects/↑ risk of hypoglycemia), possible interactions with agents with analgesic, anti-inflammatory, and antispasmodic effects; | **Dose:** Insufficient evidence; | **Monitor:** Blood glucose; | **Notes:** Traditionally used to treat liver diseases, rheumatism, and diabetes.

carrageenan (*Chondrus crispus*) | **Uses:** HIV infection (prevention), hyperlipidemia; | **Preg:** Not recommended due to insufficient evidence and possible adverse immune effects in infants; | **CIs:** Allergy/hypersensitivity; Infants; | **ADRs:** abdominal cramping, abnormal vaginal discharge, bleeding, ↑ cancer risk, diarrhea, dysuria, genital swelling, hypoglycemia, hypotension, immune system changes, inflammation, vaginal burning and itching; | **Interactions:** antiangiogenic agents (additive effects), anticoagulants/antiplatelets (↑ risk of bleeding), antidiabetic agents (additive effects/↑ risk of hypoglycemia), antihypertensive agents (additive effects/↑ risk of hypotension), antilipemic agents (additive effects), ophthalmic agents (↑ delivery), oral agents (↓ absorption); | **Dose:** General: decoctions of 15.5 g herb. Intravaginal: 5 mL carrageenan gel 3 times weekly; | **Monitor:** Blood glucose, blood pressure, coagulation panel; | **Notes:** The Irish moss popularly used as a ground cover (*Sagina subulata*) is not the same as the Irish moss discussed here (*Chondrus crispus*).

carrot (*Daucus carota*) | **Uses:** Antioxidant, diarrhea (acute), vitamin A deficiency; | **Preg:** Based on traditional use, carrot is likely safe in food amounts in pregnant or breastfeeding patients. Other uses are not recommended due to lack of sufficient evidence; | **CIs:** Allergy/hypersensitivity; | **ADRs:** asthma, carotenemia, diarrhea, extensive caries of primary teeth, throat swelling, urticaria; | **Interactions:** Antidiabetic agents (additive effects/↑ risk of hypoglycemia), laxatives (additive effects); | **Dose:** 100 g grated carrots daily for 60 days; | **Monitor:** Blood glucose, serum minerals and vitamins (particularly carotenoids); | **Notes:** Compulsive carrot eating is a rare condition in which the patient craves carrots. According to a case report, withdrawal symptoms include nervousness, cravings, insomnia, water brash, and irritability.

cascara sagrada *(Rhamnus pushiana)* | **Uses:** Bowel cleansing, constipation; | **Preg:** Not recommended due to insufficient evidence; | **CIs:** Allergy/hypersensitivity; Pregnancy, Lactation, Chronic use, Concomitant laxatives; | **ADRs:** abdominal discomfort, albuminuria, ascites, breathlessness, cachexia, cathartic colon, cholestatic hepatitis, colic, colorectal adenoma (noncancerous tumor) or carcinoma (cancerous tumor), cramps, DEPENDENCE, ELECTROLYTE IMBALANCES, fecal loss, finger clubbing, gastric melanosis (abnormal deposits of melanin in the stomach), headaches, hematuria, hypertension, hypokalemia, intestinal cramping, lethargy, muscle cramps, muscle weakness, paresthesias, peripheral edema, polyuria, portal hypertension, pigment spots in intestinal mucosa, spasms and tetany, vomiting (severe); | **Interactions:** Anticoagulants (↓ vitamin K absorption), cardiac glycosides (↑ risk of cardiac glycoside toxicity), corticosteroids (↑ risk of hypokalemia), diuretics (↑ risk of hypokalemia), stimulant laxatives (↑ risk of hypokalemia), warfarin (↑ effects of warfarin, ↑ INR, ↑ risk of bleeding); | **Dose:** General: 20–30 mg hyroxyanthracene derivatives daily. Constipation: up to 1 g dried bark daily at bedtime, or 2–6 mL liquid extract 3 times daily. Pediatric: Half the adult dose; | **Monitor:** Coagulation panel, electrolytes, potassium; | **Notes:** Anthraquinones in cascara may discolor the urine and interfere with diagnostic tests. Not to be confused with sea buckthorn (*Hippophae rhamnoides*).

cashew *(Anacardium occidentale)* | **Uses:** Metabolic syndrome; | **Preg:** Nuts are likely safe in food amounts in nonallergic pregnant or breastfeeding patients based on traditional use. Other uses are not recommended due to lack of sufficient evidence; | **CIs:** Allergy/hypersensitivity; | **ADRs:** anaphylaxis, asthma, severe cardiovascular symptoms; topical: blisters, contact dermatitis (including pruritic, erythematous, and maculopapular eruption), nodule formation, redness; | **Interactions:** May interact with agents with similar effects or related mechanisms of action (angiotensin II receptor inhibition, antibacterial, antidiarrheal, anti-inflammatory, astringent, antineoplastic, antiviral, calcium channel blocking, cardiac, hypolipidemic, immunomodulatory); | **Dose:** Oral: May be taken in homeopathic doses; twigs and leaves may be taken as tea; nuts (20% of diet has been consumed for weeks); | **Monitor:** Bacterial assays, blood pressure, histological tests, immune parameters, LFTs (bilirubin), viral titers; | **Notes:** The cashew nut tree is in the same family as poison ivy/oak. The fruit is high in vitamin C. The bark and leaves are primarily used medicinally, whereas the seeds are eaten as food.

cassava | **Uses:** Insufficient clinical evidence; | **Preg:** Likely safe in amounts found in food; not recommended in medicinal amounts due to insufficient evidence; | **CIs:** Allergy/hypersensitivity, Raw roots and leaves (cyanogenic glycosides); | **ADRs:** ↑ risk of cyanide toxicity (raw roots and leaves); | **Interactions:** Antidiabetic agents (altered effects); | **Dose:** Insufficient evidence; | **Monitor:** Blood glucose; | **Notes:** Cassava is a source of starch. It contains cyanogenic glucosides, linamarin, and lotaustralin. Traditionally, it has been used for cancer. Cassava may increase ovulation.

castor oil *(Ricinus communis)* | **Uses:** Bowel cleansing, colonoscopy preparation, contraception, dry eyes, labor induction; | **Preg:** Avoid use; | **CIs:** Allergy/hypersensitivity, Intestinal obstruction, Pregnancy; | **ADRs:** abdominal pain, cramps, diarrhea, dysmenorrhea, electrolyte abnormalities, fainting, headache, hypertension, insomnia, intestinal gas, irritation, loss of appetite, muscle cramps, pruritus, swelling of face, lips, and tongue, nausea/vomiting, taste aversion, urticaria, weakness; | **Interactions:** Antihypertensives (altered effects), digoxin (↑ absorption of digoxin), diuretic (↑ risk of electrolyte abnormalities), P-glycoprotein substrates (↑ effects of substrates), laxatives (additive effects); | **Dose:** General: 15–60 mL castor oil PO. Bowel cleansing: 30 mL castor oil with at least 600 mL of water PO. Colonoscopy preparation: 60 mL PO the night before the examination in combination with light, low-residue meals and 250 mL/h water for 8–10 hours on the day before the examination with only water consumed after 8 p.m. Contraception: 2.3–2.5g PO with water after 4–5 days of menstruation. Dry eyes, optic: 1.2% emulsion administered tid. Labor induction: 60 mL PO single dose; | **Monitor:** Electrolytes; | **Notes:** Caution is advised when taking castor oil seeds due to the ricin (a chemical warfare agent) content.

catnip *(Nepeta cataria)* | **Uses:** Insect repellent; | **Preg:** Not recommended due to insufficient evidence; | **CIs:** Allergy/hypersensitivity, Menorrhagia, Pelvic inflammatory disease; | **ADRs:** altered consciousness and central nervous system depression; | **Interactions:** CNS depressants (additive sedation), diuretics (additive effects/↑ risk of electrolyte imbalances); | **Dose:** Infusion: 2–3 tsp dried herb in tea 3 times daily. Tincture: 2–4 mL 3 times daily. Topical, essential oil: 23 or 468 mcg/cm^2. Oral, capsules: 380 mg twice daily; | **Monitor:** Insufficient evidence; | **Notes:** May be psychoactive in cats.

cat's claw *(Uncaria tomentosa, Uncaria guianensis)*

| **Uses:** Allergies, anti-inflammatory, cancer, immune stimulant, osteoarthritis, rheumatoid arthritis; | **Preg:** Not recommended due to insufficient evidence and traditional use as an abortifacient; | **CIs:** Allergy/hypersensitivity, Pregnancy, Autoimmune disorders, Transplant patients, | **ADRs:** abdominal discomfort, bleeding, bradycardia, bruising, ↓ estrogen or progesterone levels, diarrhea, dizziness, dyspnea, headache, hormonal changes, kidney disease/inflammation/failure, miscarriage, nausea, neuropathy, pruritus, tachycardia, transplant organ rejection, urticaria, vomiting, ↓ wound healing; | **Interactions:** Analgesic effects (additive effects), anticoagulants/antiplatelets (↑ risk of bleeding), antidiabetic agents (additive effects/↑ risk of hypoglycemia), antihypertensive agents (additive effects/↑ risk of hypotension), antilipemic agents (additive effects), antineoplastic agents (altered effects), CYP450 3A4 substrates (inhibits CYP3A4), diagnostic radiopharmaceuticals (altered effects), estrogens (↓ effects), hepatotoxic agents (↑ risk of liver damage), immunosuppressants (↓ effects), nephrotoxic agents (↑ risk of kidney damage), progesterone (↓ effects), photosensitizers (↑ risk of photosensitivity); | **Dose:** General: 250–1,000 mg 1–3 times daily (up to 9 capsules) or 500–600 mg once daily; 20 mg of cat's claw containing only pentacyclic oxindole alkaloids up to 3 times daily. Infusion: 1–25 g of root bark as tea 3 times daily. Tincture: 1–2 mL 2–3 times daily; 20–40 drops up to 5 times daily. Freeze-dried extract: 100 mg daily; | **Monitor:** Coagulation panel, estrogen, lipid profile, progesterone, WBC count; | **Notes:** There are more than 30 species in the genus *Uncaria*.

catuaba *(Trichilia catigua, Erythroxylum vacciniifolium)*

| **Uses:** Insufficient evidence; | **Preg:** Not recommended due to insufficient evidence; | **CIs:** Allergy/hypersensitivity; | **ADRs:** insufficient evidence; | **Interactions:** Antidepressants (altered effects); | **Dose:** Capsules: 1–2 g PO qd; tea: 1–3 cups of tea made from the bark of catuaba; | **Monitor:** N/A; | **Notes:** Brazilian folk medicine has used catuaba teas and infusions as an aphrodisiac, especially in men.

C

cedar (*Cedrus* spp.) | **Uses:** Alopecia areata; | **Preg:** Not recommended due to insufficient evidence; | **CIs:** Allergy/hypersensitivity; | **ADRs:** allergic dermatitis, allergic symptoms, alveolitis alergica (inflammation of the alveoli in the lungs caused by inhaling dust), asthma, bronchitis, conjunctivitis, organic dust toxic syndrome (ODTS), rhinitis, ↑ risk of adenocarcinoma and squamous cell cancers (malignant tumors), ↑ risk of Hodgkin's disease, ↑ risk of lung cancer; | **Interactions:** Insufficient evidence; | **Dose:** Insufficient evidence; | **Monitor:** Insufficient evidence; | **Notes:** Cedar (*Cedrus* spp.) should not be confused with *Cryptomeria japonica* (Japanese cedar), *Thuja* spp. (northern white cedar, eastern white cedar, western red cedar, cedarleaf), or *Juniperus* spp. (mountain cedar or eastern red cedar) as they are not closely related.

cedar leaf oil | **Uses:** Insufficient evidence; | **Preg:** Not recommended due to insufficient evidence and traditional use as an abortifacient; | **CIs:** Allergy/hypersensitivity, Pregnancy; | **ADRs:** abdominal pain, arrhythmia, bleeding, diarrhea, gastric irritation, gastroenteritis, hepatotoxicity, SEIZURES, skin irritation, vomiting; | **Interactions:** Anticonvulsants (↓ effects of anticonvulsants), antineoplastic agents (synergistic or antagonistic effects), DRUGS THAT LOWER SEIZURE THRESHOLD (↑ risk of seizures), hepatotoxic agents (↑ risk of liver damage), immunosuppressants (altered effects); | **Dose:** Eyedrops: 1–30 gtts in eye. Liquid extract: 2–4 mL. Testicular injection: 1/8 oz of thuja mixed with 1 oz of warm water; | **Monitor:** LFTs, seizures; | **Notes:** Cedar leaf oil is derived from *Thuja occidentalis*, and contains thuja, a neurotoxin.

celery (*Apium graveolens*) | **Uses:** Mosquito repellent; | **Preg:** Based on traditional use, celery is likely safe in food amounts in pregnant or breastfeeding patients. Other uses are not recommended due to lack of sufficient evidence; | **CIs:** Allergy/hypersensitivity; High amounts of psoralen-containing foods; | **ADRs:** ANAPHYLACTIC SHOCK, atopic dermatitis, celery-dependent exercise-induced anaphylaxis, contact dermatitis, laryngeal edema, nephritis, oral allergy syndrome, photosensitivity, sedation, urticaria; | **Interactions:** Anticoagulants/antiplatelets (↑ risk of bleeding), antihypertensive agents (additive effects/↑ risk of hypotension), antilipemic agents (additive effects), antispasmodic agents (additive effects), beta blockers (may ↑ risk of food-induced anaphylactic shock), CNS depressants (additive sedation), diuretics (additive effects), CYP450 substrates (altered drug levels), levothyroxine (↓ effects of levothyroxine), photosensitizers (↑ risk of photosensitivity); | **Dose:** Insufficient evidence; | **Monitor:** Coagulation panel, lipid profile, thyroid hormones, renal function panel; | **Notes:** Allergy to celery is fairly common because celery contains an allergen similar to the birch pollen allergen.

cesium | **Uses:** Cancer; | **Preg:** Not recommended due to insufficient evidence; | **CIs:** Allergy/hypersensitivity, Prolonged QT interval; | **ADRs:** diarrhea, nausea, QT PROLONGATION WITH TORSADES DE POINTES, ventricular tachycardias; | **Interactions:** Antineoplastic agents (additive effects), corticosteroids (↓ potassium levels), diuretics (↓ potassium levels), EDTA (altered cesium effects), QT-PROLONGING AGENTS (risk of prolonged QT interval); | **Dose:** 3–6 g PO in 3 divided doses with meals; | **Monitor:** EKG, potassium levels; | **Notes:** Cesium is structurally related to potassium. It may also be referred to as "high pH therapy" because it may increase the pH of tumor cells, which are considered acidic.

chaga mushroom *(Inonotus obliquus)* | **Uses:** Insufficient evidence; | **Preg:** Not recommended due to insufficient evidence; | **CIs:** Allergy/hypersensitivity; | **ADRs:** reduced blood glucose; | **Interactions:** Anticoagulants/antiplatelets (↑ risk of bleeding), antidiabetic agents (↑ risk of hypoglycemia); | **Dose:** Beverage: 10 drops PO bid. Powdered extract: 2–10 g PO qd. Tea: 1 tsp of crushed chaga in one cup of water PO tid; | **Monitor:** Blood glucose, coagulation panel; | **Notes:** Chaga mushrooms have been used in folk medicine since the 16th century as a remedy for cancer, gastritis, ulcers, and tuberculosis of the bones.

chamomile *(Matricaria recutita,* syn. *Matricaria suaveolens, Matricaria chamomilla, Anthemis nobilis, Chamaemelum nobile, Chamomilla chamomilla, Chamomilla recutita)* | **Uses:** Cardiovascular disorders, common cold, dermatitis, diarrhea (children), eczema, gastrointestinal disorders, hemorrhagic cystitis, hemorrhoids, infantile colic, insomnia, oral mucositis, quality of life in cancer patients, wound healing, vaginitis; | **Preg:** Not recommended due to insufficient evidence and possible estrogenic and abortifacient effects; | **CIs:** Allergy/hypersensitivity, Hormone-sensitive cancers/disorders; | **ADRs:** allergic conjunctivitis, asthma, bleeding, bruising, confusion, drowsiness, dyspnea, hypotension, miscarriage, pruritus, skin rash, urticaria, uterine contractions, vomiting (if taken at large doses); | **Interactions:** Analgesics (additive effects), anticoagulants/antiplatelets (↑ risk of bleeding), antidiabetic agents (additive effects/↑ risk of hypoglycemia), antihypertensive agents (additive effects/↑ risk of hypotension), anti-inflammatory agents (additive effects), antilipemic agents (additive effects), calcium channel blockers (additive effects), CNS depressants (additive sedation), CYP450 1A2 and 3A4 substrates (inhibits CYP1A2 and 3A4, ↑ drug levels), estrogens (competition for estrogen receptors); | **Dose:** Tea: up to 8 g dried flower. Capsules: up to 1,600 mg daily. Tincture: up to 15 mL (1:5 in alcohol). Liquid extract: up to 4 mL. Topical: 1% fluid extract or 5% tincture, or 5 g/L in a bath. Cream: 2%–10% chamomile extract; | **Monitor:** Blood glucose, blood pressure, coagulation panel, creatinine, estrogens, lipid profile; | **Notes:** The FDA has approved Hungarian chamomile flower oil (*Matricaria chamomilla*), chamomile flower oil (*Anthemis nobilis*), and Roman chamomile flower extract (*Anthemis nobilis*) either as food additives or Generally Regarded as Safe (GRAS).

C

chaparral *(Larrea tridentata)* | **Uses:** Cancer; | **Preg:** Contraindicated due to potential abortifacient effects and known toxicity; | **CIs:** Allergy/hypersensitivity, Oral use; | **ADRs:** abdominal pain, anorexia, bleeding, blood pressure changes, blood sugar changes, bruising, cancer, dark urine, diarrhea, dyspnea, fatigue, fever, HEPATOTOXICITY, light-colored stools, menstrual changes, nausea, nephrotoxicity, pruritus, swelling of lips/mouth/throat, thyroid hormone level changes, urticaria, weight loss, yellow skin or eyes; | **Interactions:** Anticoagulants/antiplatelets (↑ risk of bleeding), antidiabetic agents (additive effects/↑ risk of hypoglycemia), HEPATOTOXIC AGENTS (↑ risk of liver damage), MAO inhibitors (↑ risk of hypertensive crisis); | **Dose:** No standard or well-studied doses; may be toxic; | **Monitor:** Blood glucose, coagulation panel, creatinine, LFTs; | **Notes:** The FDA has issued warnings linking hepatitis with chaparral use. Nordihydroguaiaretic acid (NDGA), a constituent of chaparral, may have beneficial antioxidant, antiviral, and antifungal effects; however, it may also be responsible for its hepatotoxic and nephrotoxic effects.

chasteberry *(Vitex agnus-castus)* | **Uses:** Corpus luteum deficiency/luteal phase deficiency, cyclic mastalgia, hyperprolactinemia, irregular menstruation, premenstrual dysphoric disorder (PMDD), premenstrual syndrome (PMS); | **Preg:** Not recommended due to hormonal effects; traditionally used to prevent miscarriage; | **CIs:** Allergy/hypersensitivity; Hormone-sensitive conditions, Pregnancy, Lactation (↓ prolactin); | **ADRs:** acne, agitation, alopecia, circulatory disorders, depression, diaphoresis, diarrhea, dyspepsia, eczema, epistaxis, fatigue, fibroid growth, flatulence, headache, hot flashes, ↑ intraocular pressure, mastalgia, menstrual bleeding, menstrual cycle changes, nausea, palpitations, ↓ prolactin secretion, pelvic disease, polyuria, pulmonary edema, rash, seizure, skin eruptions, tachycardia, urticaria, vaginitis, vertigo, vomiting, weight gain, xerostomia; | **Interactions:** Antipsychotic agents (interfere with effects/due to dopaminergic effects), dopamine agonists (potentiates effects of dopamine agonists), dopamine antagonists (interfere with effects), estrogens (interfere with effects); | **Dose:** Commercial extract (dry): up to 40 mg daily. Commercial extract (liquid): 1.8 mL daily. Fruit extract: up to 160 mg 3 times daily. Dried fruit: up to 600 mg daily. Tincture (1:5 g/mL): up to 0.2 mL daily; | **Monitor:** Estrogens; | **Notes:** To date, clinical trials have found that treatment with chasteberry has been well tolerated, with minimal side effects.

cherry *(Prunus africana, Prunus emarginata, Prunus serotina)* | **Uses:** Muscle strains/pain (exercise-induced muscle damage prevention); | **Preg:** Based on traditional use, cherry is likely safe in food amounts in pregnant or breastfeeding patients. Other uses are not recommended due to lack of sufficient evidence; | **CIs:** Allergy/hypersensitivity; | **ADRs:** cough, dyspnea, gastrointestinal upset, mucosal irritation, urticaria; | **Interactions:** Oral agents (altered absorption), agents with anti-inflammatory, antineoplastic, or gastrointestinal effects (due to similar effects); | **Dose:** Tart cherry juice: 12 oz twice daily for 8 days; | **Monitor:** Inflammatory markers, nitric oxide, uric acid; | **Notes:** Cherry includes members of the *Prunus* genus, which contains several species that have been used both as food and medicine. Traditionally used for treating gout, BPH, and other disorders.

chervil *(Anrhriscus cerefolium)* | **Uses:** Insufficient evidence; | **Preg:** Not recommended due to insufficient evidence; | **CIs:** Allergy/hypersensitivity; | **ADRs:** Insufficient evidence; | **Interactions:** anticoagulants/antiplatelets (↑ risk of bleeding), antihypertensives (↑ risk of hypotension); | **Dose:** Insufficient evidence; | **Monitor:** Blood pressure, coagulation panel; | **Notes:** Chervil has been used as an eyewash to refresh the eyes. Historically, chervil has been used as an expectorant, aromatic, bitter tonic, and digestive stimulant. The use of chervil has also been noted for its blood-thinning and antihypertensive properties.

chia *(Salvia hispanica)* | **Uses:** Cardiovascular disease prevention/atherosclerosis; | **Preg:** Based on traditional use, chia is likely safe in food amounts in pregnant or breastfeeding patients. Other uses are not recommended due to lack of sufficient evidence; **CIs:** Allergy/hypersensitivity; **ADRs:** bleeding, gastrointestinal upset, hypoglycemia, hypotension; **Interactions:** Anticoagulants/antiplatelets (↑ risk of bleeding), antidiabetic agents (additive effects/↑ risk of hypoglycemia), antihypertensive agents (additive effects/↑ risk of hypotension), antilipemic agents (additive effects), antineoplastic agents (additive effects); **Dose:** Up to 41 g daily by mouth for 12 weeks; **Monitor:** Blood glucose, blood pressure, coagulation panel, lipid profile; **Notes:** *Salvia hispanica* seeds are used in a type of collectible terra cotta figurine known as the Chia Pet.

C

chickweed (*Stellaria* spp.) **Uses:** Insufficient clinical evidence; **Preg:** Not recommended due to insufficient evidence; **CIs:** Allergy/hypersensitivity; **ADRs:** allergic contact dermatitis, atopic dermatitis/eczema, erythema multiforme, photosensitivity; **Interactions:** Antineoplastic agents (additive effects), photosensitizers (↑ risk of photosensitivity), vasodilators (additive effects); **Dose:** Insufficient evidence; **Monitor:** Insufficient evidence; **Notes:** Common chickweed (*Stellaria media*) is a wild plant that has traditionally been collected for human consumption.

chicory *(Cichorium intybus)* **Uses:** Chronic hepatitis; **Preg:** Not recommended due to insufficient evidence and traditional use as an abortifacient; **CIs:** Allergy/hypersensitivity, Pregnancy/lactation; **ADRs:** abdominal bloating and pains, abortifacient, anorexia, contact dermatitis, contraception, emmenagogue, flatulence, intestinal gas, myalgic encephalomyelitis, occupational asthma, skin rash, weight loss; **Interactions:** Calcium (↑ absorption), CYP450 substrates (altered drugs levels); **Dose:** General: 10 g daily, or up to 700 mg/kg. Short- and long-chain fructans: up to 30 g daily. Inulin: up to 14 g daily; **Monitor:** Calcium levels; **Notes:** Traditionally, chicory juice was used as part of a remedy for headache. The leaves were used as a vegetable. The root was ground and used as a caffeine-free coffee substitute. Use with caution in patients with gallstones.

chitosan (deacetylated chitin biopolymer) **Uses:** Crohn's disease, dental caries, hyperlipidemia, obesity/weight loss, periodontitis, renal failure, wound healing; **Preg:** Not recommended due insufficient evidence; **CIs:** Allergy/hypersensitivity, Shellfish allergy; **ADRs:** ↓ absorption of fat-soluble vitamins (vitamins A, D, E, and K), bleeding,

↓ blood sugar, constipation, diarrhea, ↓ fat absorption, headache, nausea, skin itching, steatorrhea, stomach upset, swollen heels and wrists, throat dryness; | **Interactions:** Anticoagulants/antiplatelets (↑ risk of bleeding), antidiabetic agents (additive effects/↑ risk of hypoglycemia), antihypertensive agents (additive effects/↑ risk of hypotension), antilipemic agents (additive effects); | **Dose:** Up to 6 g daily for 8 weeks; | **Monitor:** Blood glucose, coagulation panel, lipid profile, urea/creatinine; | **Notes:** Chitosan is used as a substitute for synthetic polymer in many applications in the cosmetic and textile industries.

C

chlorella (*Chlorella* spp.) | **Uses:** Fibromyalgia, glioma, hypertension, skin cancer, surgery adjunct, ulcerative colitis, vaccine adjunct; | **Preg:** Not recommended due to insufficient evidence; there is clinical evidence that chlorella supplementation during pregnancy may reduce total toxic dioxin levels in breast milk; | **CIs:** Allergy/hypersensitivity; | **ADRs:** abdominal cramping, fatigue, flatulence, green-discolored feces, manganese-induced parkinsonism, nausea, occupational asthma, photosensitivity; | **Interactions:** Anticoagulants (high vitamin K/↓ anticoagulant activity of warfarin), immunosuppressants (interfere with effects), photosensitivity (↑ risk of photosensitivity), agents with similar effects (antihypertensive, antilipemic, antineoplastic, photosensitizing); vaccines (↑ antibody response); | **Dose:** Tablets: 10 g daily for 2 months. Liquid: 100 mL daily for 2 months; | **Monitor:** Antibody titers, coagulation panel, toxin/heavy metal levels, lipid profile; | **Notes:** *Chlorella* spp. are single-cell green algae that have resistance mechanisms against toxic metals; thus, chlorella could be used to detoxify water (e.g., the absorption of arsenic from water).

chlorophyll | **Uses:** Cancer (laser therapy adjunct), fibrocystic breast disease, herpes (simplex and zoster), odor reduction from incontinence/bladder catheterization, pancreatitis (chronic), pneumonia (active destructive), poisoning (reduce Yusho symptoms), protection from aflatoxins, rheumatoid arthritis, tuberculosis; | **Preg:** Not recommended due to insufficient evidence; | **CIs:** Allergy/hypersensitivity; | **ADRs:** abdominal cramping, diarrhea, food intolerance, green discoloration of the urine, green stools, nausea, photosensitivity, pseudo-jaundice, pseudoporphyria (group of rare, inherited blood disorders in which cells fail to change chemicals to the substance that gives blood its color); | **Interactions:** Antidiabetic agents (additive effects/↑ risk of hypoglycemia), antilipemic agents (additive effects); agents with similar effects (antineoplastic, antioxidant, antiviral, detoxifying, photosensitizing); **Dose:** General: 75–300 mg have been taken daily by mouth for up to 4 months. Infusion: 5–20 mg daily, or 0.25% solution intravenously. Infusion of 5–20 mg water-soluble chlorophyll-a daily for 1–2 weeks followed by intermittent administration thereafter has been used. Infusion of 0.25% chlorophyll solution in physiological sodium chloride solution administered by intravenous (via needle) drip has been studied; **Monitor:** Diagnostic tests, toxin levels, WBC count; **Notes:** Chlorophyll is a chemoprotein that contributes to the green pigmentation in plants; it can be obtained from numerous plants.

C

chocolate *(Theobroma cacao)* **Uses:** Antioxidant, cardiovascular health, constipation, (cocoa husks; children with idiopathic chronic constipation), hypercholesterolemia, HTN, insect repellant, prevention of blood clots, skin conditions, wound healing; **Preg:** Safe in amounts found in food, chocolate products provide 2–35 mg caffeine, pregnant women should not consume more than 200 mg/day of caffeine; **CIs:** Allergy/hypersensitivity; **ADRs:** bloating, constipation, flatulence, gastrointestinal upset, headache, IBS, irritability, nausea, nervousness, sleep disturbances, tremor; high consumption may cause eczema, renal calculi, tachyarrhythmias; **Interactions:** Most interactions are based on the caffeine in chocolate: anticoagulants/antiplatelets (↑ risk of bleeding), antidiabetic agents (altered glucose control), antihypertensives (altered effects), beta agonists (↑ inotropic effects of beta agonists), caffeine (additive effects), calcium (↓ absorption of chocolate), cimetidine (↑ effects of caffeine), clozapine (↑ effects of clozapine), CNS depressants (interfere with effects), dipyridamole (inhibits dipyridamole-induced vasodilation), disulfiram (↑ effects of caffeine), ergot derivatives (↑ the absorption of ergotamine), estrogens (↑ effects of caffeine), fluconazole (↑ effects of caffeine), grapefruit juice (↑ effects of caffeine), inotropes (↑ inotropic effects), iron (inhibits iron absorption), lithium (↑ risk of lithium toxicity), mexiletine (↑ effects of caffeine), MAOIs (↑ risk of hypertensive crisis), phenylpropanolamine (↑ blood pressure), quinolones (↑ effects of caffeine), theophylline (↑ risk of theophylline toxicity), verapamil (↑ effects of caffeine); **Dose:** Chocolate providing 88–446 mg total flavanols PO qd; **Monitor:** Blood glucose, blood pressure, coagulation panel; **Notes:** Complicating recommendations of chocolate intake are the varying flavonoid contents of commercial cocoa products. Chocolate flavonoids are contained in the highest amounts in dark chocolate.

choline | **Uses:** Acute viral hepatitis, allergic rhinitis, asthma, brain injuries (craniocerebral), coma, hepatic steatosis, ischemic stroke, muscle mass/body mass, nutritional supplement, Parkinson's disease, postsurgical recovery, schizophrenia, total parenteral nutrition; | **Preg:** Likely safe in amounts within recommended adequate intake (AI) parameters in pregnant or breastfeeding patients. Other uses are not recommended due to lack of sufficient evidence; | **CIs:** Allergy/hypersensitivity; | **ADRs:** agitation, anorexia, cold, constipation, cough, diaphoresis, diarrhea, epilepsy, fish odor, headache, hypotension, insomnia, nausea, paranoia, respiratory depression, salivation, skin rash (severe), steatorrhea, vertigo, vomiting; | **Interactions:** Carnitine (↓ carnitine excretion/↑ effects), lithium (↑ choline), dopamine agonists (↑ effects), methotrexate (↓ methotrexate-induced fatty liver), pentazocine (↓ effects), scopolamine (↓ effects), succinylcholine and choline precursors (↑ effects); | **Dose:** Recommended daily intake—men (18–70+ years): 550 mg daily; women (19–70+ years): 425 mg daily; women up to 18 years: 400 mg daily—not to exceed 3 g daily; pregnant women: 450 mg daily; breastfeeding women: 550 mg daily. Should not exceed 3.5 g daily for adults and 3 g for those under 18 years; | **Monitor:** Blood pressure; | **Notes:** Pure choline is rarely used because of its undesirable side effects of fishy odor. Therefore, lecithin or purified phosphatidylcholine is more commonly used.

chondroitin sulfate | **Uses:** Bladder control, coronary artery disease (secondary prevention), interstitial cystitis, iron absorption enhancement, ophthalmological uses, osteoarthritis, psoriasis; | **Preg:** Not recommend due to insufficient evidence. Chondroitin has a similar structure to heparin, which is contraindicated in pregnancy or during breastfeeding; | **CIs:** Allergy/hypersensitivity, Prostate cancer (or ↑ risk for prostate cancer) due to possible ↑ risk of recurrence or spread; | **ADRs:** alopecia, angina, bleeding, bone marrow suppression, constipation, diarrhea, dyspnea, edema, euphoria, eyelid edema, gastrointestinal upset/pain, headache, hypertension, ↑ LFTs, nausea/vomiting, photosensitivity, rash, throat and chest constriction, tremor, urticaria, worsening of asthma symptoms; | **Interactions:** Anticoagulants/antiplatelets (↑ risk of bleeding), hyaluronidase (may degrade chondroitin sulfate), NSAIDs (↑ risk of bleeding), photosensitizers (↑ risk of photosensitivity), iron (↑ absorption); | **Dose:** General: 200–400 mg in divided or once-daily dosing; up to 2,000 mg daily; | **Monitor:** Coagulation panel, iron; | **Notes:** There is a general consensus that chondroitin (with or without its partner agent glucosamine) may arrest or even reverse degenerative osteoarthritis.

chromium (Cr) **Uses:** Athletic conditioning, bipolar disorder, cardiovascular disease, cognitive function, depression, diabetes/prediabetes, glucose intolerance in polycystic ovary syndrome, hyperlipidemia, immunosuppression, myocardial infarction, obesity, osteoporosis, Parkinson's disease, schizophrenia, Turner's syndrome; **Preg:** May be safe when used orally in recommended doses; **CIs:** Allergy/hypersensitivity, Renal/hepatic insufficiency; **ADRs:** anemia, asthma, cough, diarrhea, gastrointestinal upset, headache, hypoglycemia, immunosuppression (when combined with copper), inflammation of the nose, insomnia, interstitial nephritis, irritability, kidney damage, liver damage, lung cancer, mood changes, muscle damage, myocardial damage, nausea, perforated nasal passage, rhabdomyolysis, skin problems/changes, stomach ulcers, thrombocytopenia, tubular necrosis, urticaria, vomiting; **Interactions:** Alcohol (↑ liver and kidney toxicity of hexavalent chromium), antacids (↓ chromium levels), anticoagulants and NSAIDs (↑ chromium absorption), antidiabetes agents (additive effects/↑ risk of hypoglycemia), antiobesity agents (additive effects), calcium (↓ bone resorption), chromium-containing agents (↑ risk of chromium toxicity), CNS depressants (interfere with effects), CNS stimulants (additive effects), corticosteroids (↓ chromium levels), copper (↓ immune function), CYP450 substrates (altered drugs levels), H2-blockers (↓ chromium levels), insulin, iron (competes with iron for binding), levothyroxine (↓ levothyroxine levels), lithium (↑ risk of hypoglycemia), nicotinic acid (↓ blood glucose), proton pump inhibitors (↓ chromium levels), vitamin C (↑ chromium absorption), zinc (↓ absorption of chromium and zinc); **Dose:** Adequate dietary intake of chromium in the United States is 50–200 mcg daily. Clinical studies typically use 150–1,000 mcg daily of chromium picolinate or chromium chloride. Chromium-enriched yeast: 150–400 mcg PO daily; **Monitor:** Blood glucose, blood pressure, calcium levels, chromium levels, iron, lipid profile, LFTs, renal function test; **Notes:** Chromium is an essential trace element that exists naturally in trivalent and hexavalent states. Trivalent chromium (chromium/Cr III), typically found in foods and supplements, appears to have very low toxicity and a wide margin of safety. Hexavalent chromium (chromic oxide, chromate) is a known toxin; long-term occupational exposure may lead to skin problems, perforated nasal septum, and lung cancer.

chrysanthemum (*Chrysanthemum* spp.) **Uses:** Cancer (precancerous lesions), diabetes; **Preg:** Not recommended due to insufficient evidence and possible toxicity; **CIs:** Allergy/hypersensitivity; **ADRs:** actinic reticuloid, asthma, contact dermatitis, convulsions, corneal erosions, DEATH, eczema (localized and seasonal to generalized and persistent), hyperexcitation, photosensitivity dermatitis, pollinosis, pyrethrin poisoning, rhinoconjunctivitis, urticaria; | **Interactions:** Anti-inflammatory agents (additive effects), antidiabetic agents (additive effects/↑ risk of hypoglycemia), photosensitizers (↑ risk of photosensitivity), agents with possible similar effects (analgesic, antibiotic, antifungal, antigout, antineoplastic, antiviral); | **Dose:** Jiangtangkang (a Chrysanthemum product): 8 g, 3 times per day for 6 months; | **Monitor:** Blood glucose, viral load, WBC count; | **Notes:** Not to be confused with tansy (*Tanacetum vulgare*), sometimes classified as *Chrysanthemum vulgare*.

chrysin | **Uses:** Insufficient evidence; | **Preg:** Not recommended due to insufficient evidence; | **CIs:** Allergy/hypersensitivity; | **ADRs:** insufficient evidence; | **Interactions:** Androgens (increases androgens levels), anticoagulants/antiplatelets (↑ risk of bleeding), antihypertensives (↑ risk of hypotension), aromatase inhibitors (additive effects), cephalosporins (increases cephalosporin level), CYP450 1A2 (inhibits CYP1A2 isoenzymes), glucuronidated drugs (increases clearance of UGT1A1 substrates); | **Dose:** 50–2,000 mg PO qd; | **Monitor:** Bilirubin, blood pressure, hormone panel, coagulation panel, immune panel, lipid profile; | **Notes:** Chrysin is a flavonoid typically extracted from the passion flower. Chrysin's efficacy may be limited when administered orally due to its poor absorption in the small intestine.

chymotrypsin | **Uses:** Burns, cataracts, digestion, edema, fractures (anti-inflammatory), hemorrhoids, immunomodulation, skin conditions; | **Preg:** Not recommended due to insufficient evidence; | **CIs:** Allergy/hypersensitivity; | **ADRs:** oral: dyspnea, edema, loss of consciousness, urticaria; ophthalmic: corneal edema, filamentary keratitis, intraocular pressure, iridoplegia, striation, uveitis; | **Interactions:** Insufficient evidence; | **Dose:** IM: 5,000 USP units 1–3 times/day. Ophthalmic: 1:5,000 or 1:10,000 in 0.9% NaCl injected to irrigate cannula. Oral (6:1, trypsin:chymotrypsin): 100,000–200,000 units PO qid; | **Monitor:** N/A; | **Notes:** Chymotrypsin is a pancreatic enzyme that is important for the digestion of proteins in the intestines.

cinnamon (*Cinnamomum* spp.) | **Uses:** Allergic rhinitis, angina, bacterial infection, candidiasis (oral), coronary heart disease, diabetes (type 2), *Helicobacter pylori* infection, lung cancer, metabolic syndrome; | **Preg:** Likely safe in food amounts in pregnant or breastfeeding patients based on traditional use. Other uses are not recommended due to lack of sufficient evidence; **CIs:** Allergy/hypersensitivity; **ADRs:** allergic hypersensitivity, asthma, cheilitis, chronic respiratory symptoms, dermatitis, hepatotoxicity, gingivitis, glossitis, oral lesions, orofacial granulomatosis, perioral dermatitis, squamous cell carcinoma, stomatitis, thrombocytopenia, urticaria; **Interactions:** Clinical studies have produced insufficient evidence of clinical interactions involving cinnamon; may possibly interact with agents with similar effects (antibiotic, anticoagulant, antifungal, antioxidant, antispaspodic, antiviral, cardiovascular, immunomodulating), antidiabetic agents (↑ risk of hypoglycemia), CYP450 substrates (altered drug levels), hepatotoxic agents (↑ risk of liver damage); **Dose:** Candidiasis: 8 lozenges daily for 1 week; solution made by cooking 250 g of cinnamon in 2,000 mL of water on medium heat until there was 500 mL of solution (solution defined as 50% cinnamon solution), then gargle with 20–30 mL of solution 4–6 times a day. Diabetes (type 2): up to 6 g daily for 40 days. *Helicobacter pylori* infection: 80 mg extract daily for 4 weeks (lack of effect); **Monitor:** Blood glucose, coagulation panel, LFTs; **Notes:** Does not include *Cinnamomum camphora*, or the camphor tree, which can be lethal to humans in large doses, or *Cinnamomum kotoense*, which is an ornamental species.

CLA (conjugated linoleic acid) **Uses:** Cancer, diabetes, exercise performance enhancement, hypercholesterolemia, HTN, immune function, obesity/weight loss; **Preg:** Safe when used appropriately; **CIs:** Allergy/hypersensitivity, liver disorders; **ADRs:** abdominal distention, diarrhea, dyspepsia, nausea, weight gain; **Interactions:** Anticoagulants/antiplatelets (↑ risk of bleeding), antidiabetic agents (altered effects), antihypertensives (↑ risk of hypotension), antilipemic agents (additive effects), immunosuppressants (altered effects), vitamin A (↑ vitamin A storage in tissues); **Dose:** 3–6 g PO qd; **Monitor:** Blood glucose, blood pressure, coagulation panel, lipid profile; **Notes:** CLA is a fatty acid naturally found in beef and dairy products in the diet. The estimated daily intake of CLA is 0.35 g daily for women and 0.43 g daily for men, predominantly from milk, milk products, and meat. CLA oil contains 9 calories/g; CLA powder is 7.9 calories/g.

clay **Uses:** Encopresis, gastrointestinal disorders, mercuric chloride poisoning, protection from aflatoxins; **Preg:** Not recommended due to ↑ risk of toxemia; **CIs:** Pregnancy, Lactation, Wilson's disease, Renal insufficiency, Immune disorders;

ADRs: anemia, anorexia, blood chemistry imbalance, bowel obstruction, cardiomegaly, chronic bronchitis, constipation, DEATH, dermatitis, dyspepsia, dyspnea, flatulence, hepatomegaly, hookworm infections, hypercalcemia, hypermagnesemia, hypokalemia, lead poisoning, microorchidism (small testes), myopathy (due to severe hypokalemia), neurolathyrism, neurological damage, polyuria, respiratory tract infection, splenomegaly, tetanus, thrombocytopenia, vomiting; **Interactions:** Cimetidine (↓ absorption), potassium-depleting agents (↑ risk of hypokalemia), quinine (↓ bioavailability); **Dose:** Irritable bowel syndrome: 3 g beidellitic montmorillonite (purified clay containing a double aluminum and magnesium silicate) twice daily for 8 weeks; 3 sachets dioctahedral smectite (natural adsorbent clay) daily for 8 weeks; **Monitor:** Iron, LFTs, potassium, renal function tests; **Notes:** Chronic clay eating (pica or geophagia) is associated with numerous adverse effects.

cleavers *(Galium aparine)* **Uses:** Insufficient clinical evidence; **Preg:** Not recommended due to insufficient evidence and possible hormonal effects; **CIs:** Allergy/hypersensitivity; **ADRs:** contact dermatitis, hormonal effects; **Interactions:** May interact with agents with similar effects (antigout, anti-inflammatory, antineoplastic, diuretic, laxative, hormonal); **Dose:** Dried herb: 2–4 g 3 times daily. Fluid extract: 2–4 mL 3 times daily. Tincture (5:1 25%) 4–10 mL 3 times daily; **Monitor:** Hormone panel; **Notes:** Cleavers is an ingredient in Hoxsey formula.

clove *(Syzygium aromaticum,* syn. *Eugenia aromaticum)* **Uses:** Fever, mosquito repellent, premature ejaculation, toothache; **Preg:** Likely safe in amounts found in food; not recommended in medicinal amounts due to insufficient evidence; **CIs:** Allergy/hypersensitivity, Bleeding disorders; **ADRs:** Aphthous ulcers, ASPIRATION PNEUMONITIS (FATAL), bleeding, bronchospasm, burning, cheilitis, CNS depression, contact dermatitis, damage to dental pulp or supporting periodontium, dermatitis, disseminated intravascular coagulopathy (DIC), dyspnea, epistaxis, erectile dysfunction (sporadic; delayed ejaculation), fever, gum sensitivity, hemoptysis, hepatotoxicity, hypoglycemia, hypohidrosis, irritation, lacrimation, local tissue irritation, lung damage, metabolic acidosis, painful sensations, pleural effusion, proteinuria, rash, respiratory infection, seizures, urinary abnormalities, urticaria, uveitis; **Interactions:** Analgesics (additive effects), anticoagulants/antiplatelets (↑ risk of bleeding), antidiabetic agents (additive effects/↑ risk of hypoglycemia), anti-inflammatory agents (additive effects), antipyretics (additive effects), CYP450 substrates (altered drug levels), agents that have similar effects (antifungal, antihistamine, antineoplastic, cardiovascular, hepatotoxic, nephrotoxic); | **Dose:** General: Maximum 2.5 mg/kg body weight daily. Topical: 2:3 clove:glycerin mixture; 0.1 mL clove oil per 30 cm^2 skin; | **Monitor:** Blood glucose, coagulation panel, LFTs, renal function tests; | **Notes:** Not to be confused with baguacu, black plum, *Eugenia cumini*, *Eugenia edulis*, *Eugenia jambolana*, *Eugenia umbelliflora*, Jamun, java apple, java plum, *Syzygium cordatum* extract, *Syzygium cumini*, *Syzygium samarangense*, water apple, or wax apple. Clove oil (eugenol) is widely used as a flavoring agent in food, pharmaceuticals, and mouthwashes. Eugenol is also used as an anesthetic and antiseptic agent in various dental products.

club moss ***(Lycopodium clavatum)*** | **Uses:** Insufficient clinical evidence; | **Preg:** Not recommended due to insufficient evidence; | **CIs:** Allergy/hypersensitivity; | **ADRs:** cramping, dizziness, nausea, occupational asthma; | **Interactions:** May interact with agents with similar effects effects (cholinergic, anti-inflammatory, antineoplastic, cholinesterase inhibition); | **Dose:** Insufficient evidence; | **Monitor:** Vital signs; | **Notes:** Not to be confused with *Lycopodium selago*, a huperzine A–containing species with potent anticholinesterase inhibiting activity, as ingestion of *Lycopodium selago* may result in cholinergic toxicity.

coconut oil | **Uses:** Dehydration, diabetes mellitus, diarrhea, dry skin, hyperlipidemia, HTN, infant development, lice, hepatoprotection, psoriasis; | **Preg:** Safe in amounts found in food; | **CIs:** Allergy/hypersensitivity; | **ADRs:** allergic reactions, ↑ cholesterol levels (large amounts); | **Interactions:** Antidiabetic agents (additive effects/↑ risk of hypoglycemia), antihypertensives (↑ risk of hypotension), antilipemic agents (altered effects); | **Dose:** Insufficient evidence; | **Monitor:** Blood glucose, blood pressure, lipid profile; | **Notes:** Topically, coconut oil does not block UVA or UVB radiation.

codonopsis ***(Codonopsis pilosula)*** | **Uses:** Insufficient evidence; | **Preg:** Not recommended due to insufficient evidence and antifertility activity observed in rats; | **CIs:** Allergy/hypersensitivity, Pregnancy; | **ADRs:** contraceptive activity, diarrhea, infertility; | **Interactions:** Anticoagulants/antiplatelets (↑ risk of bleeding), antacids/H2 antagonists/proton pump inhibitors (interfere with effects), fertility agents (interfere with effects), laxatives (additive effects), oral agents (↓ absorption); | **Dose:** Decoction: 3–9 g; some conditions may require dosages up to 30 g/day. Tea: 12–15 g of codonopsis added to 3-4 cups water, boiled until the volume is reduced by one-half, and cooled, then taken in 2 doses on an empty stomach; | **Monitor:** Coagulation panel; | **Notes:** Codonopsis is known as "poor man's ginseng."

coenzyme Q10 (CoQ10) | **Uses:** Age-related macular degeneration, Alzheimer's disease, angina, asthma, breast cancer, cancer, cardiomyopathy (dilated, hypertrophic), cardioprotection (during surgery), chemotherapy toxicity (anthracycline), chronic fatigue syndrome, cocaine dependence, coenzyme Q10 deficiency, congestive heart failure, coronary heart disease, exercise performance, fertility (increasing sperm count), Friedreich's ataxia, HIV/AIDS, hyperlipidemia/adjunct to statin therapy, hypertension, Kearns-Sayre syndrome, migraine, mitochondrial encephalomyopathies, mitral valve prolapse (children), muscular dystrophies, myelodysplastic syndrome, myocardial infarction, Parkinson's disease, periodontal disease, postoperative recovery (adjuvant), prostate cancer, renal failure, tinnitus; | **Preg:** Not recommended due to insufficient evidence; | **CIs:** Allergy/hypersensitivity, underlying medical conditions; | **ADRs:** bleeding, contusion, diarrhea, dizziness, dyspnea, fatigue, flu-like symptoms, gastrointestinal upset, headache, heartburn, hyper-/hypoglycemia, hypotension, insomnia, irritability, ↑ liver enzymes, loss of appetite, nausea, Photosensitivity, pruritus, rash, thrombosis, thyroid hormone alterations, vomiting; | **Interactions:** Antidepressants (↓ coenzyme Q10 levels), antidiabetic agents (altered effects), antihypertensives (↑ risk of hypotension), antilipemic agents (additive effects), beta-blockers (↓ coenzyme Q10 levels), clonidine (↓ coenzyme Q10 levels), corticosteroids (↓ effects), diuretics (↓ coenzyme Q10 levels), doxorubicin (↓ effectiveness), fenofibrate (↑ coenzyme Q10 levels), HMG-CoA reductase inhibitors (↓ coenzyme Q10 levels), hydralazine (↓ coenzyme Q10 levels), immunosuppressants (altered effects), methyldopa (↓ coenzyme Q10 levels), smoking (↓ coenzyme Q10 levels), thyroid hormones (altered effects), warfarin (↓ anticoagulant effects), zidovudine (↓ zidovudine-associated myopathy); | **Dose:** General: 20 mg daily PO; studies have used up to 1,200 mg daily PO; | **Monitor:** Blood glucose, blood pressure, coagulation panel, conenzyme Q10 levels, immune parameters, lactate, LFTs, lipid profile, T_4/T_8 ratio; | **Notes:** Coenzyme Q10 (CoQ10), also known as ubiquinone, is endogenously produced and serves as a cofactor in oxidative respiration for the Krebs cycle and the electron transport chain. Long-term studies have shown moderate CoQ10 doses to be generally safe in otherwise wealthy individuals; few or minor adverse effects have been reported.

coleus *(Coleus forskohlii)* **Uses:** Asthma, breathing aid for intubation, cardiomyopathy, cardiopulmonary bypass, depression, erectile dysfunction, glaucoma, lactation stimulant, schizophrenia; **Preg:** Not recommended due to insufficient evidence and possible anti-implantation effects observed in animals; **CIs:** Allergy/hypersensitivity, Concurrent use with vasodilators (e.g., nitrates); **ADRs:** bleeding, bradycardia, contusion, cough, dyspepsia, dyspnea, hyper-/hypoglycemia, hyper-/hypotension, milky film over eyes (from eyedrop preparations), miscarriage, pruritus, rash, restlessness, sedation, skin pigment changes, sore throat, tachycardia, thyroid hormone alterations, tremor, ulcers, upper respiratory tract irritation; **Interactions:** Anticoagulants/antiplatelets (↑ risk of bleeding), antidiabetic agents (altered effects), antihypertensives (↑ risk of hypotension), cardiac glycosides, CYP450 substrates (altered drug levels), VASODILATORS (additive effects); agents with similar effects or mechanism of action (abortifacient, analgesic, bronchodilatory, antidepressant, antihistamine, antineoplastic, cardioactive, gastrointestinal, antacid, neurologic, thyroid hormones); **Dose:** Extract: 50 mg standardized extract (18% forskolin) 1–3 times daily; or 250 mg 1% forskolin extract 1–3 times daily. Liquid: 2–4 mL standardized extract (10%–20% forskolin) 2–3 times daily. Dried root: 2–10 mg taken 2–3 times daily. Eyedrops: 50 mcL forskolin suspension eyedrops (1%) applied to the cornea in healthy people. Intravenous: 0.5 mcg/kg/min and increased at 15-min intervals to 1, 2, and 3 mcg/kg/min up to 1 hour. Single-dose inhalation: forskolin powder (10 mg) from a Spinhaler; **Monitor:** Blood glucose, blood pressure, coagulation panel, heart rate, hormone panel; **Notes:** Although most studies have used the isolated forskolin extract, it is believed that the whole coleus plant may be more effective, due to the presence of multiple compounds that may act synergistically. Generally, coleus appears to be well tolerated with few adverse effects.

collagen (type II) **Uses:** Insufficient clinical evidence; **Preg:** Not recommended due to insufficient evidence; **CIs:** Allergy/hypersensitivity; **ADRs:** insufficient evidence; **Interactions:** Immunosuppressants (altered effects); **Dose:** Oral, capsules: 500 mg PO qd, preferably with orange juice q a.m. on an empty stomach; wait 20 min before eating; **Monitor:** N/A; **Notes:** Collagen type II or chicken collagen is used for pain syndromes such as arthritis and back pain.

C

colloidal silver | **Uses:** Insufficient clinical evidence; | **Preg:** Not recommended due to insufficient evidence; | **CIs:** Allergy/hypersensitivity, Oral use; | **ADRs:** argyria (silver salts deposit in the skin), coma, DEATH, fatigue, gastrointestinal distress, headache, renal damage, seizures, skin irritation; | **Interactions:** Levothyroxine (↓ absorption), pencillamine (↓ absorption), quinolones (↓ absorption), tetracyclines (↓ absorption); | **Dose:** Insufficient evidence; | **Monitor:** Insufficient evidence; | **Notes:** The FDA issued a final ruling in August 1999 establishing that all over-the-counter (OTC) drug products containing colloidal silver ingredients or silver salts for internal or external use are not generally recognized as safe and effective and are misbranded. This rule was issued because colloidal silver has been marketed for many serious disease conditions, and the FDA is not aware of any substantial scientific evidence that supports the use of OTC colloidal silver ingredients or silver salts for these diseases or conditions.

coltsfoot *(Tussilago farfara)* | **Uses:** Insufficient clinical evidence; | **Preg:** Not recommended due to insufficient evidence; | **CIs:** Allergy/hypersensitivity; | **ADRs:** HEPATOTOXIC due to pyrrolizidine alkaloid content; | **Interactions:** Anticoagulants/antiplatelets (↑ risk of bleeding), HEPATOTOXIC AGENTS (↑ risk of liver damage), may interact with agents with similar effects (antiasthma, antihypertensive, antitussive, calcium channel blocking, expectorant); | **Dose:** Insufficient evidence; | **Monitor:** Blood pressure, coagulation panel, LFTs; | **Notes:** Coltsfoot is considered to be unsafe due to hepatotoxic pyrrolizidine constituents.

comfrey (*Symphytum* spp.) | **Uses:** Inflammation, myalgia, pain; | **Preg:** Not recommended due to insufficient evidence and known toxicity; | **CIs:** Allergy/hypersensitivity, Oral ingestion (due to hepatotoxic pyrrolizidine alkaloids); | **ADRs:** abdominal pain, acute pneumonitis, ascites, Budd-Chiari syndrome, cancer, cardiovascular disease, damage to Disse's space, DEATH, extravasation of red blood cells, hemorrhagic necrosis, hepatomegaly, HEPATOTOXIC (due to pyrrolizidine alkaloid content), jaundice, obstructive ileus, phytobezoar, portal hypertension (severe), sinusoid damage, skin redness, vascular congestion, venous endophlebitis; | **Interactions:** Aminopyrine N-demethylase–metabolized agents; CYP450 3A4 substrates (CYP3A4 inducers can ↑ toxic metabolites), HEPATOTOXIC AGENTS (↑ risk of liver damage), anti-inflammatory agents; | **Dose:** Not recommended due to safety concerns; | **Monitor:** Blood pressure, heart rate, LFTs, WBC count; | **Notes:** Comfrey is known to be toxic, carcinogenic, and potentially fatal; sale is prohibited in the United States and several countries.

copper | **Uses:** Age-related macular degeneration, Alzheimer's disease (prevention), arthritis, cancer, copper deficiency, enamel protection, heart disease (prevention), immune system function, marasmus, Menkes' kinky hair disease, osteoporosis/osteopenia, plaque prevention, schizophrenia, sideroblastic anemia, skin rejuvenation, systemic lupus erythematosus (SLE), trimethylaminuria; | **Preg:** The daily U.S. recommended dietary allowance (RDA) is 1,000 mcg for pregnant women. Copper is potentially unsafe when used orally in higher doses. It is unclear if copper supplementation is necessary during pregnancy to maintain adequate levels; | **CIs:** Allergy/hypersensitivity; Hypercupremia and associated conditions (cutaneous leishmaniasis, sickle cell disease, unipolar depression, breast cancer, epilepsy, measles, Down syndrome, controlled fibrocalculous pancreatic diabetes), Disrupted copper metabolism (Wilson's disease, Indian childhood cirrhosis, or idiopathic copper toxicosis); | **ADRs:** abdominal pain (high amounts), anemia, anxiety, arthralgias, coma (high amounts), DEATH (high amounts), decreased concentration, depression, diarrhea (high amounts), discolored skin/hair, fatigue, gingivitis, hypertension, insomnia, liver/kidney/neurological damage (high amounts), myalgias, pleural damage, postpartum psychosis, ↑ risk of pelvic infection, seizure, skin irritation, stuttering, vomiting (high amounts), weakness, weight gain; | **Interactions:** Antacids (↓ copper absorption), anticoagulants (essential for certain coagulation factors), anticonvulsants (↓ copper metabolism), antipsychotic agents (↑ copper levels), estrogens (↑ copper levels), calcium (↑ bone generation), ethambutol (chelates copper/↓ copper levels), hepatotoxic agents (↑ risk of liver damage), nephrotoxic agents (↑ risk of kidney damage), nifedipine (↓ copper levels), penicillamine (↑ copper excretion/↓ copper levels), trientine (chelates copper/↓ copper levels), zidovudine (↓ copper levels); | **Dose:** The daily U.S. recommended dietary allowance (RDA) for adults is 900 mcg; 1,000 mcg for pregnant women; and 1,300 mcg for nursing women. Up to 10,000 mcg daily appears to be safe for consumption in adults and is the tolerable upper level; | **Monitor:** Blood pressure, markers of copper status, coagulation panel, complete blood count, folate, hemoglobin, homocysteine, iron, lipid panel, serum diamine oxidase; | **Notes:** Copper supplements are available as copper acetate, copper amino acid chelates, copper gluconate, copper sebecate, copper sulfate, cuivre, cupric oxide, cupric sulfate, elemental copper, inorganic copper, and organic copper. Copper is use to make some intrauterine devices (IUDs).

C

C

coptis formula | **Uses:** Diabetes; | **Preg:** Not recommended due to insufficient evidence; | **CIs:** Allergy/hypersensitivity; | **ADRs:** insufficient evidence; | **Interactions:** Antidiabetic agents (additive effects/↑ risk of hypoglycemia); | **Dose:** Insufficient evidence; | **Monitor:** Blood glucose; | **Notes:** Coptis formula contains coptis, rhubarb, skullcap, phellodendra, gypsum, gardenia, forsythia, chrysanthemum, schizonepeta, angelica, viticis, cnidium, Ledebouriella, mint, inula, platycodon, and licorice.

coral | **Uses:** Bone reconstruction (graft); | **Preg:** Not recommended due to insufficient evidence; | **CIs:** Allergy/hypersensitivity, Kidney disease; | **ADRs:** infection, nephrotoxicity, wound irritation; | **Interactions:** Calcium (altered effects); | **Dose:** Insufficient clinical evidence; | **Monitor:** Calcium levels, renal function tests; | **Notes:** Coral calcium is listed by the U.S. Food and Drug Administration (FDA) as Generally Recognized as Safe (GRAS). Solid coral blocks serve as bone graft substitutes in clinical orthopedics.

cordyceps *(Cordyceps sinensis)* | **Uses:** Aging, asthma, bronchitis, chemoprotection, cirrhosis, exercise performance enhancement, hepatitis B, hyperlipidemia, immunosuppression, renal failure (chronic), sexual dysfunction; | **Preg:** Not recommended due to insufficient evidence and possible hormonal effects; | **CIs:** Allergy/hypersensitivity, Autoimmune disease; | **ADRs:** angina, anorexia, bleeding, diarrhea, drowsiness, ↑ estrogen/progesterone levels, gastrointestinal upset, nausea, palpitations, wheezing, urticaria, xerostomia; | **Interactions:** Hepatotoxic agents (improves drug-induced hepatotoxicity), immunosuppressants (↓ immunosuppressant effects), nephrotoxic agents (improves drug-induced nephrotoxicity); may interact with agents with similar effects or mechanisms of action (anticoagulant, antibiotic, antidepressant, antidiabetic, antihypertensive, anti-inflammatory, antilipemic, antineoplasic, corticosteroid induction, hormonal); | **Dose:** Fermented extract: 3–9 g daily by mouth for up to 8 weeks; | **Monitor:** Blood glucose, creatinine, hormone levels, lipid profile, LFTs, renal function tests, WBC count; | **Notes:** Owing to the increasing popularity of *Cordyceps sinesis*, some supplements have been adulterated or substitute other species of cordyceps.

corn poppy *(Papaver rhoeas)* | **Uses:** Insufficient clinical evidence; | **Preg:** Not recommended due to insufficient evidence; | **CIs:** Allergy/hypersensitivity; | **ADRs:** contact urticaria; | **Interactions:** CNS depressants (additive sedation), iron (chelates iron), morphine (↓ morphine withdrawal), | **Dose:** Insufficient evidence; | **Monitor:** Iron; | **Notes:** Corn poppy (*Papaver rhoeas*) is well known for its showy red flowers, and should not be confused with the opium poppy (*Papaver somniferum*).

C

cornflower *(Centaurea cyanus)* | **Uses:** Urolithiasis recurrence; | **Preg:** Not recommended due to insufficient evidence; | **CIs:** Allergy/hypersensitivity, Concurrent urolithiasis treatment; | **ADRs:** insufficient evidence; | **Interactions:** May interact with agents with similar effects or mechanisms of action (anti-inflammatory, antiurolithiasis); | **Dose:** Insufficient evidence; | **Monitor:** Insufficient evidence; | **Notes:** Cornflowers are often used as an ingredient in tea and are sometimes used as a garnish.

corydalis (*Corydalis* spp.) | **Uses:** Angina, arrhythmia, parasites, *Helicobacter pylori* infection, pain (cold induced); | **Preg:** Not recommended due to insufficient evidence and potential cytotoxicity; | **CIs:** Allergy/hypersensitivity, Pregnancy; | **ADRs:** arrhythmia, sedation; | **Interactions:** May interact with agents with similar effects or mechanisms of action (analgesic, antiarrhythmic, antibiotic, antineoplastic, antiretroviral, cardiovascular, sedative); | **Dose:** Up to 6.5 g raw extract; | **Monitor:** Bacterial cultures, heart rate, viral load; | **Notes:** Corydalis is commonly used in traditional Chinese medicine (TCM) preparations for gastrointestinal disorders.

couch grass *(Elytrigia repens,* syn. *Triticum repens, Agropyron repens, Elymus repens)* | **Uses:** Ulcerative colitis; | **Preg:** Not recommended due to insufficient evidence; | **CIs:** Allergy/hypersensitivity; | **ADRs:** atopic dermatitis, coughing, dyspnea, hypokalemia, nasal itching, throat swelling; | **Interactions:** May interact with agents with similar effects or mechanisms of action (antihypertensive, diuretic); | **Dose:** Decoction: 8 g dried root 3 times daily. Liquid extract (1:1 in 25% alcohol): up to 8 mL 3 times daily. Tincture (1:5 in 40% alcohol): up to 15 mL 3 times daily; | **Monitor:** Blood pressure, electrolytes; | **Notes:** Traditionally used for urinary tract conditions.

cow parsnip *(Heracleum maximum)* | **Uses:** Insufficient clinical evidence; | **Preg:** Not recommended due to insufficient evidence; | **CIs:** Allergy/hypersensitivity, Pregnancy,

UV light therapy; | **ADRs:** photosensitivity, skin irritation and rash; | **Interactions:** Photosensitizers (↑ risk of photosensitivity); | **Dose:** Insufficient evidence; | **Monitor:** Insufficient evidence; | **Notes:** Although cow parsnip is considered an invasive weed in western North America, it is considered endangered in Kentucky.

C

cowhage *(Mucuna pruriens)* | **Uses:** Hyperprolactinemia, Parkinson's disease; | **Preg:** Not recommended due to insufficient evidence; | **CIs:** Allergy/hypersensitivity, Lactation (may ↓ prolactin secretion), Oral/topical use of hair of cowhage bean pod; | **ADRs:** acute toxic psychosis, gastrointestinal effects, pruritus; | **Interactions:** Anesthesia (↑ risk of cardiac arrhythmia), antidiabetic agents (additive effects/↑ risk of hypoglycemia), antipsychotic agents (↑ risk of hypoglycemia), kava (↓ effectiveness of cowhage), levodopa (additive effects/due to L-dopa content), dopaminergic agents, MAOIs (↑ risk of hypertensive crisis), METHYLDOPA (additive hypotensive effects), tricyclic antidepressants (↓ absorption of cowhage), vitamin B_6 (↓ effectiveness of cowhage); | **Dose:** 30 g cowhage preparation for 1 week, up to 9 sachets cowhage derivative (7.5 g/satchet); | **Monitor:** Coagulation panel, blood glucose, ketones, LFTs, prolactin levels, uric acid; | **Notes:** Used in Ayurveda to treat Parkinson's disease.

cowslip *(Primula veris)* | **Uses:** Bronchitis (combination product, Bronchipret), sinusitis (combination product, Sinupret); | **Preg:** Not recommended due to insufficient evidence; | **CIs:** Allergy/hypersensitivity; | **ADRs:** allergic reaction, gastrointestinal distress, ↓ red blood cells; | **Interactions:** May interact with agents with similar effects or mechanisms of action (anticonvulsant, anti-inflammatory, antiarrhythmic, hemolytic); | **Dose:** Insufficient evidence; | **Monitor:** RBC count; | **Notes:** Used in Danish folk medicine to treat epilepsy and convulsions, and as a sedative.

cramp bark *(Viburnum opulus)* | **Uses:** Insufficient clinical evidence; | **Preg:** Not recommended due to insufficient evidence and purported effects on the uterus; | **CIs:** Allergy/hypersensitivity; | **ADRs:** insufficient evidence; | **Interactions:** May interact with agents with similar effects or mechanisms of action (antibiotic, antiulcer, antispasmodic, astringent, antihypertensive, immunomodulatory); | **Dose:** Insufficient evidence; | **Monitor:** WBC count; | **Notes:** Traditionally, cramp bark has been used to treat asthma, cramps, colic, or painful menstruation.

C

cranberry *(Vaccinium macrocarpon)* | **Uses:** Antibacterial, antifungal, antioxidant, antiviral, cancer (prevention), dental plaque, gastric ulcer, memory loss, radiotherapy adverse effects, renal calculi, urinary tract infection (treatment/prevention), urinary odor reduction (with incontinence/bladder catheterization), urine acidification, urostomy care; | **Preg:** Likely safe in food amounts in pregnant or breastfeeding patients based on traditional use. Other uses are not recommended due to lack of sufficient evidence; | **CIs:** Allergy/hypersensitivity, Aspirin allergy, Bladder cancer, Nephrolithiasis; | **ADRs:** ↑ bladder cancer risk, bleeding, ↑ blood glucose (sweetened cranberry preparations), contusion, diarrhea, nausea, nephrolithiasis, vaginal yeast infections, vomiting; | **Interactions:** Antacids (↓ effects), antibiotics (additive effects), anticoagulants/antiplatelets (↑ risk of bleeding), antidiabetic agents (juice, may alter effects); CYP450 2C9 substrates (inhibits CYP2C9), warfarin (↑ risk of bleeding), salicylates (↑ salicylate levels), vitamin B_{12} (juice, ↑ absorption vitamin B_{12}); | **Dose:** Juice cocktail: 500 mL daily. Unsweetened 100% juice: 15–30 mL. Capsules: 200–800 mg once daily or in divided doses; | **Monitor:** Blood glucose, coagulation panel, LFTs, renal function tests; | **Notes:** Cranberry is widely used to prevent urinary tract infection. It was previously thought to acidify the urine; however, evidence suggests that the proanthocyanidin constituent prevents bacterial adhesion.

cranesbill | **Uses:** Insect repellant; | **Preg:** Not recommended due to insufficient evidence; | **CIs:** Allergy/hypersensitivity; | **ADRs:** gastrointestinal upset; | **Interactions:** Antidiarrheals (additive effects), antineoplastic agents (additive effects), antiviral agents (additive effects), anxiolytics (additive effects), cholinesterase inhibitors (additive effects); | **Dose:** Oral: 1,200 mg PO 2–3 times/day. Tea: boil 1–2 tsp (5–10 g) for 10–15 min in 2 cups (500 mL) of water, for 3 or more cups/day. Tincture: ½ tsp or 3 mL PO tid. Topical: apply oil to skin as insect repellant; | **Monitor:** N/A; | **Notes:** Cranesbill (also known as geranium) gets its name from the appearance of the seed heads, which have the same shape as the bill of a crane.

creatine | **Uses:** Apnea (of prematurity), athletic performance, congestive heart failure, chronic obstructive pulmonary disease (COPD), depression, dialysis, enhanced muscle mass/strength, GAMT deficiency, Huntington's disease, hyperornithinemia, hyperlipidemia, ischemic heart disease, McArdle's disease, memory, mitochondrial disorders, multiple sclerosis, muscular dystrophy, myocardial infarction (heart attack), osteoporosis, surgery adjunct, spinal cord injury, | **Preg:** Not recommended due to insufficient evidence; | **CIs:** Allergy/hypersensitivity, Renal dysfunction; | **ADRs:** abdominal discomfort, aggression, anxiety, atrial fibrillation, ↑/↓ cholesterol levels, dehydration, depression, diarrhea, edema, electrolyte imbalances, fever, headache, heat intolerance, hepatic dysfunction, hypertension, irritability, lightheadedness, muscle cramping, pruritus, purpuric dermatosis, RENAL DYSFUNCTION, seizure, syncope, tachycardia, urinary incontinence, water retention, weight gain; | **Interactions:** Caffeine (↑ risk of adverse effects), carbohydrates (↑ creatine levels), cimetidine (competes with creatine for renal excretion), CNS stimulants (↑ risk of adverse effects), ephedra (↑ risk of adverse effects), ergotamine (↓ creatine effects), hepatotoxic agents (↑ risk of liver damage), indomethacin (additive effects), NEPHROTOXIC AGENTS (↑ risk of kidney damage), nifedipine (synergistic effects); may interact with agents with similar effects or mechanisms of action (antidiabetic, anti-inflammatory, antineoplasic, diuretic); | **Dose:** General: Up to 400 mg/kg body weight, or up to 25 g daily PO; | **Monitor:** Albumin, ammonia, blood glucose, CBC, cortisol, creatine (serum), creatine kinase, creatinine, electrolytes, homocysteine, LFTs, lipid profile, renal function tests; | **Notes:** The U.S. Food and Drug Administration (FDA) has warned consumers to consult with their physicians before beginning creatine supplementation.

cumin ***(Cuminum cyminum)*** | **Uses:** Insufficient evidence; | **Preg:** Likely safe in amounts found in food; not recommended in medicinal amounts due to insufficient evidence; | **CIs:** Allergy/hypersensitivity; | **ADRs:** contact dermatitis, hepatocellular carcinoma, hypoglycemia, respiratory problems; | **Interactions:** Anticoagulants/antiplatelets (↑ risk of bleeding), antidiabetic agents (↑ risk of hypoglycemia) antifungal agents (additive effects), antilipemic agents (additive effects), opiates (↓ effects of opiates), rifampin (↑ bioavailability of rifampin); | **Dose:** Insufficient evidence; | **Monitor:** Blood glucose, LFTs; | **Notes:** Caution is warranted in patients with liver damage because cumin contains aflatoxin B1, which has been associated with hepatocellular carcinoma.

cyclo-hispro | **Uses:** Insufficient evidence; | **Preg:** Not recommended due to insufficient evidence; | **CIs:** Allergy/hypersensitivity; | **ADRs:** insufficient evidence; | **Interactions:** Alcohol (↓ concentrations of alcohol), amphetamines (↑ effects), antidiabetic agents (↑ risk of hypoglycemia), ketamine (antagonistic effects); | **Dose:** 200–300 mg (of powdered prostate extract containing cyclo-hispro) PO 2–4 times/day; **Monitor:** Blood glucose; **Notes:** Cyclo-hispro is a metabolite of a thyrotropin-releasing hormone, which occurs in large quantities in the prostate gland. Cyclo-hispro is marketed as stimulating healthy metabolism of glucose. It also enhances the intestinal absorption of zinc.

D

cypress ***(Cupressus*** **spp.)** **Uses:** Insufficient evidence; **Preg:** Not recommended due to insufficient evidence; **CIs:** Allergy/hypersensitivity; **ADRs:** anemia, liver failure, renal failure, skin sensitivity, thrombocytopenia; **Interactions:** Anticoagulants/antiplatelets (↑ risk of bleeding), immunosuppressants (altered effects); **Dose:** Insufficient evidence; **Monitor:** Insufficient evidence; **Notes:** Cypress essential oil has been used as a fragrance and in aromatherapy. There is little evidence about this herb.

daio-kanzo-to **Uses:** Constipation; **Preg:** Not recommended due to insufficient evidence; **CIs:** Allergy/hypersensitivity; **ADRs:** insufficient evidence; **Interactions:** Insufficient evidence; **Dose:** 0.5–1.5g daily PO as needed; **Monitor:** Insufficient evidence; **Notes:** Daio-kanzo-to is a Kampo formula that includes a mixture of rhubarb and licorice. Traditionalists consider it a safe remedy for habitual constipation and other abdominal symptoms.

daisy ***(Bellis perennis)*** **Uses:** Bleeding (postpartum); **Preg:** Not recommended due to insufficient evidence and possible adverse effects on fetal growth; **CIs:** Allergy/hypersensitivity to the Asteraceae/Compositae family, Pediatric use (due to possible ↓ growth); **ADRs:** growth retardation, hemolysis, respiratory allergies, thrombosis; **Interactions:** Anticoagulants/antiplatelets (altered effects); **Dose:** General, tea: 1 cup of tea (2 tsp of dried herb steeped in 300 mL of boiling water for 20 mintues, strained) 2–4 times daily; **Monitor:** Coagulation panel; serum iron; **Notes:** Considered to be the archetypal species of daisy; not to be confused with oxeye daisy (*Chrysanthemum leucanthemum*) or other species with "daisy" as the common name. Generally well tolerated in extremely dilute homeopathic preparations.

damiana ***(Turnera diffusa)*** **Uses:** Obesity, sexual dysfunction (female); **Preg:** Not recommended due to insufficient evidence and traditional use as an abortifacient; **CIs:** Allergy/hypersensitivity, Pregnancy, Alzheimer's disease, Parkinson's disease, Psychiatric disorders (e.g., schizophrenia);

ADRs: diarrhea, erotic dreams, hallucinations, headaches, insomnia, mood changes; **Interactions:** Antidiabetic agents (additive effects/↑ risk of hypoglycemia), progesterone (additive effects); **Dose:** General: 2–4 g dried leaf (directly or as tea) 2–3 times daily; **Monitor:** Blood glucose, progesterone; **Notes:** Damiana has been reported as one of the top six highest progesterone receptor–binding herbs commonly consumed.

D

dandelion *(Taraxacum officinale)* **Uses:** Inflammation, antioxidant, cancer, colitis, diabetes, diuretic, hepatitis B, urinary tract infections; **Preg:** Not recommended due to insufficient evidence; **CIs:** Allergy/hypersensitivity; **ADRs:** anorexia, asthma, bleeding, bowel obstruction, contusion, cough, diarrhea, dyspepsia, dyspnea, eczema, edema of lips/mouth/throat, gastrointestinal upset, hepatotoxicity, hypoglycemia, photosensitivity, pruritus, rhinoconjunctivitis, skin rash (redness), vomiting; **Interactions:** Anticoagulants/antiplatelets (↑ risk of bleeding), CYP450 1A2 substrates (inhibits CYP1A2, ↑ drug levels), ciprofloxacin (↓ absorption), diuretics (additive effects), estrogens (additive effects), glucuronidated agents (induce UDP-glucuronosyltransferase/↑ drug levels), lithium (↑ risk of toxicity/due to ↓ sodium), potassium-depleting agent (↑ risk of hypokalemia), quinolones (↓ quinolone levels); **Dose:** General, decoction, infusion: 2–8 g of the dried root. Fluid extract, leaf: 4–8 mL of a 1:1 extract in 25% alcohol. Tincture, root: 1 or 2 tsp of a 1:5 tincture in 45% alcohol; **Monitor:** Coagulation panel, electrolytes, estrogens, urine tests; **Notes:** Dandelion has been used traditionally to treat numerous disorders.

danshen *(Salvia miltiorrhiza)* **Uses:** Asthmatic bronchitis, burns, cardiovascular disease, chronic hepatitis B, cirrhosis, diabetic foot, dialysis (peritoneal), glaucoma, hyperlipidemia, ischemic stroke, kidney disease, liver fibrosis, obesity, prostatitis, syncope, tinnitus; **Preg:** Not recommended due to insufficient evidence and possible ↑ bleeding and miscarriage risks; **CIs:** Allergy/hypersensitivity, Concurrent use with anticoagulants/antiplatelets, Concurrent use with digoxin; **ADRs:** abdominal discomfort, aggravated brain injury, altered mental status, angina, anorexia, bleeding, bradycardia, contusion, convulsions, drowsiness, dyspnea, dystonia, miscarriage, pruritus; **Interactions:** Alcohol (↓ effects), ANTICOAGULANTS/ANTIPLATELETS (↑ risk of bleeding), antihypertensives (additive effects/↑ risk of hypotension), DIGOXIN (↑ risk of arrhythmias), nitrates (↓ tolerance), P-glycoprotein substrates (altered drug levels), steroids (additive effects); may interact with agents with similar effects or mechanisms of action (antibiotic, anti-inflammatory, antilipemic, antineoplastic, benzodiazepines, cardiovascular, immunosuppressant, inotropic, sedative); **Dose:** Insufficient evidence; **Monitor:** Blood pressure, atrial natriuretic peptide (ANP), CD4 count, coagulation panel, creatine kinase, intraocular pressure (IOP), lipid profile, LFTs, pulmonary function tests; **Notes:** Danshen should not be confused with sage or other members of the *Salvia* genus. Danshen is often used in combination with other products in traditional medicine.

date palm *(Phoenix dactylifera)* **Uses:** Wrinkles; **Preg:** Likely safe in food amounts in pregnant or breastfeeding patients based on traditional use. Other uses are not recommended due to lack of sufficient evidence; **CIs:** Allergy/hypersensitivity; **ADRs:** allergic rhinitis, bony pseudotumors, bronchial asthma, *Cladosporium cladosporioides* and *Sporobolomyces roseus* infections, encephalitis, oral allergy syndrome, rhinoconjunctivitis, synovitis, wheezing; **Interactions:** Insufficient evidence; **Dose:** Topical: 5% date palm kernel cream, applied twice daily to the eye area for 5 weeks; **Monitor:** Insufficient evidence; **Notes:** Foreign body puncture wounds due to date palm thorns or thorn fragments, some causing systemic illness and requiring surgical removal, have been reported.

deer velvet **Uses:** Aerobic fitness, sexual dysfunction (libido, erectile dysfunction); **Preg:** Not recommended due to insufficient evidence and possible hormonal effects; **CIs:** Allergy/hypersensitivity, Hormone-sensitive conditions; **ADRs:** both deer antler powder and extract have been well tolerated in available clinical studies; **Interactions:** Androgens (additive effects), estrogens (additive effects); **Dose:** Four 250-mg capsules daily for 12 weeks (no effect); **Monitor:** Hormonal levels, LFTs; **Notes:** Deer velvet, also referred to as antler velvet, refers to antlers that have been removed in the growth stage, when they are covered in soft velvet-like hair.

dehydroepiandrosterone (DHEA) **Uses:** Addison's disease, adrenal insufficiency, Alzheimer's disease, atrichia pubis, cardiovascular disease, cervical cancer, chronic fatigue syndrome, cocaine withdrawal, critical illness, Crohn's disease, depression, HIV/AIDS, infertility, menopausal symptoms, muscle strength, myotonic dystrophy, labor induction, obesity, osteoporosis, psoriasis, rheumatoid arthritis, schizophrenia, septicemia, sexual dysfunction/libido/erectile dysfunction, Sjögren's syndrome, skin aging, systemic lupus erythematosus, vaginal atrophy; | **Preg:** Contraindicated due to potential adverse effects to developing fetuses; | **CIs:** Allergy/hypersensitivity; Pregnancy, Lactation, Hormone-sensitive conditions or concomitant hormonal agents; | **ADRs:** acne, aggression, agitation, amenorrhea, arrhythmias, bleeding, blood pressure changes, breast tenderness, contusion, cholesterol level changes, Cushing's syndrome, delusions, dyspnea, emotional changes, fatigue, headache, hepatotoxicity, hirsutism, hormone changes, hyper-/hypoglycemia, insomnia, irritability, male breast development/growth, mania, masculinization in women (greasy skin, facial hair, hair loss, ↑ sweating, weight gain around waist, deeper voice), miscarriage, nasal congestion, nervousness, pruritis, psychosis, skin rash, ↑ risk of prostate/breast/ovarian cancer, testicular wasting (in men), thrombosis, thyroid hormone changes; weight gain, | **Interactions:** Alcohol (may ↑/↓ effects of DHEA), amlodipine (↑ DHEA sulfate [DHEAS]), antiestrogens (interfere with effects), antidiabetic agents (altered effects), antipsychotic drugs (↓ DHEAS), benfluorex (↑ DHEA), beta-adrenergic antagonists (↑ DHEAS secretion), budesonide (↓ DHEAS), canrenoate (↑ DHEA), corticosteroids (↓ DHEA production), CYP450 3A4 (inhibits CYP3A4/↑ drug levels), danazol (↑ DHEAS), dexamethasone (↓ DHEA and DHEAS), diltiazem (↑ DHEA), estrogens (↓ DHEA and DHEAS), ethanol (↓ DHEA), gefitninib (↓ DHEA and DHEAS), growth hormone (↑ DHEAS), insulin (↓ DHEAS), metformin (↓ DHEA), methylphenidate (↑ DHEA and DHEAS), metopirone (↑ DHEA and DHEAS), nitrendipine (↓ DHEAS), progesterone (↓ DHEA and DHEAS), thyroid hormones (altered effects), triazolam (↑ triazolam concentration/inhibits CYP450 3A4), vaccines (↓ antibody development); | **Dose:** General: 5–200 mg daily PO for 3 months. Topical: 5%–10% cream applied to the thighs or buttocks. Parenteral: 10 mg twice weekly for induction of labor; 200 mg daily for dementia; | **Monitor:** ACTH, antibody titers, antidiuretic hormone, blood glucose, body mass index (BMI), coagulation panel, cortisol, lipid profile, estrogens, glucagon, immune parameters, insulin, growth hormone, progesterone, prolactin, sex hormones, thyroid hormone, testosterone; | **Notes:** DHEA is an endogenous hormone (made in the human body), and secreted by the adrenal gland. DHEA serves as a precursor to male and female sex hormones (androgens and estrogens). DHEA levels decrease after age 30, as well as in certain medical conditions or with concomitant medications. Use cautiously in patients with diabetes, hyperlipidemia, liver dysfunction, psychiatric disorders, and polycystic ovarian syndrome.

desert parsley *(Lomatium dissectum)* | **Uses:** Insufficient clinical evidence; | **Preg:** Not recommended due to insufficient evidence; | **CIs:** Allergy/hypersensitivity; | **ADRs:** nausea, rash, urticaria; | **Interactions:** Anticoagulants/antiplatelets (↑ risk of bleeding); may interact with agents with related effects or mechanisms of action (antifungal, antiviral); | **Dose:** Lomatium isolates (resin removed): 1–3 mL daily. Tea: 1–2 tsp dried herb 3 times daily. Tincture: 1–3 mL (10–30 drops) 1–4 times daily; | **Monitor:** Coagulation panel; | **Notes:** Desert parsley has been used by many Native American tribes to treat a wide variety of infections, mainly of the lungs.

devil's claw *(Harpagophytum procumbens)* | **Uses:** Appetite stimulant, cancer, digestive tonic, low back pain, osteoarthritis, rheumatoid arthritis; | **Preg:** Not recommended due to insufficient evidence; | **CIs:** Allergy/hypersensitivity; Gallstones, Peptic ulcer disease, Pregnancy; | **ADRs:** abdominal pain, allergic skin reactions, anorexia, arrhythmia, bleeding, contusion, diarrhea, dysmenorrhea, dyspnea, gallstones, ↑ gastric acid secretion, headache, hemodynamic instability, hypogeusia, hypoglycemia, nausea, pruritus, skin rash, tinnitus, vomiting; | **Interactions:** Analgesics (additive effects), antacids/H2-blockers/proton pump inhibitors (↓ effectiveness), antidiabetic agents (additive effects/↑ risk of hypoglycemia), antilipemic agents (additive effects), CYP450 2C19/2C9/3A4 (inhibits CYP2C19/2C9/3A4, ↑ drug levels), laxatives (additive effects), warfarin (may cause purpura/over-anticoagulation); | **Dose:** Liquid extract (1:1 in 25% ethanol): up to 0.25 mL 3 times daily. Decoction: 1.5 g daily. Tincture (1:10 in 25% ethanol): up to 3 mL daily. Crude extract: up to 9 g daily. Tablets: up to 1,200 mg standardized to 50–100 mg harpagosides. Capsules: up to 2,610 mg daily; | **Monitor:** Blood glucose, blood pressure, coagulation panel, lipid profile, uric acid; | **Notes:** Potentially active chemical constituents of devil's claw include iridoid glycosides (2.2% total weight), harpagoside (0.5%–1.6%), 8-p-coumaroylharpagide, 8-feruloylharpagide, 8-cinnamoylmyoporoside, pagoside, acteoside, isoacteoside, 6′-O-acetylacteoside, 2,6-diacetylacteoside, cinnamic acid, caffeic acid, procumbide, and procumboside.

devil's club *(Oplopanax horridus)* | **Uses:** Diabetes; | **Preg:** Not recommended due to insufficient evidence and traditional use as a uterine stimulant; | **CIs:** Allergy/hypersensitivity; Pregnancy, Lactation; | **ADRs:** allergic reaction, diarrhea, hypoglycemia, weight gain; | **Interactions:** Antidiabetic agents (additive effects/↑ risk of hypoglycemia);

Dose: Decoction: Up to ½ glass daily, or 125 mL before meals. Extract: 1.5 mL per pound body weight. Tincture: up to 30 drops 3 times daily; **Monitor:** Blood glucose; **Notes:** Devil's club is most commonly used as a general tonic and for treating infections.

D

DHA (docosahexaenoic acid) **Uses:** ADHD, age-related macular degeneration, Alzheimer's disease/dementia, angina, asthma, CAD, depression, diabetes, dyslexia, dysmenorrhea, dyspraxia, eczema, hyperlipidemia, HTN, IBD, IgA nephropathy, infant development, maternal health, nephrotic syndrome, lupus, obesity, plaque psoriasis, prevention of cyclosporine toxicity, prevention of graft failure (after heart bypass surgery), psychiatric disorders, PTCA (prevention of restinosis), psoriasis, RA, stroke prevention; **Preg:** Likely safe; **CIs:** Allergy/hypersensitivity; **ADRs:** abdominal bloating, atrophic gastritis, belching, bleeding, contusion, diarrhea, epistaxis, fishy taste, flatulence, indigestion, ↑ LDL, nausea, vitamin A and D toxicity (with fish liver oil [e.g., cod liver oil]), vitamin E deficiency (long-term use, fish oil); **Interactions:** Anticoagulants/antiplatelets (↑ risk of bleeding), antidiabetic agents (altered effects), antihypertensives (↑ risk of hypotension), antilipemic agents (altered effects); **Dose:** Oral, general: 1,000–2,000 mg PO qd. Do not exceed more than 3 g PO qd due to increased risk of bleeding. General, algae-derived: 200 mg PO qd. Dyslexia (vision problems): 480 mg PO qd. Hyperlipidemia: 4 g PO qd. Infant development (maternal ingestion): 200 mg PO qd. Maternal health: 200 mg PO qd. Intravenous: 4.2 g plus EPA 4.2 g daily IV; **Monitor:** Blood glucose, coagulation panel, lipid profile; **Notes:** Ratio of omega-6 to omega-3 fatty acids should be between 1:1 and 4:1. DHA/EPA ratio of 2:1 produces optimal growth in fish. Take with meals to minimize GI upset.

digitalis *(Digitalis purpurea*, foxglove) **Uses:** Insufficient evidence; **Preg:** Avoid use; **CIs:** Allergy/hypersensitivity, Oral use/self-medication, Ventricular fibrillation; **ADRs:** toxic effects: cardiac effects, gastrointestinal distress, headache, nausea/vomiting, psychiatric disturbances (altered mental status, confusion, disorientation, hallucinations), visual disturbances (yellow halos around lights), weakness; **Interactions:** Activated charcoal (bind/remove digitalis), analgesics (additive effects), antacids (↓ effectiveness of digitalis), antiarrhythmic agents (altered effects), anticoagulants/antiplatelets (↑ risk of bleeding), antidepressant agents (additive effects), antihypertensives (altered effects), anti-inflammatory agents (additive effects), antilipemic agents (additive effects), antineoplastic agents (altered effects), beta blockers (altered effects), calcium channel blockers (altered effects), calcium (↑ risk of arrhythmias), carob (↑ risk of toxicity), CNS depressants (altered effects), DIGOXIN (↑ risk of toxicity), diphenoxylate (↑ digoxin absorption), diuretics (↑ risk of hypokalemia and toxicity), gossypol (↑ risk of toxicity), immunosuppressants (altered effects), laxatives (↑ risk of hypokalemia and toxicity), licorice (↑ risk of toxicity), macrolides (↑ risk of toxicity), magnesium (↓ levels of digitalis), QUININE (↑ risk of toxicity), propantheline (↑ digitalis absorption), rifampin (↓ levels of digitalis), succinylcholine (↑ risk of arrhythmias), sulfasalazine (↓ effectiveness of digitalis), sympathomimetics (↑ risk of arrhythmias), tetracyclines (↑ risk of toxicity), thyroid hormones (↓ effectiveness of digitalis), vasodilators (altered effects); | **Dose:** Insufficient evidence; | **Monitor:** Blood pressure, coagulation panel, EKG, heart rate, potassium, thyroid hormones; | **Notes:** Avoid using digitalis (foxglove) without medical supervision. Digitalis (foxglove) contains cardiac glycoside toxins, which are considered poisonous. Digoxin-specific Fab fragments have been used in case reports to treat digitalis (foxglove) poisoning.

dill *(Anethum graveolens)* | **Uses:** Hyperlipidemia; | **Preg:** Likely safe in amounts found in food; not recommended due to insufficient evidence; | **CIs:** Allergy/hypersensitivity; | **ADRs:** phytophotodermatitis, pruritus, swelling of tongue/throat; | **Interactions:** Antidiabetic agents (↑ risk of hypoglycemia), anti-inflammatory agents (additive effects), antilipemic agents (additive effects); CNS depressants (↑ sedation), CYP450 3A4 substrates (inhibits CYP3A4); | **Dose:** Oral, infusion: 1–2 tsp of dill steeped in a cup of boiling water for 10 minutes, left to cool, and sipped slowly. Oral, tincture: ½–1 tsp up to 3 times/day. Topical: mix dill tea with petroleum jelly, apply to affected area (frequency/duration unknown); | **Monitor:** Blood glucose, lipid profile; | **Notes:** Traditionally, dill has been used to treat ailments of the digestive tract and alleviate insomnia.

dimethyl sulfoxide (DMSO) | **Uses:** Amyloidosis, diabetic ulcers, extravasation, gastritis, herpes zoster, inflammatory bladder disease, interstitial cystitis, intracranial pressure, pressure ulcers (prevention), reflex sympathetic dystrophy, rheumatoid arthritis, surgical skin flap ischemia, tendopathy; | **Preg:** Not recommended due to insufficient evidence; | **CIs:** Allergy/hypersensitivity; | **ADRs:** agitation, anorexia, diarrhea, dizziness, dysuria, encephalopathy, eosinophilia, facial flushing, flu-like symptoms, halitosis, headache, hematuria, hemolysis, hypotension, myocardial infarction, nausea, sedation, seizure, skin irritation/rash, stroke, urine discoloration, vomiting; | **Interactions:** Sulindac (↓ effectiveness, ↓ metabolism, ↑ risk of peripheral neuropathy); may potentiate the effects of oral, injectable, and topical drugs; may interact with agents with related effects or mechanisms of action (analgesic, antiarthritic, antihistamine, cholinesterase inhibition); | **Dose:** Oral: 2–15 g daily PO. Amyloidosis: 7–15 g PO daily. Gastritis: 500 mg PO qid with 400 mg cimetidine PO bid. Topical: up to 100% applied to affected skin; | **Monitor:** Blood glucose, LFTs, renal function tests; | **Notes:** Industrial-grade DMSO may contain impurities and is not safe for medical use, because DMSO readily crosses the skin and may ↑ absorption of impurities and other substances. Use cautiously in patients with diabetes, intracranial pressure, liver dysfunction, and renal dysfunction.

D

dogwood (*Cornus* spp.) | **Uses:** Fertility, postmenopausal symptoms; | **Preg:** Not recommended due to insufficient evidence and possible hormonal effects; | **CIs:** Allergy/hypersensitivity, Pregnancy, Lactation, Concomitant hormonal agents; | **ADRs:** insufficient evidence; | **Interactions:** May interact with agents with related similar effects or related mechanisms of action (antidiabetic, antilipemic, antineoplastic, antioxidant, antiretroviral, contraceptive, estrogenic, hormonal); | **Dose:** Insufficient evidence; | **Monitor:** Hormones (estrogens, estradiols, FSH), viral load, lipid profile; | **Notes:** According to secondary sources, the name dogwood is said to originate from "dagwood," denoting the historical use of the hard-wooded stems for making "dags" (daggers).

dolomite | **Uses:** Insufficient evidence; | **Preg:** Not recommended due to insufficient evidence; | **CIs:** Allergy/hypersensitivity, Heart block, Renal insufficiency; | **ADRs:** cardiac arrest, cardiac arrhythmias, constipation, diarrhea, gastrointestinal distress, hypermagnesemia, hypotension, nausea/vomiting, renal calculi, respiratory problems, seizures, weakness; | **Interactions:** Bisphosphonates (↓ absorption of bisphosphonates), boron (↑ magnesium levels), calcium (↑ risk of constipation), estrogens (↑ calcium absorption), levothyroxine (↓ levothyroxine absorption), magnesium (↑ risk of diarrhea), quinonlones (↓ quinolone absorption), potassium-sparing diuretics (interfere with effects), sotalol (↓ absorption of sotalol), tetracycline (↓ absorption of tetracyclines), THIAZIDE DIURETICS (↓ calcium excretion), vitamin D (↑ absorption of oral calcium); **Dose:** Secondary references on dietary supplements have recommended a dose of 45–483 mg of magnesium daily, 1,000 mg of calcium daily up to age 50, and 1,200 mg of calcium daily after the age of 50. However, it is unclear if dolomite is a safe and effective means of fulfilling daily requirements for calcium or magnesium; **Monitor:** Calcium levels, hormone panel, lead levels, vitamin D levels; **Notes:** Dolomite is a sedimentary carbonate rock or mineral composed of calcium magnesium carbonate crystals. Dolomite rock (or dolostone) is primarily composed of the mineral dolomite. Dolomitic limestone (or magnesium limestone) is limestone that is partially replaced by dolomite. Dolomite, which is soluble and usable by the body, is commonly used as a calcium supplement. Dolomite may be contaminated with lead and other heavy metal contaminants.

dong quai *(Angelica sinensis)* **Uses:** Amenorrhea, angina, arthritis, CAD, dysmenorrhea, pulmonary hypertension, kidney disease, menopausal symptoms, menstrual migraine headache, neuralgia, thrombocytopenia; **Preg:** Not recommended due to insufficient evidence, traditional use as an abortifacient and uterine stimulant effects; **CIs:** Allergy/hypersensitivity, Concurrent use with anticoagulants/antiplatelets, Pregnancy, Lactation; **ADRs:** arrhythmia, asthma, bleeding, bloating, diaphoresis, diarrhea, dizziness, fever, gastrointestinal upset, headache, hot flashes, hyper-/hypotension, insomnia, irritability, lightheadedness, ↑ male breast size, ↓ menstrual flow, nausea, nephrotoxicity, photosensitivity, skin rash, vomiting, weakness; **Interactions:** ANTICOAGULANTS/ANTIPLATELETS (↑ risk of bleeding); may interact with agents with similar effects or related mechanisms of action (hormonal, photosensitizing, antiarrhythmic, antidepressant, anticancer); **Dose:** Oral: powdered/dried root/root slices, fluid extract/tincture, decoctions, dried leaf tinctures and extracts. Topical: diluted essential oil; **Monitor:** Blood pressure, coagulation panel, heart rate, hormone panel; **Notes:** Although dong quai is accepted as being safe as a food additive in the United States and Europe, its safety in medicinal doses is unclear.

durian **Uses:** Anthelmintic (traditional), aphrodisiac (traditional); **Preg:** Insufficient available evidence; traditionally, pregnant women are advised not to consume durian; **CIs:** Allergy/hypersensitivity, Concurrent alcohol consumption; **ADRs** flatulence, hypertension, irritation of the mouth, ↑ insulin levels; **Interactions:** ALCOHOL (altered effects), antihypertensives (↓ effects of antihypertensives), insulin (additive effects/↑ risk of hypoglycemia); | **Dose:** The roots may be boiled with *Hibiscus rosa-sinensis, Nephelium longan, Nephelium mutabile,* and *Artocarpus integrifolia* to make a decoction for oral consumption. Topically, durian may be found in lotion or boil in water for bathing; | **Monitor:** Blood glucose, blood pressure, insulin levels; | **Notes:** Uncooked seeds should be avoided.

eastern hemlock *(Tsuga canadensis)* | **Uses:** Insufficient clinical evidence; | **Preg:** Not recommended due to insufficient evidence and known toxicity; | **CIs:** Allergy/hypersensitivity; | **ADRs:** dermatitis, gastrointestinal upset, liver necrosis, nephrotoxicity; | **Interactions:** Diuretics (additive effects/↑ risk of electrolyte imbalances), may interact with oral agents due to high tannin content and cause precipitation; | **Dose:** Safe doses or maximum duration of eastern hemlock has not been clinically established; | **Monitor:** Electrolytes, LFTs, renal function tests; | **Notes:** Not related to poison hemlock (*Conium* spp.) used by Socrates to commit suicide.

echinacea *(Echinacea angustifolia; Echinacea pallida; Echinacea purpurea)* | **Uses:** URIs (prevention and treatment); cancer; immune system modulation; radiation-associated leukopenia; uveitis; vaginal yeast infections; | **Preg:** Recommended doses of oral preparations may be safe (except tinctures); parenteral administration is not advised; | **CIs:** Hypersensitivity to echinacea, its constituents, or any members of the Asteraceae/Compositae family (e.g., ragweed, chrysanthemums, marigolds, daisies), Concurrent use with amoxicillin, anesthesia; | **ADRs:** abdominal pain, ALLERGIC REACTIONS, atrial fibrillation, dizziness, drowsiness, erythema nodosum, gastrointestinal upset, headache, hepatitis, kidney failure, leukopenia, hepatotoxicity, mild nausea or vomiting, rash, reduced penetration of sperm, sore throat, thrombotic thrombocytopenic purpura (TTP), urticaria; | **Interactions:** AMOXICILLIN (may cause life-threatening reactions), anesthetics (altered effects), antineoplastic agents (altered effects), caffeine (↑ caffeine levels), corticosteroids (altered effects), cytochrome P450 substrates (inhibits CYP1A2; inhibits or induces CYP3A4), disulfiram (with tinctures) (↑ risk of disulfiram reactions), econazole nitrate (synergistic effects), hydrophilic agents (altered effects), immunosuppressants (interfere with effects), hepatotoxic agents (↑ risk of liver damage), metronidazole (↑ risk of disulfiram reactions), midazolam (↓ effectiveness), and herbs and supplements with similar effects; | **Dose:** Oral, adults: For URI prevention, a 1.5-mL tincture containing the equivalent of 300 mg *Echinacea angustifolia* root, taken 3 times daily either for a 7-day course before experimental infection or starting on the day of experimental infection and continuing for 5 days. For URI treatment, 500–1,000 mg 3 times daily, for 5–7 days. Oral, children: Dose recommendations in children are often weight based; | **Monitor:** Immune function, symptom improvement in patients with URI, LFTs; | **Notes:** Discontinue if allergic reaction occurs; the German Commission E warns against the use of echinacea in patients with AIDS/HIV, collagen vascular diseases, multiple sclerosis, or tuberculosis, owing to theoretical adverse effects on immune function, although no specific trial data support this assertion.

elder *(Sambucas nigra)* | **Uses:** Bronchitis, influenza, hyperlipidemia, sinusitis; | **Preg:** Not recommended due to insufficient evidence and risks of cyanide toxicity and miscarriage; | **CIs:** Allergy/hypersensitivity; | **ADRs:** abdominal cramps, birth defects, bradycardia, convulsions, cyanide poisoning, diarrhea, dizziness, dyspnea, gastrointestinal upset, headache, hyper-/hypoglycemia, miscarriage, polyuria, skin rash, tachycardia, vomiting, weakness; | **Interactions:** Doxycycline (additive effects), anti-inflammatory agents (additive effects), antineoplastic agents (additive effects), caffeine and other methylxanthines (↓ xanthine oxidase), decongestants (additive effects), immunosuppressants (interfere with effects); may interact with agents with similar effects or related mechanisms of action (antibiotic, antidiabetic, diuretic, laxative); | **Dose:** Oral: 3–5 g dried flowers (as tea) 3 times daily; 2 tablets Sinupret 3 times daily; up to 60 mL extract syrup (Sambucol) daily in divided doses for 5 days. Topical: elder flower cream applied to hands at bedtime; | **Monitor:** Blood glucose, heart rate, vital signs; | **Notes:** The flowers and berries (blue/black only) are used most often medicinally. The bark, leaves, seeds, and raw/unripe fruit contain the cyanogenic glycoside sambunigrin, which is potentially toxic.

elecampane *(Inula helenium)* | **Uses:** Insufficient clinical evidence; | **Preg:** Not recommended due to insufficient evidence; | **CIs:** Allergy/hypersensitivity, Pregnancy, Lactation; | **ADRs:** contact dermatitis; | **Interactions:** CNS depressants (additive sedation), may interact with agents with similar effects or related mechanisms of action (antibiotic, antidiabetic, antifungal, antihypertensive, antineoplastic, antioxidant, antiparasitic, antispasmodic, cardiovascular, laxative, sedative); | **Dose:** Decoction: Up to 4 g in tea 3 times daily for 10 days. Alantolactone: 300 mg (200 mg for children) daily for 5-day intervals (separated by 10 days). Tincture: up to 25 drops (12 drops for children) daily; | **Monitor:** Blood glucose, blood pressure; | **Notes:** Elecampane is approved for use in alcoholic beverages in the United States. Traditionally, elecampane is used as an antifungal, antiparasitic, and general antimicrobial agent, as well as an expectorant for coughs, colds, and bronchial ailments.

E

emu oil | **Uses:** Cosmetic uses; | **Preg:** Not recommended due to insufficient evidence; | **CIs:** Allergy/hypersensitivity; | **ADRs:** restless legs syndrome; | **Interactions:** May interact with anti-inflammatory agents due to similar effects; | **Dose:** Insufficient evidence; | **Monitor:** Insufficient evidence; | **Notes:** Emu oil is the refined and deodorized oil rendered from the back fat of the emu (*Dromaius novaehollandiae*). Emu oil is used topically for dermatological purposes; oral use is frequently recommended for reducing hypercholesterolemia.

English ivy ***(Hedera helix)*** | **Uses:** Asthma (children), COPD; | **Preg:** Not recommended due to insufficient evidence; | **CIs:** Allergy/hypersensitivity; | **ADRs:** allergic contact dermatitis, allergic rhinoconjunctivitis, asphyxia, asthmatic bronchitis, DEATH, severe blistering dermatitis; | **Interactions:** May interact with agents with similar effects or related mechanisms of action (antineoplastic, antioxidant); | **Dose:** Insufficient evidence; | **Monitor:** Insufficient evidence; | **Notes:** Used as a landscaping groundcover; also considered a noxious weed in some areas. Growing English ivy indoors has been recommended to filter carbon dioxide and carbon monoxide out of the air.

EPA (eicosapentaenoic acid) | **Uses:** ADHD, age-related macular degeneration, Alzheimer's disease, angina, anorexia, arrhythmias, asthma, bipolar disorder, borderline personality disorder, CAD, cancer (prevention), cardiovascular events (secondary prevention), colon cancer, cyclosporine toxicity (prevention), cystic fibrosis, depression, diabetes, dysmenorrhea, eclampsia, eczema, hayfever, HTN, Huntington's disease, hyperlipidemia, infant eye/brain development, inflammatory bowel disease, IgA nephropathy, intrauterine growth, lupus, menopausal symptoms, nephrotic syndrome, obesity, OCD, perioperative infections (prevention), prevention of restenosis and graft failure in heart bypass, prostate cancer, psoriasis, rheumatoid arthritis, schizophrenia, stroke; | **Preg:** Likely safe; | **CIs:** Allergy/hypersensitivity, Active bleeding; | **ADRs:** abdominal bloating, acid reflux, back pain, bleeding, ↓ blood pressure, ↑ colon cancer in patients with familial adenomatous polyposis (FAP), contusion, diarrhea, epigastric discomfort, epistaxis, eructation, fishy taste, heartburn, intestinal gas, ↑ LDL, myalgia, nausea, pruritus, ↑ risk of viral infections, vitamin A and D toxicity (with fish liver oil [e.g. cod liver oil]), vitamin E deficiency (long-term use, fish oil); | **Interactions:** Anticoagulants/antiplatelets (↑ risk of bleeding), antidiabetic agents (↑ risk of hypoglycemia), antihypertensives (↑ risk of hypotension); antilipemic agents (additive or antagonistic effects); | **Dose:** Oral, general: 169–563 mg EPA in fish oil; anorexia: 1 g ethyl-EPA PO qd; borderline personality disorder: 1 g PO qd; cancer: 2 g PO qd; depression: 1 g PO bid; Huntington's disease: 2 g ethyl-EPA PO qd; menopausal symptoms: 500 mg ethyl-EPA PO tid; OCD: 2 g PO qd with SSRI; plaque psoriasis: 1,800 mg ethyl-EPA PO qd; schizophrenia: 1–3 g PO qd. Intravenous: 4.2 g EPA plus 4.2 g DHA; | **Monitor:** Blood glucose, coagulation panel, lipid profile; | **Notes:** Ratio of omega-6 to omega-3 fatty acids should be between 1:1 and 4:1. DHA/EPA ratio of 2:1 produces optimal growth in fish. Take with meals to minimize GI upset.

E

ephedra *(Ephedra sinica)* | **Uses:** Asthma, allergic rhinitis, hypertension, obesity, sexual arousal; | **Preg:** Contraindicated due to established risks; | **CIs:** Use should be avoided due to established risks and ban by the FDA; | **ADRs:** acute coronary artery thrombosis, agitation, anorexia, anxiety, arrhythmia, auditory/visual hallucinations, bradycardia/asystole, cardiogenic pulmonary edema, cardiomyopathies, cardiorespiratory arrest, cerebral infarction, cerebrovascular accidents, confusion, constipation, contact dermatitis, coronary artery spasm, coronary atherosclerosis, DEATH, degeneration of muscle tissue, delirium, diaphoresis, diuresis, dizziness, dyspnea, dysuria, eosinophilia-myalgia syndrome, erythroderma, euphoria, excitation, exfoliative dermatitis, flare, ↓ gastric emptying, headache, heart damage, hepatitis, hepatotoxicity, hyperactive reflexes, hyper/hypoglycemia, HYPERTENSION, hypokalemia, insomnia, intracerebral hemorrhage, irritability, ischemic stroke, mania, mood disorder, multiorgan failure, myalgia, MYOCARDIAL INFARCTION, myocarditis, myoglobinuric kidney failure, nausea, nervousness, obsessive-compulsive disorder, palpitations, paranoid psychosis, parkinsonism, permanent disability, psychosis, renal calculi, respiratory depression, restlessness, rhabdomyolysis, satiety, SEIZURE, STROKE, suicide attempt, syncope, tachycardia, tachypnea, transient cortical blindness, tremors, urinary retention, uterine contractions, vertigo, vomiting, weakness, weight loss, xerostomia; | **Interactions:** Acidifying agents (↑ ephedrine excretion), alcohol, alkaline agents (↓ ephedrine excretion), anesthetics (↓ effectiveness), alpha blockers (↓ ephedrine effects), may interact with agents with similar effects or related mechanisms of action (androgenic, arrhythmic, bronchodilatory, hypoglycemic, antigout, antilipemic, antiobesity, neurologic), antihypertensive agents (antagonistic effects), CNS STIMULANTS (additive effects), diuretics (additive effects), ergot derivatives (↑ hypertension), MAO inhibitors (↑ risk of hypertensive crisis), methylxanthines (↑ stimulatory adverse effects), phenothiazines (↓ effects of ephedra), QT-PROLONGING DRUGS (risk of ventricular arrhythmias), steroids (↑ clearance, ↓ effectiveness), thyroid hormones (additive effects); | **Dose:** Avoid use; | **Monitor:** Blood glucose, blood pressure, heart rate, lipid profile, LFTs, pulmonary function tests, thyroid hormones, urine tests (may cause false-positive amphetamine/methamphetamine test results); | **Notes:** The FDA banned the sale of ephedra in the United States, effective April 2004. Ephedrine, found in ephedra, can also be used as a starting material for the illegal manufacture of "speed" or methamphetamine.

E

Essiac | **Uses:** Cancer; | **Preg:** Not recommended due to insufficient evidence and possible fetal toxicities of individual components; | **CIs:** Allergy/hypersensitivity, Pregnancy, Electrolyte imbalance, Intestinal obstruction, Fever, Appendicitis, Hemorrhoids, Hepatic dysfunction, Use longer than 2 weeks, Renal calculi, Xerostomia; | **ADRs:** bradycardia, DEATH, diarrhea, discoloration of urine, electrolyte imbalances, fluoride poisoning, GI upset, hepatotoxicity, hyper-/hypoglycemia, hypotension, intestinal cramping, mouth/throat burning, nausea, nephrotoxicity, oxalic acid toxicity/poisoning, renal calculi, ↑ risk of head and neck cancers, seizure, throat swelling, vomiting; | **Interactions:** Alkaloid agents (↑ risk of precipitation), ACE inhibitors (↓ creatinine, additive effects), antacids (↓ rhubarb effects), antibiotics (additive effects), antiplatelet agents (additive effects), antipsychotic agents (↓ needed doses), chemotherapy (↓ effects), chlorhexidine (additive effects, ↓ gingivitis), cisplatin (↓ toxicity), corticosteroids (↓ corticosteroid-induced lung injury), CYP450 substrates (altered drug levels), digoxin (↑ risk of digoxin toxicity), nifedipine (additive effects), oral contraceptives (altered effects), may interact with agents with similar effects or related mechanisms of action (antiarrhythmic, diuretic, estrogenic, hepatotoxic, hypoglycemic, laxative, nephrotoxic); | **Dose:** Insufficient evidence; instructions for tea preparation and dosing vary from product to product; | **Monitor:** Calcium, coagulation panel, electrolytes, iron, renal function tests, LFTs; | **Notes:** Traditional Essiac blend contains burdock (*Arctium lappat*), sorrel (*Rumex acetosa*), slippery elm (*Ulvus rubra* or *Ulvus fulva*), and rhubarb (*Rheum officinale*). Although the major constituents appear to be sorrel and burdock, precise amounts of the different herbs are proprietary secrets.

eucalyptus (*Eucalyptus* spp.) | **Uses:** Arthritis, asthma, decongestant/cough suppressant, dental plaque/gingivitis (mouthwash), headache (applied to the skin), skin ulcers, smoking cessation, tick repellant (topical), with decongestant/cough suppressant/expectorant; | **Preg:** When used in amounts found in foods; | **CIs:** Allergy/hypersensitivity, Porphyria, Ingestion (undiluted oil), When used topically in children due to increased risk of neurotoxicity; | **ADRs:** abdominal pain, abnormal heartbeat, ataxia, bleeding, ↓ brain functions and reflexes, bronchospasm, cardiovascular collapse, circulation problems, CNS depression/excitation, coma, cough, DEATH (> 3.5 mL of undiluted oil), dizziness, drowsiness, dyspnea, headache, hepatotoxicity, hyperactivity, hypoglycemia, hypotension, hypoventilation, multiorgan failure, nausea, neurotoxicity (topical, children), pneumonitis, pupilliary constriction, seizures, skin rash/burning, speech impairment (slurring), tachycardia, vertigo, vomiting; | **Interactions:** 5-Fluorouracil (↑ topical permeation), amphetamine (↓ levels), antidiabetic agents (additive effects/↑ risk of hypoglycemia), antihypertensive agents (additive effects/↑ risk of hypotension), CYP450 1A2/2C9/2C19/3A4 substrates (inhibits CYP1A2/2C9/2C19/3A4 enzyme/↑ drug levels), pentobarbital (↓ effects), may interact with agents with similar effects or related mechanisms of action (antibiotic, antidiabetic, antifungal, anti-inflammatory, antineoplastic, antiparasitic, antiviral, appetite stimulatory, expectorant, choleretic, insect repellant, sedation and CNS depression, vasodilatory); | **Dose:** Oral: 1,8-cineol (eucalyptol) 200 mg tid; | **Monitor:** Blood glucose, vital signs; | **Notes:** Eucalyptus oil is commonly used as a decongestant/expectorant in URIs or inflammation, and in various musculoskeletal conditions. The oil is found in numerous over-the-counter cough and cold lozenges, inhalation vapors, topical ointments, and mouthwashes.

euphorbia (*Euphorbia* spp.) | **Uses:** Chronic bronchitis, eczema, epilepsy, inflammation (oral); | **Preg:** Not recommended due to insufficient evidence; | **CIs:** Allergy/hypersensitivity, Infectious/inflammatory GI disorders; | **ADRs:** acute keratouveitis, African Burkitt's lymphoma, asthma, conjunctivitis, contact dermatitis, Epstein-Barr virus (EBV), eye injury, eye irritation, GI tract irritation, nausea, skin rash, vomiting; | **Interactions:** May interact with agents with similar effects or related mechanisms of action (antidiabetic, anticonvulsant, antioxidant, antitussive, antiarthritic, hormonal, pulpal devitalizing); | **Dose:** Oral: 50 mg pulverized plant 3 times daily by mouth for up to 6 weeks; | **Monitor:** Blood glucose, hormone levels; | **Notes:** More than 2,000 species of *Euphorbia* exist; all contain latex and are poisonous. Natives in many cultures used various *Euphorbia* species as arrow poison.

E

evening primrose *(Oenothera biennis)* | **Uses:** Atopic dermatitis, breast cancer, breast cysts, bronchitis, chronic fatigue syndrome, diabetes, diabetic neuropathy, eczema, ichthytosis vulgaris, mastalgia, multiple sclerosis, obesity/weight loss, osteoporosis, pre-eclampsia, Raynaud's phenomenon, rheumatoid arthritis; | **Preg:** Not recommended due to insufficient evidence; | **CIs:** Allergy/hypersensitivity, Epilepsy/seizure disorders, Concurrent use with anticoagulants/antiplatelets; | **ADRs:** abdominal pain, diarrhea, headache, hypotension, nausea, seizures/↓ seizure threshold, skin rash; | **Interactions:** Anesthesia (↑ risk of seizures), ANTICOAGULANTS/ANTIPLATELETS (↑ risk of bleeding), drugs that lower seizure threshold (↑ risk of seizures), CYP450 substrates (altered drug levels), phenothiazines (↑ risk of seizures); may interact with agents with similar effects or related mechanisms of action (anesthetic, antiarthritic, antidepressant, antihypertensive, antineoplastic, antiobesity, antiviral, gastrointestinal, neurological); | **Dose:** Oral: 3–8 g daily in divided doses; | **Monitor:** Blood pressure, coagulation panel, lipid profile; | **Notes:** The U.S. Food and Drug Administration (FDA) lists evening primrose oil as Generally Recognized as Safe (GRAS).

eyebright *(Euphrasia officinalis)* | **Uses:** Anti-inflammatory, conjunctivitis, hepatoprotection; | **Preg:** Not recommended due to insufficient evidence; | **CIs:** Allergy/hypersensitivity; | **ADRs:** confusion, constipation, cough, diaphoresis, dyspnea, insomnia, ↑ expectoration, headache, hoarseness of the throat, ↑ IOP, lacrimation, nasal congestion, nausea, pruritus, photophobia, polyuria, toothache, redness and swelling of the eye, sneezing, vision changes, yawning; | **Interactions:** CYP450 substrates (altered drug levels), may interact with agents with similar effects or related mechanisms of action (antidiabetic); | **Dose:** General: 2–4 g dried herb 3 times daily PO. Ophthalmic: One drop Euphrasia 1–5 times daily for up to 17 days. May also use an eyebright-soaked compress; | **Monitor:** Blood glucose, IOP, LFTs; | **Notes:** The expert German Commission E suggests that eyebright has not been proven safe and effective, and does not recommend topical application for hygienic reasons. The Council of Europe lists eyebright as a natural source for food flavoring. In the United Kingdom, eyebright is included on the General Sale List. The U.S. Food and Drug Administration (FDA) has not evaluated eyebright for a Generally Recognized as Safe (GRAS) status.

fennel *(Foeniculum vulgare)* | **Uses:** Colic, cough, dysmenorrhea, photoprotection; | **Preg:** Contraindicated; | **CIs:** Allergy/hypersensitivity (including allergies to celery, carrot, or mugwort), Hormone-sensitive conditions, Lactation, Pregnancy; | **ADRs:** asthma, dyspnea, photosensitivity, rash, rhinoconjunctivitis, seizures, sinus inflammation, | **Interactions:** Anticoagulants/antiplatelets (↑ risk of bleeding), antiestrogens (↓ effects), ciprofloxacin (↓ effectiveness of ciprofloxacin), estrogens (additive effects); | **Dose:** Up to 20 g equivalent as tea, oil, fruit, tincture, syrup, and extracts; | **Monitor:** Coagulation panel, bacterial assays, estrogens; | **Notes:** Some languages do not differentiate between anise and fennel.

F

fenugreek *(Trigonella foenum-graecum)* | **Uses:** Diabetes (types 1 and 2), hyperlipidemia, lactation stimulant; | **Preg:** Avoid supplemental use due to possible abortifacient effects; | **CIs:** Allergy/hypersensitivity, Children, Lactation, Pregnancy; | **ADRs:** abdominal distention, bleeding, contusion, cough, diarrhea, dizziness, dyspepsia, dyspnea, facial edema, flatulence, hypoglycemia, hypokalemia, miscarriage, numbness, premature birth, pruritus, rhinorrhea, shock, skin rash, sneezing, swelling of face/lips/mouth/throat, syncope, thyroid hormone changes, watery eyes, wheezing; | **Interactions:** Alcohol (↓ alcohol hepatotoxicity), analgesics (additive effects), anticoagulants/antiplatelets (↑ risk of bleeding), antidiabetic agents (additive effects/↑ risk of hypoglycemia), antilipemic agents (additive effects), antineoplastic agents (additive effects), cardiac glycosides (↑ risk of toxicity from cardiac glycosides), estrogens (additive effects), laxatives (additive effects), oral drugs (↓ absorption by fenugreek fiber), potassium-depleting agents (↑ risk of hypokalemia), thyroid hormones (altered effects); | **Dose:** Debitterized powdered seed: up to 100 g daily by mouth in divided doses. Seed powder: up to 25 g seed powder daily by mouth in divided doses; | **Monitor:** Blood glucose, coagulation panel, lipid profile, potassium, thyroid function panel, urinalysis; | **Notes:** False diagnoses of maple syrup urine disease have occurred following ingestion of fenugreek.

feverfew *(Tanacetum parthenium)* | **Uses:** Migraine headache prevention, rheumatoid arthritis; | **Preg:** Not recommended due to insufficient evidence and traditional use as an abortifacient; | **CIs:** Allergy/hypersensitivity, Pregnancy; | **ADRs:** allergic reaction (severe), anxiety, arthralgia, bleeding, bleeding gums, bloating, constipation, contusion, diarrhea, digestion problems, dysgeusia, dyspepsia, fatigue, flatulence, headache (rebound), hepatotoxicity, insomnia, lip edema, muscle stiffness, nausea, photosensitivity, stomatitis, tachycardia, tongue irritation; | **Interactions:** Anticoagulants/antiplatelets (↑ risk of bleeding), antidepressants (altered effects/feverfew may worsen depression symptoms), paclitaxel (↑ chemotherapeutic activity), CYP450 1A2/2C9/2C19/2D6/3A4 substrates (inhibits CYP450 1A2/2C9/2C19/2D6/3A4 enzymes/↑ drug levels), may interact with agents with similar effects or related mechanisms of action (abortifacient, antiangiogenic, antibiotic, anesthetic, antifungal, antihistamime, anti-inflammatory, antineoplastic, gastrointestinal, neurologic, photosensitizing, vasodilatory); | **Dose:** Oral: Up to 250 mg (standardized to 0.2% parthenolide) daily PO; | **Monitor:** Coagulation panel; | **Notes:** Feverfew appears to be well tolerated in clinical trials, with a mild and reversible side effects profile. Feverfew may cause bleeding, and patients should discontinue use of feverfew 2 weeks before surgery. Do not abruptly stop the use of the herb in chronic users, as there is a risk of a withdrawal syndrome, characterized by rebound, headache, anxiety, fatigue, muscle stiffness, and joint pain.

fig *(Ficus carica)* | **Uses:** Diabetes (type 1); | **Preg:** Fruit is likely safe in food amounts in pregnant or breastfeeding patients based on traditional use. Other uses (including fig leaf) are not recommended due to lack of sufficient evidence; | **CIs:** Allergy/hypersensitivity; | **ADRs:** anaphylaxis, asthma, conjunctivitis, gallbladder empyemas, hemolytic anemia, IgE-mediated respiratory diseases, obstructive ileus, occupational allergy, perennial asthma, photodermatitis, retinal hemorrhage, rhinitis; | **Interactions:** Anticoagulants/antiplatelets (↑ risk of bleeding), antidiabetic agents (additive effects/↑ risk of hypoglycemia); | **Dose:** Decoction: 13 g leaf as tea, taken daily PO; | **Monitor:** Blood glucose, coagulation panel; | **Notes:** Traditionally, figs have been used to treat constipation, bronchitis, hyperlipidemia, eczema, psoriasis, vitiligo, and diabetes.

flax *(Linum usitatissimum)* | **Uses:** ADHD, breast cancer (flaxseed only), constipation (flaxseed only), diabetes (flaxseed only), cardiovascular disease, hypertension, hyperlipidemia, HIV/AIDS, mastalgia (flaxseed only), menopause (flaxseed only), obesity, pregnancy (spontaneous delivery), prostate cancer (flaxseed only), renal disease (flaxseed only), xerophthalmia; | **Preg:** Not recommended due to insufficient evidence and potential risk of spontaneous delivery; **CIs:** Allergy/hypersensitivity; Hormone-sensitive conditions, Hypertriglyceridemia, Raw/unripe flaxseed; **ADRs:** abdominal discomfort, anaphylaxis, bleeding, bowel obstruction, constipation, diarrhea, dyspnea, headache, hormone changes, hypoglycemia, hypotension, malaise, mania, nausea, ↑ risk of prostate cancer, pruritus, skin rash, sneezing, stuffy nose, seizures, tachypnea, vomiting, watery eyes; **Interactions:** Acetaminophen (↓ absorption of acetaminophen), antibiotics (interfere with the effects of flaxseed), anticoagulants/antiplatelets (↑ risk of bleeding), antidiabetic agents (↑ risk of hypoglycemia), antiestrogens (mixed effects), antihypertensives (↑ risk of hypotension), estrogens (mixed effects), antilipemic agents (additive effects), furosemide (↓ absorption of furosemide), ketoprofen (↓ absorption of ketoprofen), metoprolol (↓ absorption of metoprolol), oral agents (↓ absorption by flaxseed); may interact with agents with similar effects or related mechanisms of action (anti-inflammatory, antiobesity, cardiovascular, cognitive, diuretic, antineoplastic, gastrointestinal, laxative, mood stabilizing, antiulcer, muscle relaxant); **Dose:** Oil: Up to 2 g daily PO for up to 180 days. Powder/flour: Up to 60 g daily PO, in divided doses with liquid, for up to 4 weeks; **Monitor:** Alkaline phosphatase, blood glucose, coagulation panel, inflammatory markers, lipid profile, prostate-specific antigen, RBC, triglycerides; **Notes:** Flaxseed oil contains the ALA component of flaxseed, not the fiber or lignan components. Therefore, flaxseed oil may share the purported lipid-lowering properties of flaxseed but not the proposed laxative or anticancer abilities.

folate (folic acid) **Uses:** Alzheimer's disease, arsenic poisoning, cancer, chronic fatigue syndrome, cognitive function, end-stage renal disease, depression, diabetes, folate deficiency, gingival hyperplasia (phenytoin induced), gingivitis (pregnancy related), hearing loss, hyperhomocysteinemia, megaloblastic anemia (due to folate deficiency), methotrexate toxicity, neural tube birth defects, nitrate tolerance, pre-eclampsia, prevention of pregnancy complications, stoke, vitiligo, **Preg:** U.S. Recommended Dietary Allowance (RDA): 600 mcg for pregnant women; **CIs:** Allergy/hypersensitivity to product ingredients, Seizure disorders; **ADRs:** abdominal bloating/cramps, alopecia, altered sleep patterns, anaphylaxis, aphthous ulcers, bitter taste, bronchospasm, confusion, diarrhea, erythema, excitability, flatulence, malaise, impaired judgment, irritability, myelosuppression, nausea, neurological damage, overactivity, pruritus, psychotic behavior, rash, restenosis, seizure, skin flushing; stomatitis, urine discoloration, urticaria, vivid dreaming, zinc

F

depletion; | **Interactions:** 5-fluorouracil antibiotics (additive effects), antifungal agents (additive effects), (↑ risk of toxicity of 5-FU); alcohol (↑ folate requirement), antibiotics (additive effects), antifungal agents (additive effects), green tea (↓ activity of folic acid), capecitabine (↑ risk of toxicity of capecitabine), methotrexate (↓ efficacy of methotrexate), phenytoin/fosphenytoin (↑ risk of seizures), primidone (↑ risk of seizures), pyrimethamine (antagonizes antiparasitic effects/↓ folate levels), trimethoprim (inhibits enzyme involved in conversion of folic acid to its active form); drugs that deplete folic acid: alkaline agents, aminosalicylic acid, antacids, antibiotics, aspirin, bile acid sequestrants, carbamazepine, chloramphenicol, cycloserine, diuretics, estrogens, H2 blockers, metformin, methotrexate, methylprednisolone, NSAIDs, pancreatic enzymes, pentamidine, phenobarbital, phenytoin, proton pump inhibitors, pyrimethamine, sulfasalazine, triamterene, trimethoprim, valproic acid, zinc; | **Dose:** U.S. Recommended Dietary Allowance (RDA): 400 mcg for adults, 500 mcg for breastfeeding women, 600 mcg for pregnant women, 65 mcg for infants 0–6 months old, 80 mcg for infants 7–12 months, 150 mcg for children 1–3 years, 200 mcg for children 4–8 years, 300 mcg for children 9–13 years old; | **Monitor:** Folate levels, MCV; | **Notes:** Folate occurs naturally in food, and folic acid is the synthetic form of this vitamin. Large amounts of folate may mask the symptoms of pernicious, aplastic, or normocystic anemia.

fo-ti ***(Polygonum multiflorum)*** | **Uses:** Insufficient clinical evidence; | **Preg:** Not recommended due to insufficient evidence; | **CIs:** Allergy/hypersensitivity, Hepatic disorders; | **ADRs:** abdominal pain, arrhythmia, asthenia, diarrhea, hallucinations, HEPATOXICITY, hypokalemia, nausea, paresthesia, rash, vomiting, weakness, urine discoloration; | **Interactions:** Antidiabetic agents (additive effects/↑ risk of hypoglycemia), cytochrome P450 1A2/2C9/2C19/2D6/3A4 substrates (inhibits CYP 1A2/2C9/2C19/2D6/3A4 /↑ drug levels), digoxin (↑ cardiotoxicity, due to hypokalemia), diuretics (↑ risk of hypokalemia), estrogens (additive effects), hepatotoxic agents (↑ risk of liver damage), potassium-depleting agents (↑ risk of hypokalemia), stimulant laxatives (↑ risk of hypokalemia); | **Dose:** Capsules: 560 mg 2–3 times daily by mouth with water at mealtimes. Dried herb: 9–15 g daily by mouth. Tea: 1 tsp or 5 g root boiled in 1 cup of water, taken PO. Topical: Cream or ointment applied to affected area 3–4 times daily. | **Monitor:** Blood glucose, LFTs, potassium, urinalysis; | **Notes:** Fo-ti is NOT recommended for oral use due to risk of liver damage. Fo-ti is used traditionally to prevent aging, or taken by mouth for its laxative effect and heart disease prevention. It is used topically for acne, athlete's foot, dermatitis, razor burn, and scrapes.

fumitory | **Uses:** Biliary dyskinesia, IBS; | **Preg:** Not recommended due to insufficient evidence; | **CIs:** Allergy/hypersensitivity; | **ADRs:** acute hepatitis; flushing, GI upset, glaucoma; | **Interactions:** Anticoagulants/antiplatelets (↑ risk of bleeding), antifungal agents (potentiate effects), anti-inflammatory agents (additive effects), antineoplastic agents (alter effects), antiviral agents (potentiate effects), cholinesterase inhibitors (potentiate effects), CNS depressants (additive sedation); | **Dose:** Capsules: 250–1,500 mg PO in 3 divided doses; tincture: (1:5 in 25% alcohol) in doses of 1–2 mL 3 times daily has been administered for "skin problems"; | **Monitor:** Coagulation panel, LFTs; | **Notes:** Fumitory is commonly used as an antispasmodic and to treat skin disease. An Austrian *Fumaria officinalis* preparation, Oddibil, is marketed as a treatment for cholecystopathy (biliary dyskinesia).

G

fuzheng jiedu tang | **Uses:** Insufficient evidence; | **Preg:** Not recommended due to insufficient evidence; | **CIs:** Allergy/hypersensitivity to any of the constituents; | **ADRs:** insufficient evidence; | **Interactions:** Insufficient evidence; | **Dose:** Insufficient evidence; | **Monitor:** LFTs; | **Notes:** Fuzheng jiedu tang is a mixture of five Japanese herbs mixed in set proportions used for fatigue, to boost immunity, and to help relieve the symptoms. Based on review, fuzheng jiedu tang has not demonstrated benefit in patients with hepatitis B or C.

galactooligosaccharide | **Uses:** Allergic disorders (prevention), atopic dermatitis (prevention), bone loss (prevention), colic, constipation, hyperlipidemia, immune modulation; | **Preg:** Safe in amounts found in food; | **CIs:** Allergy/hypersensitivity; | **ADRs:** diarrhea, flatulence; | **Interactions:** Alcohol (↓ effects of galactooligosaccharides), caffeine (↓ effects of galactooligosaccharides), calcium (↑ calcium absorption); | **Dose:** 3–20 g PO qd; | **Monitor:** calcium levels; | **Notes:** Galactooligosaccharides are considered prebiotics (promote the growth of intestinal flora). Galactooligosaccharides are believed to mimic the oligosaccharides found naturally in human breast milk, which may contribute to the known health benefits of breastfeeding.

gamma linolenic acid (GLA) | **Uses:** Acute respiratory distress syndrome, atopic dermatitis, ADHD, cancer treatment, diabetic neuropathy, immune system improvement, hypertension, mastalgia, menopausal hot flashes, migraine, osteoporosis, pre-eclampsia, premenstrual syndrome (PMS), pruritus, rheumatoid arthritis, Sjögren's syndrome, ulcerative colitis; | **Preg:** Likely safe in amounts found in foods in pregnant or breastfeeding patients based on traditional use. Other uses are not recommended due to lack of sufficient evidence; | **CIs:** Allergy/hypersensitivity; | **ADRs:** abdominal bloating, bleeding, flatulence, gastrointestinal upset, nausea, seizures, vomiting; | **Interactions:** Anticoagulants/antiplatelets (↑ risk of bleeding), antineoplastic agents (additive effects), ceftazidime (↑ effects), drugs that lower seizure threshold (↑ risk of seizures), cyclosporine (additive effects); | **Dose:** Up to 6 g daily PO; | **Monitor:** Coagulation panel, lipid profile; | **Notes:** Gamma linolenic acid (GLA) is a dietary omega-6 fatty acid found in many plant oil extracts.

G

gamma oryzanol | **Uses:** Gastritis, hyperlipidemia, hypothyroidism, menopausal symptoms, prevention of restenosis after coronary angioplasty (PTCA), skin conditions; | **Preg:** Not recommended due to insufficient evidence and possible growth hormone repression; | **CIs:** Allergy/hypersensitivity; | **ADRs:** insufficient evidence; | **Interactions:** Anticoagulants/antiplatelets (↑ risk of bleeding), antidiabetic agents (additive effects/↑ risk of hypoglycemia), antilipemic agents (additive effects), thyroid hormones (altered effects); | **Dose:** Oral: up to 500 mg daily according to manufacturer's instructions; | **Monitor:** Coagulation panel, lipid profile, GH, hormone panel, TSH; | **Notes:** Gamma oryzanol is a mixture of ferulic acid esters of sterol and triterpene alcohols found primarily in rice bran oil, corn, and barley oils. It is used as a body-building aid, specifically to increase testosterone levels, and to stimulate the release of endorphins (pain-relieving substances made in the body).

garcinia *(Garcinia cambogia)*, **hydroxycitric acid** (HCA) | **Uses:** Exercise performance, obesity; | **Preg:** Not recommended due to insufficient evidence; | **CIs:** Allergy/hypersensitivity; | **ADRs:** gastrointestinal discomfort, headache, nausea; rhabdomyolysis associated with a combination product containing garcinia; | **Interactions:** Antidiabetic agents (additive effects/↑ risk of hypoglycemia), HMG-CoA reductase inhibitors (↑ risk of rhabdomyolysis); | **Dose:** 250–1,500 mg daily PO in divided doses; | **Monitor:** Blood glucose, body weight, creatine kinase, peak expiratory flow rate; | **Notes:** The principal active constituent of garcinia rind is hydroxycitric acid, a potent competitive inhibitor of the enzyme ATP citrate lyase.

garden cress *(Lepidium sativum)* | **Uses:** Insufficient evidence; | **Preg:** Likely safe in amounts found in food; medicinal use is not recommended due to insufficient evidence; seeds may be unsafe to consume during pregnancy due to traditional use as an abortifacient; | **CIs:** Allergy/hypersensitivity; | **ADRs:** GI irritation; | **Interactions:** Vitamin C (↑ amounts); | **Dose:** Insufficient evidence; | **Monitor:** N/A; | **Notes:** Garden cress contains high amounts of vitamin C. It has been traditionally used for cough and poor immune function. It may be added to soups and sandwiches for flavor.

G

gardenia *(Gardenia jasminoides)* | **Uses:** Insufficient evidence; | **Preg:** Not recommended due to insufficient evidence; | **CIs:** Allergy/hypersensitivity; | **ADRs:** ↓ blood sugar, diarrhea, sedation; | **Interactions:** Antidiabetic agents (↑ risk of hypoglycemia), antimalarial agents (additive effects), antineoplastic agents (additive effects), CNS depressants (additive effects), laxatives (additive effects); | **Dose:** Oral, decoction: use 3–12 g/day PO. Topical, poultice: apply several times/day; | **Monitor:** Blood glucose; | **Notes:** Gardenia is used to protect the liver, although clinical trials are lacking.

garlic *(Allium sativum)* | **Uses:** Anticoagulant, atherosclerosis, BPH, cancer (prevention), common cold, corns, familial hypercholesterolemia, hyperlipidemia, hypertension, myocardial infarction (prevention), peripheral vascular disease, preelampsia, tick repellant, tinea corporis, tinea cruris, tinea pedis, URI, warts; | **Preg:** Likely safe in food amounts in pregnant or breastfeeding patients based on traditional use; other uses are not recommended due to lack of sufficient evidence; | **CIs:** Allergy/hypersensitivity, Children (large amounts), Concurrent use with isoniazid, NNRTIs, or protease inhibitors, IBD, Pregnancy (medicinal amounts), Lactation (medicinal amounts); | **ADRs:** anorexia, bleeding, bromidrosis, burning inside the mouth, chills, constipation, contusion, diaphoresis, diarrhea, dizziness, dyspepsia, dyspnea, fever, flatulence, halitosis, hyper-/hypoglycemia, hypotension, intestinal gas, nausea, pruritus, rhinorrhea, skin burns (topical), thyroid changes, urticaria, uterine spasms, vomiting; | **Interactions:** Anticoagulants/antiplatelets (↑ risk of bleeding), antidiabetic agents (altered effects), antihypertensive agents (additive effects/↑ risk of hypotension), antilipemic agents (additive effects), contraceptives (↓ effectiveness), cyclosporine (↓ effectiveness), cytochrome P450 2E1 and 3A4 substrates (inhibits CYP2E1; induces/inhibits 3A4), ISONIAZID (↓ isoniazid levels), NON-NUCLEOSIDE REVERSE TRANSCRIPTASE INHIBITORS (↓ levels of NNRTIs), PROTEASE INHIBITORS (SAQUINAVIR, ↓ levels of protease inhibitors); | **Dose:** Oral: 600–900 mg garlic powder (standardized to 1.3% allicin) daily in divided doses; 3–5 mg allicin daily (equivalent of 2–5 g fresh garlic, 2–5 mg garlic oil, 300–1,000 mg extract, or 2–4 mL tincture); | **Monitor:** Blood glucose, coagulation panel, lipid profile, urinary allylmercapturic acid; | **Notes:** Garlic can result in urinary excretion of allylmercapturic acid (*N*-acetyl-S-allyl-L-cysteine), which may interfere with urinary monitoring of workers for industrial exposure to allyl halides.

gelatin | **Uses:** Hair growth, infant mortality, joint pain, skin care; | **Preg:** Not recommended due to insufficient evidence; | **CIs:** Allergy/hypersensitivity; | **ADRs:** abdominal fullness, allergic reactions, belching, bloating, hypotension, unpleasant taste, urticaria, wheezing; | **Interactions:** Enhances absorption: anxiolytics, anticonvulsants, antifungals, anti-inflammatory agents, diuretics; | **Dose:** 2–12 g/day PO; | **Monitor:** N/A; | **Notes:** Gelatin is used in various edible and food products, as well as pharmaceutical and nutraceutical products. Common examples of foods that contain gelatin are gelatin desserts, jelly, trifles, aspic, marshmallows, and confectioneries such as peeps and gummy bears. Gelatin may be used as a stabilizer, thickener, or texturizer in foods, finishing agent, ice cream, jams, yogurt, cream cheese, fruit juices, wine, beer, and margarine.

gentiana lutea | **Uses:** Insufficient evidence; | **Preg:** Not recommended due to insufficient evidence; | **CIs:** Allergy/hypersensitivity; | **ADRs:** allergic skin reactions, diarrhea, GI upset, hypotension, nausea/vomiting; | **Interactions:** Antihypertensives (↑ risk of hypotension); | **Dose:** Boil one tsp of powdered root in 2 pints of water in covered container for 20 min; tincture (1:5 prepared in 45% alcohol): ¼–½ tsp (1–3 mL) PO qd, 20 min before meals; | **Monitor:** Blood pressure; | **Notes:** Gentian has traditionally been used to stimulate the gallbladder and the liver, and to treat indigestion associated with anorexia.

germanium (Ge) | **Uses:** Hepatitis B, multiple myeloma; | **Preg:** Inorganic germanium should be avoided; organic germanium not recommended due to insufficient evidence. Embryonic resorption and malformation has been observed in animals; | **CIs:** Allergy/hypersensitivity; Inorganic germanium, ORAL USE, Pregnancy, Lactation; | **ADRs:** asthenia, ataxia, blurred vision, confusion, DEATH, depression, diarrhea, dizziness, fatigue, HEPATIC STEATOSIS, LACTIC ACIDOSIS, MYOPATHY, nausea, brain and lung damage, rash, RENAL FAILURE, tremors; | **Interactions:** May ↑ 5-fluorouracil toxicity, may ↑ morphine analgesia; | **Dose:** Germanium sesquioxide: 150–1,000 mg daily PO; | **Monitor:** Insufficient evidence; | **Notes:** Organic germanium compounds such as spirogermanium and carboxyethyl germanium sesquioxide are most commonly used therapeutically; inorganic germanium compounds (germanium dioxide, germanium citrate lactate, and elemental germanium) are potentially toxic and should not be confused with organic germanium. There have been multiple cases of renal failure, hepatic steatosis, and death in individuals using germanium.

G

giant knotweed | **Uses:** Insufficient evidence; | **Preg:** Not recommended due to insufficient evidence; | **CIs:** Allergy/hypersensitivity, Hormone-sensitive conditions; | **ADRs:** insufficient evidence; | **Interactions:** Anticoagulants/antiplatelets (↑ risk of bleeding), CYP450 1A, 2E1, 3A4 substrates (↑ levels of drugs metabolized by these enzymes), estrogens (↑ estrogenic effects), immunosuppressants (altered effects); | **Dose:** Insufficient evidence; | **Monitor:** Coagulation panel, estrogen levels; | **Notes:** Giant knotweed (or hu zhang) is a rich source of trans-resveratrol and may be used as an immune stimulant. It may also have estrogenic effects.

ginger (*Zingiber* officinale) | **Uses:** Antiplatelet agent, hyperemesis gravidarum, labor, migraine, motion sickness/sea sickness, nausea and vomiting (chemotherapy induced), nausea and vomiting (postoperative), obesity, osteoarthritis, rheumatoid arthritis, urinary disorders (post-stroke); | **Preg:** Controversial; not recommended by some due to possible abortifacient, emmenagogic, mutagenic, and antiplatelet effects; however, there is evidence supporting its safety and efficacy in treating pregnancy-induced nausea and vomiting; | **CIs:** Allergy/hypersensitivity; | **ADRs:** abdominal bloating/discomfort, arrhythmias, bowel obstruction, burning sensation of the tongue (transient), CNS depression, conjunctivitis, dermatitis, drowsiness, dyspepsia, flatulence, gastrointestinal symptoms (mild), halitosis, hyper-/hypotension, hypoglycemia, intestinal gas, nausea, oral/esophageal irritation, urge incontinence; | **Interactions:** Anticoagulants/antiplatelets (↑ risk of bleeding), antidiabetic agents (↑ insulin levels/↑ risk of hypoglycemia), antihypertensive agents (↑ risk of hypotension), calcium channel blockers (↑ risk of hypotension), CNS depressants (↑ risk of sedation), CYP450 substrates (altered drug levels), P-glycoprotein substrates (altered drug levels); agents with similar effects or related mechanisms of action (gastric acid inducing, antiarrhythmic, antiarthritic, antiemetic, anti-inflammatory, antilipemic, antihypertensive, antihistamine, antineoplastic, antiobesity, antitussive, beta blocking, gastrointestinal, immunosuppressant, vasodilatory); | **Dose:** Oral: up to 4 g daily (powder, tablets, or fresh-cut ginger) in divided doses; | **Monitor:** Blood glucose, blood pressure, coagulation panel, heart rate; | **Notes:** The rhizomes and stems of ginger have assumed significant roles in Chinese, Japanese, and Indian medicine since the 1500s. The oleoresin of ginger is often contained in digestive, antitussive, antiflatulent, laxative, and antacid compounds.

G

ginkgo *(Ginkgo biloba)* | **Uses:** Claudication (peripheral vascular disease), dementia (multi-infarct and Alzheimer's type), cerebral insufficiency, acute hemorrhoidal attacks, acute ischemic stroke, age-associated memory impairment (AAMI), altitude (mountain) sickness, asthma, cardiovascular disease, reducing adverse effects of chemotherapy, chronic cochleovestibular disorders, chronic venous insufficiency, cocaine dependence, decreased libido and erectile dysfunction (drug related), depression, seasonal affective disorder (SAD), diabetic neuropathy, dyslexia, gastric cancer, glaucoma, Graves' disease (adjunct), macular degeneration, memory enhancement (healthy patients), mood and cognition (postmenopausal women), multiple sclerosis, PMS, pulmonary interstitial fibrosis, Raynaud's disease, retinopathy, schizophrenia, tinnitus, vertigo, vitiligo; | **Preg:** Caution due to the risk of increased bleeding; | **CIs:** Hypersensitivity to ginkgo, Bleeding disorders, Concurrent use with anticoagulants/antiplatelets and ibuprofen, Seizure disorders, Infertility, Surgery; | **ADRs:** asthenia, BLEEDING, diarrhea, dizziness, gastrointestinal upset, headache, hyper-/hypotension, hypotonia, infertility, nausea, rash, restlessness, SEIZURE, vomiting; | **Interactions:** AGENTS THAT LOWER THE SEIZURE THRESHOLD (↑ risk of seizures), aged foods (e.g., wine and cheese), alprazolam (↓ effectiveness), anticonvulsants (↓ effectiveness), ANTICOAGULANTS/ANTIPLATELETS (↑ risk of bleeding), antidepressants (↑ risk of seizures and hypomania), antidiabetic agents (additive effects/↑ risk of hypoglycemia), antipsychotic drugs (↑ risk of seizures and hypomania), IBUPROFEN (↑ risk of bleeding), drugs used for erectile dysfunction, antihypertensive agents (additive effects/↑ risk of hypotension), CYP450 3A4/2C9/2C19/2D6/1A2 substrates (ginkgo may induce or inhibit CYP450 3A4/2C9/2C19/ 2D6/1A2; altered drug levels), efavirenz (↓ levels of efavirenz), trazadone (↑ risk of coma), St. John's wort (↑ risk of hypomania); herbs or supplements with similar effects; | **Dose:** 80–240 mg divided into 2 or 3 doses has been taken PO daily; | **Monitor:** Blood glucose, blood pressure, coagulation panel, S/S of hypoglycemia; | **Notes:** May alter insulin requirements (effects depend on patient status); uncooked ginkgo seeds contain ginkotoxin, which can cause seizures; monitor INR in individuals using warfarin and ginkgo, adjust dose, if necessary, due to increased risk of bleeding with concurrent use.

ginseng (*Panax* spp.) | **Uses:** Aplastic anemia, ADHD, birth outcomes, cancer (chemotherapy adjunct), cancer (prevention), cardiovascular disease, chronic hepatitis B, congestive heart failure, CAD, dementia, diabetes, diabetic kidney disease, exercise performance, fatigue, stress, fistula, hepatoprotection, hyperlipidemia, hypertension, ITP, immunostimulant, intracranial pressure, intrauterine growth retardation, menopausal symptoms, mental performance, MRSA, neurological disorders, postoperative recovery (breast cancer), premature ejaculation, radiation therapy side effects, renal disease, respiratory disorders, sexual dysfunction/libido/erectile dysfunction, viral myocarditis; | **Preg:** Not recommended due to unclear safety evidence and possible hormonal and toxic effects to the embryo; | **CIs:** Allergy/hypersensitivity; | **ADRs:** angina, anorexia, arrhythmia, blurred vision, ↑ breast growth, breast tenderness, confusion (high doses), delayed ejaculation, diarrhea, dizziness, drowsiness, epistaxis, erectile dysfunction, fever, GI discomfort, headache, hyper-/hypoglycemia, insomnia, irritation and burning, leg edema, ↑ libido, mania (in bipolar disorder), menstrual changes (excess bleeding, cessation of menstruation in younger women, cycle alterations), mydriasis (high doses), pain (mild), nausea, nervousness, seizures (after high doses), skin disturbances, swelling, tachycardia, throat irritation, vomiting, water retention; | **Interactions:** Alcohol (↓ alcohol levels), analgesics (↑ effects of aspirin/↓ effects of morphine), anticoagulants/antiplatelets (alters effects/may ↑ clearance of warfarin), antidepressants (↑ risk of adverse effects associated with MAOIs), antidiabetic agents (↑ risk of hypoglycemia), antihypertensives (↓ effects), antilipemic agents (additive effects), antineoplastic agents (↑ effects of paclitaxel, ↓ cisplatin-induced nausea, ↑ effects of mitomycin C), antipsychotics (↑ effects), antiviral agents (additive effects), caffeine (additive effects), CNS stimulants (additive effects), CYP450 2D6/2C9/ 3A4 substrates (inhibits or induces 2D6/2C9/ 3A4), digoxin (↑ effects), hepatotoxic agents (↑ risk of liver damage), immunosuppressants

(↓ effects), influenza vaccine (↑ effects), nifedipine (↑ nifedipine concentration), protease inhibitors (↓ effects), sildenafil (additive effects); may interact with agents with similar effects or related mechanisms of action (ACE inhibition, antidementia, antiarrhythmic, appetite suppressant, estrogenic, gastrointestinal, glucocorticoid, hormonal, immunomodulatory, sedative, radioprotective, sodium channel blocking, sympathomimetic, vasodilatory); | **Dose:** Short-term use: up to 2 g daily. Long-term use: up to 1 g dried root daily; | **Monitor:** Blood alcohol, blood glucose, blood pressure, coagulation panel, antibody titers, cortisol, hormones, heart rate, hemoglobin, lipid profile, LFTs, sperm count, urinalysis; | **Notes:** Not to be confused with Siberian ginseng (*Eleutherococcus senticosus*). Use with caution in individuals with autoimmune disease, bleeding disorders, cardiovascular conditions, diabetes, hormone-sensitive conditions, insomnia, organ transplant patients, and psychiatric disorders.

globe artichoke *(Cynara scolymus)* | **Uses:** Alcohol-induced hangover, antioxidant, choleretic, dyspepsia, hyperlipidemia, irritable bowel syndrome; | **Preg:** Likely safe in food amounts in pregnant or breastfeeding patients based on traditional use. Other uses are not recommended due to lack of sufficient evidence; | **CIs:** Allergy/hypersensitivity, Bile duct obstruction; | **ADRs:** allergic rhinitis, asthma, ↑ bile flow, chest tightness, cough, diarrhea, dyspnea, flatulence, ↑ hunger, nausea, nephrotoxicity, pruritus, urticaria; | **Interactions:** Anticoagulant/antiplatelets (↑ risk of bleeding), antilipemic agents (additive effects); | **Dose:** Tablets/capsules: 250–750 mg cynarin daily, or dried artichoke extract 1,800–1,900 mg daily. Liquid/fluid: 3–8 mL 1:2 liquid extract daily, up to 10 mL of pressed juice from fresh leaves and flower buds of the artichoke. Tincture (1:5 g/mL): 6 mL 3 times daily. Dried leaves: 1–9 g daily. Dry extract: 0.5 g of a 12:1 (w/w) dried extract given as a single daily dose; | **Monitor:** Bilirubin, LFTs, lipid profile; | **Notes:** Cynarin, luteolin, cynardoside (luteolin-7-O-glycoside), scolymoside, and chlorogenic acid are believed to be artichoke's active constituents. The most studied component, cynarin, is concentrated in the leaves.

glucomannan *(Amorphophallus konjac)* | **Uses:** Constipation, diabetes/glucose control, HTN, hyperlipidemia, hyperthyroidism, obesity; | **Preg:** Not recommended due to insufficient evidence; | **CIs:** Allergy/hypersensitivity; | **ADRs:** abdominal pain, asthma, flatulence, gastric discomfort, GI obstruction, hepatitis; | **Interactions:** Antidiabetic agents (↑ risk of hypoglycemia), antihypertensives (↑ risk of hypotension), antilipemic agents (additive effects), antiobesity agents (additive effects), fat-soluble vitamins (↓ absorption of vitamins A, D, E, K), glibenclamide (↓ levels of glibenclamide), immunosuppressants (altered effects), laxatives (additive effects), oral drugs (↓ absorption of oral drugs), thyroid hormones (altered effects); | **Dose:** Adults: 2–13 g PO qd; children: 1–5 g PO qd; | **Monitor:** Blood sugar, lipid profile, weight; | **Notes:** Glucomannan is a highly viscous soluble fiber. Thus, when consumed, it absorbs water in the digestive tract, reducing absorption of carbohydrates and cholesterol. Glucomannan is being studied as a way to deliver drugs to the large intestines.

glucosamine | **Uses:** Chronic venous insufficiency, diabetes, inflammatory bowel disease (Crohn's disease, ulcerative colitis), leg pain, osteoarthritis of the knee (mild–moderate), osteoarthritis (general), rehabilitation, rheumatoid arthritis, temporomandibular joint (TMJ) disorders; | **Preg:** Not recommended due to insufficient evidence; | **CIs:** Allergy/hypersensitivity; | **ADRs:** abdominal pain/upset, ↑/↓ appetite, bleeding, cataracts, constipation, diarrhea, drowsiness, dyspepsia, flatulence, hard nails, headache, hepatomegaly, hypertension, insomnia, insulin resistance (after injections), liver inflammation, nausea, palpitations, photosensitivity, proteinuria, skin reactions, tachycardia, vomiting; | **Interactions:** acetaminophen (↓ analgesia), ANTICOAGULANTS/ANTIPLATELETS (↑ risk of bleeding), antidiabetic agents (altered effects), antineoplastic agents/topoisomerase inhibitors (reduces drugs' inhibition of topoisomerase II), diuretics (additive effects); | **Dose:** Oral: 500 mg 3 times daily for up to 6 months. Intramuscular: 400 mg 2–3 times weekly. Intra-articular: 400 mg glucosamine sulfate daily. Intravenous: 400 mg daily for 7 days; | **Monitor:** Blood glucose, coagulation panel, electrolytes, urinalysis; | **Notes:** Glucosamine is an amino-monosaccharide that is naturally produced in humans. Use with caution in patients with asthma, diabetes, hypertension, or shellfish allergies.

glutamine | **Uses:** Alcoholism, athletic performance, burns, cancer (adjunct), catabolic wasting, chemotherapy (prevention of adverse effects), critical illness, cystinuria, diarrhea, fibromyalgia, HIV (adjunct), HIV wasting, IBD, immune enhancement, muscular dystrophy, oral mucositis, PUD, post-surgical healing, short-bowel syndrome, surgery, TPN adjunct; | **Preg:** Not recommended due to insufficient evidence; | **CIs:** Allergy/hypersensitivity; | **ADRs:** gritty taste; | **Interactions:** Anticonvulsants (antagonistic effects), chemotherapy (altered effects), lactulose (antagonistic effects); | **Dose:** 500–4,000 mg 3 times/day. Doses up to 40 g daily have been used for HIV wasting; | **Monitor:** Ammonia levels, glutamate levels;

Notes: Glutamine is the most abundant amino acid in the human body. It is metabolized to ammonia, which may cause adverse neurological and psychiatric effects.

glyconutrients | **Uses:** ADHD, failure-to-thrive (poor weight gain/growth failure); | **Preg:** Glyconutrients are essential in cellular communication and are important for pregnant and lactating women. However, human clinical trials investigating therapeutic use of glyconutrients are currently lacking; | **CIs:** Insufficient evidence; | **ADRs:** ↓ vitamin B_{12} levels, ↓ copper levels; | **Interactions:** Preparations containing vitamin K or ubidecarenone may ↓ anticoagulants, ↑ iron absorption; | **Dose:** Insufficient evidence; | **Monitor:** Coagulation panel, lipid panel, ceruloplasmin, serum nutrients, vitamin B_{12} levels, copper levels; | **Notes:** Glyconutrients are often food and plant based; thus, there is a possible risk of allergy or reactivity with any herb or supplement that contains glyconutrients.

G

goat's rue *(Galega officinalis)* | **Uses:** Insufficient evidence; | **Preg:** Not recommended due to insufficient evidence; | **CIs:** Allergy/hypersensitivity; | **ADRs:** insufficient evidence; | **Interactions:** Anticoagulants/antiplatelets (↑ risk of bleeding), antidiabetic agents (↑ risk of hypoglycemia), antiobesity agents (additive effects), iron (interfere with effects); | **Dose:** Oral, tablets/capsules: 20–200 mg PO tid. Oral, infusion: one teaspoonful of dried leaves into a cup of boiling water, infuse for 10–15 minutes, drink 1 cup twice/day. Tincture: 20–40 drops (2–4 mL) PO 2–3 times/day; | **Monitor:** Blood glucose, coagulation panel; | **Notes:** Goat's rue was introduced into the United States in 1891 as forage for livestock and is found in Utah, Pennsylvania, and New York. It is now considered a weed and has been catalogued on the Federal Weed List in the United States. Goat's rue has been documented to increase milk production in cows by 35%–50%. It has been traditionally used to increase lactation and treat diabetes. Goat's rue has shown glycemic control and weight loss effect in animal studies.

goji (*Lycium* spp.) | **Uses:** Asthma, cancer, vision; | **Preg:** Not recommended due to insufficient evidence and traditional use as a uterine stimulant; | **CIs:** Allergy/hypersensitivity; | **ADRs:** insomnia, nausea, vomiting; | **Interactions:** Anticoagulants/antiplatelets (↑ risk of bleeding; ↑ effects of warfarin), antidiabetic agents (↑ risk of hypoglycemia), antihypertensives (↑ risk of hypotension), CYP450 2C9 substrates (inhibits 2C9/↑ drug levels), may interact with agents with similar effects or related mechanisms of action (antibiotic, antidepressant, antidiabetic, antifungal, antihypertensive, antilipemic, antineoplastic, antiviral, cardioprotective, hormonal, immunostimulatory, bone-inducing); | **Dose:** Berries: 6–15 g daily. Juice: 3–4 oz. Tea: One or more cups daily. | **Monitor:** Blood glucose, coagulation panel, hormone levels, immune parameters, LFTs, lipid profile, RBC count, WBC count; | **Notes:** Various polysaccharide components extracted from goji berries have demonstrated anticancer, antidiabetes, antihypertensive, anti-infertility, antimyelosuppressive, antioxidant, hypolipidemic, immune-stimulating, and radiosensitizing properties.

goldenrod *(Solidago virgaurea)* | **Uses:** Insufficient clinical evidence; | **Preg:** Not recommended due to insufficient evidence; | **CIs:** Allergy/hypersensitivity, Irrigation therapy in patients with edema due to kidney or heart conditions; | **ADRs:** allergic contact dermatitis, bronchial asthma, dyspepsia, rhinoconjunctivitis, uticaria; | **Interactions:** Diuretics (additive effects), may interact with agents with similar effects or related mechanisms of action (anti-inflammatory, hypotensive, sedative); | **Dose:** Infusion: 2–3 tsp dried herb in 1 cup water, gargled or consumed 3 times daily. Tincture: 0.5–2 mL fluid extract (1:1 in 25% ethanol) 2–3 times daily; | **Monitor:** Electrolytes; | **Notes:** Avoid confusion with mullein, which is also referred to as goldenrod, and with rayless goldenrod, which is a species from the same family as goldenrod.

goldenseal *(Hydrastis canadensis)* | **Uses:** Chloroquine-resistant malaria, common cold/upper respiratory tract infection, heart failure, hyperlipidemia, immune system stimulation, infectious diarrhea, narcotic concealment, trachoma; | **Preg:** Not recommended due to insufficient evidence and traditional use as an abortifacient; | **CIs:** Allergy/hypersensitivity, Hyperbilirubinemia (newborns); | **ADRs:** abdominal bloating, arrhythmias, bradycardia, dried mucous membranes, headache, hypernatremia, hypoglycemia, hypotension, irritation of the esophagus/stomach, nausea, numbness in arms/legs, photosensitivity, respiratory failure, seizure, ulcers, vomiting, ↓ WBC count; | **Interactions:** Anticoagulants/antiplatelets (↑ or ↓, effects unclear), antilipemic agents (additive effects), antimalarial agents (pyrimethamine, tetracycline, cotrimoxazole combinations; additive effects); beta blockers (altered effects), carmustine (↑ effects), CYCLOSPORINE (may ↑ serum levels via CYP450 3A4 inhibition), CYP450 2D6/3A4 substrates (inhibits 2D6/3A4 /↑ drug levels), heart rate–regulating agents (altered effects), P-glycoprotein substrates (inhibits P-gp/↑ levels of substrates), neostigmine (↓ effects), phenylephrine (↑ effects), tetracycline (↓ effects), vasopressors (altered effects), warfarin (↓ anticoagulant effects of warfarin), yohimbine (↓ effects), may interact with agents with similar effects or related mechanisms of action (antiarrhythmic, antibiotic, antidiabetic, antidiarrheal, antihistamine, antihypertensive, anti-inflammatory, antineoplastic, immunosuppressant, laxative, neurological, photosensitizing, sedative); | **Dose:** General, tablets/capsules: 0.5–1 g PO tid. Oral: 0.3–1 mL extract (1:1 in 60% ethanol), 2–4 mL tincture (1:10 in 60% ethanol). Intravenous: 0.2 mg/kg/min for 30 minutes. Ophthalmic: 2 drops 0.2% berberine tid for 3 weeks; | **Monitor:** Bilirubin, blood glucose, blood pressure, coagulation panel, lipid profile, sodium levels, urinalysis, WBC count; | **Notes:** The active ingredients of goldenseal include isoquinoline alkaloids, such as berberine, canadine, and hydrastine. Goldenseal is sometimes referred to as "Indian turmeric" or "curcuma" but should not be confused with turmeric (*Curcuma longa*).

G

gossypol | **Uses:** Contraception (female and male), cancer, endometriosis, | **Preg:** Not recommended due abortifacient effects; | **CIs:** Allergy/hypersensitivity, Concurrent potassium-depleting drugs; Consumption of alcohol, Pregnancy, Urogenital irritation; | **ADRs:** anorexia, diarrhea, dyspnea, dizziness, fatigue, fever, hair discoloration, heart failure, hepatotoxicity, HYPOKALEMIA, ileus, infertility (long-term), mucosal necrosis, mucosal sloughing, photosensitivity, reduction in testicular volume, skin burning; | **Interactions:** Alcohol (accumulation of blood levels of alcohol), beta blockers (↑ risk of potassium depletion), contraceptives (altered effects), cyclosporine (↑ risk of potassium depletion), digoxin (↑ risk of toxicity due to potassium depletion), laxatives (additive effects, ↑ risk of potassium depletion), metapyrone (altered effects), NSAIDs (↑ risk of adverse gastrointestinal effects), phenobarbital (altered effects), sulfadiazine (synergistic effects), theopylline (↓ effects of gossypol); | **Dose:** Oral: 15–70 mg PO qd. Intravaginal: 0.5 mg/mL gossypol acetic acid applied to the vagina 1 hour before intercourse; | **Monitor:** Potassium levels, LFTs; | **Notes:** Concurrent use of gossypol and potassium-depleting drugs can increase the risk of hypokalemia.

gotu kola ***(Centella asiatica)*** | **Uses:** Anxiety, atherosclerosis, chronic venous insufficiency/varicose veins, cognitive function, deep vein thrombosis (DVT), diabetic microangiopathy, keloids, liver cirrhosis, psoriasis, scarring, schistosomiasis, striae gravidarum (stretch marks), wound healing; | **Preg:** Not recommended due to insufficient evidence and possible antifertility effects; | **CIs:** Allergy/hypersensitivity; Concurrent use with CNS depressants; Pregnancy or attempting to conceive; Liver disease; | **ADRs:** allergic reactions, cancer, contact dermatitis (topical), drowsiness, fatigue, gastrointestinal upset, hepatotoxicity, hyperglycemia, hyperlipidemia, infertility, nausea, night eating syndrome, sedation; | **Interactions:** Antidiabetic agents (antagonistic effects), corticosteroids (↓ gotu kola asiaticosides), CNS DEPRESSANTS (additive sedation), CYP450 substrates (altered drug levels), hepatotoxic agents (↑ risk of hepatotoxicity), phenylbutazine (↓ asiaticoside), may interact with agents with similar effects or related mechanisms of action (antidementia, anti-inflammatory, antianxiety, antibiotic, antilipemic, antineoplastic, antiviral, diuretic, fertility agents, hormonal, sedative, vasodilatory); | **Dose:** Oral: 12 g crude herb, or up to 120 mg (in capsule form) daily; | **Monitor:** Blood glucose, LFTs, lipid profile; | **Notes:** Gotu kola is not related to the kola nut (*Cola nitida, Cola acuminata*). Gotu kola is not a stimulant and does not contain caffeine.

G

grape seed *(Vitis vinifera, Vitis coignetiae)* | **Uses:** Agitation in dementia, antioxidant, cancer, cardiovascular disease, chronic venous insufficiency, diabetic retinopathy, edema, hyperlipidemia, melasma (chloasma), night vision, ocular stress, pancreatitis, platelet aggregation inhibitor, premenstrual syndrome (PMS), radiation skin protection (UV), skin aging (postmenopausal women), vascular fragility, vision problems; | **Preg:** Not recommended due to insufficient evidence; | **CIs:** Allergy/hypersensitivity; | **ADRs:** allergic reactions, angioedema, bleeding, dizziness, dry, itchy scalp, gastritis, headache, hypertension, indigestion, nausea, urticaria; | **Interactions:** Anticoagulants/antiplatelets (↑ risk of bleeding), antihypertensive agents (mixed effects), antiemetics (antagonistic effects), CYP 1A2 substrates (induce CYP1A2/↓ drug levels), CYP450 2E1/2C9/3A4 (inhibits 2E1/2C9/3A4), *Lactobacillus acidophilus* (inhibits growth of *L. acidophilus*), methotrexate (↑ risk of methotrexate toxicity), phenacetin (↓ drug levels), vitamin C (↑ blood pressure when used with grape seed, may enhance the absorption and effectiveness of vitamin C); may interact with agents with similar effects or related mechanisms of action (ACE inhibitory, xanthine oxidase inhibitory, antilipemic, antineoplastic); | **Dose:** Up to 300 mg daily by mouth; | **Monitor:** Blood pressure, coagulation panel; | **Notes:** Pycnogenol is a patented nutrient supplement extracted from the bark of European coastal pine *Pinus maritima*. Pycnogenol consists of flavonoids, catechins, procyanidins, and phenolic acids, which are the same things found in grape seed but not the same supplement.

grapefruit *(Citrus x paradisi)* | **Uses:** Atopic eczema, cardiovascular disease, metabolic syndrome, renal calculi; | **Preg:** Likely safe in food amounts in pregnant or breastfeeding patients based on traditional use. Other uses are not recommended due to lack of sufficient evidence; | **CIs:** Allergy/hypersensitivity; | **ADRs:** enamel loss, headaches, hyper-/hypokalemia, hyper-/hypotension, pseudohyperaldosteronism (Liddle's syndrome), pruritus, ↑ or ↓ renal calculi, urticaria; | **Interactions:** Acebutolol (↓ plasma concentration of acebutolol), amiodarone (↓ metabolism and ↑ adverse effects), ARTEMETHER (↑ bioavailability), anticonvulsants (↑ bioavailability of anticonvulsant agents), antidepressants (inhibits metabolism of antidepressants), antidiabetic agents (altered effects), antineoplastic agents (reduced effectiveness of antineoplastic agents), BENZODIAZEPINES (↑ plasma levels of triazolam, midazolam, diazepam), beta blockers (↓ concentrations of beta blockers), BUSPIRONE (↑ absorption/↑ concentrations of buspirone), caffeine (↓ clearance/↑ adverse effects), CALCIUM CHANNEL BLOCKERS (↑ absorption/↑ concentrations of CCBs), CARBAMAZEPINE (↑ absorption/↑ concentrations of carbamazepine), CARVEDILOL (↑ bioavailability of carvedilol), CISAPRIDE (↑ absorption/↑ concentrations of cisapride), CLOMIPRAMINE (↑ levels of clomipramine), CYCLOSPORINE (↑ absorption/↑ concentrations of cyclosporine), CYP450 1A2/2C19/2C9 substrates (inhibit CYP450 1A2/2C19/2C9/↑drug levels), CYP450 3A4 (inhibit CYP450 3A4/↑ drug levels), DEXTROMETHORPHAN (↑ drug levels), digoxin (↑ AUC/↑ risk of adverse effects), eplerenone (↑ AUC/↑ risk of adverse effects), erythromycin (↑ absorption/↑ concentrations of erythromycin), ESTROGENS (↑ drug levels), ETOPOSIDE (↓ absorption/↓ levels of etoposide), FEXOFENADINE (↓ absorption/↓ levels of fexofenadine), HMG-CoA REDUCTASE INHIBITORS (↑ absorption/↑ concentrations of HMG-CoA reductase inhibitors), immunosuppressants (↑ absorption/↑ plasma concentrations of immunosuppressants), ITRACONAZOLE (↓ absorption/↓ levels of itraconazole), losartan (↓ effectiveness), methadone (↑ concentrations/↑ adverse effects), METHYLPREDNISOLONE (↑ concentrations), P-glycoprotein substrates (altered drug levels), PRAZIQUANTEL (↑ concentrations), QUINIDINE (↓ clearance), protease inhibitors (↑ absorption/↑ concentrations of PIs), SCOPOLAMINE (↑ absorption/↑ concentrations of scopolamine), SILDENAFIL, TERFENADINE (↑ absorption/↑ concentrations of terfenadine), theophylline (↓ levels of theophylline), vincristine (alters permeation of vincristine across blood–brain barrier), warfarin (↑ warfarin effects); | **Dose:** Oral, pectin: 5 g 3 times daily; seed extract: 150 mg 3 times daily for 1 month; juice: 8 oz 3 times daily, before meals. | **Monitor:** Blood glucose, coagulation panel, cortisol, drug levels, hematocrit, lipid panel, electrolytes; | **Notes:** Grapefruit juice is a potent inhibitor of the intestinal cytochrome P450 system (specifically, CYP3A4-mediated drug metabolism), which is responsible for the first-pass metabolism of many medications. It is via this enzyme system that grapefruit increases the drug levels of calcium channel blockers, benzodiazepines, immunosuppressants, and HMG-CoA reductase inhibitors.

gravel root *(Eupatorium purpureum)* | **Uses:** Insufficient evidence; | **Preg:** Avoid use; | **CIs:** Allergy/hypersensitivity, Oral use (due to hepatotoxic pyrrolizidine alkaloids); | **ADRs:** dehydration, diaphoresis, diarrhea, diuresis, HEPATOTOXICITY, hypokalemia, muscle weakness, vomiting; | **Interactions:** Anti-inflammatory agents (additive effects), cytochrome P450 3A4 inducers (↑ conversion of pyrrolizidine alkaloids to toxic metabolites), diuretics (↑ effects), hepatotoxic agents (↑ risk of liver damage), laxatives (additive effects/↑ risk of hypokalemia); | **Dose:** Dried root: 2–4 g PO tid. Liquid extract (1:1 in 25% alcohol): 2–4 mL PO tid. Tincture (1:5 in 40% alcohol): 1–2 mL PO tid; | **Monitor:** LFTs, potassium levels; | **Notes:** Gravel root contains hepatotoxic pyrrolizidine alkaloids.

graviola *(Annona muricata)* | **Uses:** Insufficient evidence; | **Preg:** Not recommended due to insufficient evidence; | **CIs:** Allergy/hypersensitivity, Parkinson's disease (when used orally); | **ADRs:** hypotension, nausea/vomiting; high doses: myeloneuropathy, neuronal dysfunction; | **Interactions:** Antidepressants (additive effects), antihypertensives (↑ risk of hypotension), anti-Parkinson's agents (altered effects); | **Dose:** Infusion: 150 mL boiling water poured over 2 g of dried graviola leaf and stem, steeped for 5–10 minutes, PO tid between meals; | **Monitor:** Toxic effects including MOVEMENT DISORDERS (myeloneuropathy); | **Notes:** Graviola contains compounds that may cause movement disorders and neurotoxicity. Graviola may be unsafe, particularly in high doses.

greater celandine *(Chelidonium majus)* | **Uses:** Biliary colic, cancer (general), dyspepsia, esophageal cancer, lung cancer, pancreatic cancer, tonsillitis; | **Preg:** Not recommended due to insufficient evidence and possible embryotoxic effects; | **CIs:** Allergy/hypersensitivity, Liver disease; | **ADRs:** ↓ bone mineral density (BMD), contact dermatitis, hemolytic anemia, hepatotoxicity, intravascular hemolysis, kidney failure, liver cytolysis, thrombocytopenia, weight gain; | **Interactions:** CNS depressants (additive sedation), hepatotoxic agents (↑ risk of liver damage); may interact with agents with similar effects or related mechanisms of action (monoamine oxidase inhibition, serotonergic inhibition, antidiabetic, anti-inflammatory, antineoplastic, antiretroviral, antiulcer, apoptotic, antiosteoporotic, cytotoxic, dopaminergic, immunomodulatory); | **Dose:** Oral: 1 tsp root or 2 tsp herb as tea 2–3 times daily. Intravenous/intramuscular: up to 10 mg every other day; | **Monitor:** Albumin, BMD, blood glucose, body weight, immune parameters, LFTs; | **Notes:** Ukrain (a semisynthetic anticancer drug containing greater celandine alkaloids conjugated with thiophosphoric acid), has shown some promise in clinical trials as a cancer treatment.

G

green coffee extract *(Coffea arabica, Coffea canephora, Coffea robusta)* | **Uses:** Hypertension, cardiovascular disease (prevention), glucose intolerance, obesity; | **Preg:** Not recommended due to insufficient evidence; pregnant women are recommended to limit caffeine to 300 mg daily to avoid miscarriage or fetal growth impairment; | **CIs:** Allergy/hypersensitivity; | **ADRs:** asthma, conjunctivitis, contact allergy, cough, dyspnea, headache, hyperhomocysteinemia, hyperlipidemia, hypertension, kidney problems, nausea, rhinitis, sneezing, sputum production, tachycardia (due to caffeine), UTI, weight gain, wheezing; | **Interactions:** May interact with agents with similar effects or related mechanisms of action (antidiabetic, antihypertensive, beta-adrenergic, anticholinergic); | **Dose:** Chlorogenic acid: up to 2 g daily for one week; 140 mg daily for 12 weeks; | **Monitor:** Blood glucose, blood homocysteine, blood pressure; | **Notes:** Adverse effects and interactions related to caffeine (see Caffeine) or other constituents may vary depending on their content in various green coffee extract preparations.

green tea *(Camellia sinensis)* | **Uses:** Anxiety, arthritis, asthma, cancer prevention and treatment, cardiovascular disease, common cold prevention, dental cavity prevention, diabetes, fertility, genital warts, hypertension, hyperlipidemia, hypertriglyceridemia, memory enhancement, menopausal symptoms, myocardial infarction (prevention), obesity, sun protection, viral infection; | **Preg:** Not recommended in high doses during pregnancy due to caffeine content. Caffeine may ↑ risk of miscarriage, intrauterine growth retardation, low birth weight, birth defects, ↑ risk of sudden infant death syndrome (SIDS); **CIs:** Allergy/hypersensitivity; Pregnancy and lactation (in high doses); **ADRs:** abdominal pain, agitation, angina, anxiety, arrhythmia, cancer, change in voice quality, constipation, convulsions, delirium, dizziness, dyspepsia, dysuria, excitement, flatulence, gastric irritation, heartburn, hyperglycemia, hypernatremia, hypertension, hypokalemia, inflammation, incontinence, insomnia, ↑ IOP in glaucoma patients, iron deficiency, metabolic acidosis, microcytic anemia, muscle pain, muscle spasm, nausea/vomiting/diarrhea, nervousness, palpitations, polyuria, psychosis, respiratory alkalosis, restlessness, rhabdomyolysis, seizure, skin rashes, tachycardia, tachypnea, thrombosis, tremor; **Interactions:** Adenosine (caffeine is competitive inhibitor of adenosine), alcohol (↑ caffeine concentrations), analgesics (accelerates absorption, enhances analgesic effects), antibiotics (altered effects), anticoagulants/antiplatelets (↑ risk of bleeding), antidiabetic agents (altered or interfere with effects), antihypertensives (antagonistic effects), antilipemic agents (additive effects), antineoplastics (enhance the cytotoxicity), beta blockers (antagonistic effects), bitter orange (additive stimulant effects/↑ of adverse cardiovascular effects), boronic acid–based proteasome inhibitors (blocks proteasome inhibitory action), calcium (↑ calcium excretion), cimetidine (↓ caffeine clearance), clozapine (↑ risk of toxicity of clozapine), contraceptives (↑ caffeine concentrations), CNS depressants (antagonistic effects), CNS stimulants (additive stimulant effects), creatine (↑ risk of adverse cardiovascular effects), CYP450 substrates (altered drug levels), dexamethasone (↓ caffeine levels), dipyridamole (↓ vasodilation), disulfiram (↓ clearance/↑ half-life of caffeine), diuretics (additive effects), dopaminergic drugs (additive effects), echinacea (↑ effects), ephedrine (additive stimulant effects), ergot derivatives (↑ absorption of ergot derivatives), estrogens (↑ caffeine concentrations), fluconazole (↑ caffeine effects), fluvoxamine (↑ levels of caffeine), furafylline (↑ levels of caffeine), grapefruit (↑ caffeine concentrations), haloperidol (reduced haloperidol-induced catalepsy), hydrocortisone (added beneficial effects), iron (↓ iron absorption), lithium (↑ lithium levels), magnesium (↑ excretion of magnesium), MAO inhibitors (↑ risk of hypertensive crisis), methoxsalesen (inhibitor of caffeine metabolism), mexiletine (↑ caffeine effects), nicotine (altered effects), opiates (potentiate analgesic effects), pentobarbital (antagonistic effects), phenothiazines (precipitation of fluphenazine solutions), phenylpropanolamine (↑ blood pressure/stimulant effects), phenytoin (↑ caffeine clearance), quinolones (↑ caffeine effects), riluzole (↑ risk of adverse effects of riluzole), terbinafine (↑ caffeine effects), theophylline (↑ theophylline levels), TCAs (precipitation of TCA solutions), verapamil (↑ caffeine concentrations), warfarin (↓ effects of warfarin), yohimbine (↑ risk of hypertensive crisis); | **Dose:** Heart disease prevention: 250–900 mL of tea, taken PO daily for up to 4 weeks. Mental performance: 400 mL taken 3 times daily. Dental cavity prevention: 20 mL of black tea gargled for 60 seconds daily; | **Monitor:** Blood pressure, blood glucose, ferritin, heart rate, plasma homocysteine, LFTs, renal function tests, theophylline levels, uric acid level; | **Notes:** Green tea, black tea, and oolong tea come from the same plant. Much of the adverse effects and interactions of green tea are related to caffeine content (see Caffeine).

G

green-lipped mussel *(Perna canaliculus)* | **Uses:** Asthma, osteoarthritis, rheumatoid arthritis; | **Preg:** Not recommended due to insufficient evidence and possible uterotrophic effects; | **CIs:** Allergy/hypersensitivity, Hepatitis; Pregnancy/lactation; | **ADRs:** abnormal liver function, arthritis symptoms, dyspnea, fluid retention, gout, heart failure, intestinal gas, lung dysfunction, metallic taste, nausea, neurotoxic shellfish poisoning, skin rash, stomach upset, toxic hepatitis; | **Interactions:** Pentoxifylline (↑ effects), may interact with agents with similar effects or related mechanisms of action (antiasthma, antihistamine, anti-inflammatory, corticosteroid, immunomodulating, uterotrophic); | **Dose:** Lipid extract: 200 mg daily by mouth. Powder: 1,000 mg daily PO; | **Monitor:** LFTs; | **Notes:** The green-lipped mussel (*Perna canaliculus*) is native to the New Zealand coast and is a staple in the diet of the indigenous Maori culture (particularly those who live in coastal regions). Green-lipped mussel appears to be generally well tolerated in nonallergic people.

ground ivy *(Glechoma hederacea)* | **Uses:** Insufficient clinical evidence; | **Preg:** Avoid due to possible abortifacient effects; | **CIs:** Allergy/hypersensitivity, Liver disease, Kidney disease, Pregnancy, Seizure disorders; | **ADRs:** angioedema, dyspnea, kidney irritation, liver damage, seizures; | **Interactions:** Drugs that lower seizure threshold (↑ risk of seizures), hepatotoxic agents (↑ risk of liver damage), nephrotoxic agents (↑ risk of kidney damage); possible interactions may be related to high vitamin C content (see Vitamin C); | **Dose:** Oral: Up to 4 g dried plant as tea or in tincture 3 times daily. Topical: crushed leaves applied to the skin as needed; | **Monitor:** LFTs, renal function tests; | **Notes:** Not to be confused with English ivy (*Hedera helix*), although the species have similar common names.

guar gum | **Uses:** Cholera, cholestasis (pregnancy), constipation, diabetes, diarrhea, dumping syndrome, hypercholesterolemia, IBS; | **Preg:** Likely safe when used appropriately; | **CIs:** Allergy/hypersensitivity, Esophageal/GI obstruction; | **ADRs:** abdominal discomfort, asthma, diarrhea, flatulence, heartburn, hypoglycemia itching; | **Interactions:** Antidiabetic agents (↑ risk of hypoglycemia), antilipemic agents (additive effects), digoxin (↓ rate of digoxin absorption), estrogens (↓ estrogen absorption), metformin (↓ metformin absorption), penicillin (↓ penicillin absorption), potassium (↑ potassium excretion), sodium (↑ sodium excretion); | **Dose:** 4–12 g PO qd, start with small dose and titrate up; | **Monitor:** Blood glucose, lipid profile; | **Notes:** Guar gum is a soluble dietary fiber that works as a bulk laxative.

G

guarana *(Paullinia cupana)* | **Uses:** Cognitive enhancement, mood enhancement, obesity; | **Preg:** Not recommended in high doses during pregnancy due to caffeine content. Caffeine may ↑ risk of miscarriage, intrauterine growth retardation, ↓ birth weight, birth defects, ↑ risk of sudden infant death syndrome (SIDS); | **CIs:** Allergy/hypersensitivity, Pregnancy, Lactation, Hypertension, Liver dysfunction, Arrhythmias, Breast disease, Concomitant CNS stimulants, Psychiatric disorders; | **ADRs:** adverse effects largely related to caffeine content; agitation, angina, anorexia, anxiety, arrhythmia, bleeding, blurred vision, breast disease, cancer, convulsions, delirium, dizziness, dyspepsia, dysuria, excitement, ↑ gastric emptying, gastric irritation, headache, hyperglycemia, hypernatremia, hypertension, hypokalemia, incontinence, insomnia, ↑ IOP in glaucoma patients, iron deficiency, irritability, lack of concentration, metabolic acidosis, microcytic anemia, muscle spasm, nervousness, palpitation, polyuria, psychosis, respiratory alkalosis, restlessness, rhabdomyolysis, seizure, skin rashes, tachycardia, tachypnea, thrombosis, tremor, ventricular fibrillation; | **Interactions:** The drug interactions associated with guarana are based upon the adverse effect profile of caffeine. Adenosine (caffeine is competitive inhibitor of adenosine), alcohol (↑ caffeine concentrations), analgesics (accelerates absorption, enhances analgesic effects), antibiotics (altered effects), anticoagulants/antiplatelets (↑ risk of bleeding), antidiabetic agents (altered or interfere with effects), antihypertensives (antagonistic effects), antilipemic agents (additive effects), antineoplastics (enhance the cytotoxicity), beta blockers (antagonistic effects), bitter orange (additive stimulant effects/↑ of adverse cardiovascular effects), calcium

(↑ calcium excretion), cimetidine (↓ caffeine clearance), clozapine (↑ risk of toxicity of clozapine), contraceptives (↑ caffeine concentrations), CNS depressants (antagonistic effects), CNS stimulants (additive stimulant effects), creatine (↑ risk of adverse cardiovascular effects), CYP450 substrates (altered drug levels), dexamethasone (↓ caffeine levels), dipyridamole (↓ vasodilation), disulfiram (↓ clearance/↑ half-life of caffeine), diuretics (additive effects), dopaminergic drugs (additive effects), echinacea (↑ effects), ephedrine (additive stimulant effects), ergot derivatives (↑ absorption of ergot derivatives), estrogens (↑ caffeine concentrations), fluconazole (↑ caffeine effects), fluvoxamine (↑ levels of caffeine), furafylline (↑ levels of caffeine), grapefruit (↑ caffeine concentrations), haloperidol (reduced haloperidol-induced catalepsy), hydrocortisone (added beneficial effects), iron (↓ iron absorption), lithium (↑ lithium levels), magnesium (↑ excretion of magnesium), MAO inhibitors (↑ risk of hypertensive crisis), methoxsalesen (inhibitor of caffeine metabolism), mexiletine (↑ caffeine effects), nicotine (altered effects), opiates (potentiate analgesic effects), pentobarbital (antagonistic effects), phenothiazines (precipitation of fluphenazine solutions), phenylpropanolamine (↑ blood pressure/stimulant effects), phenytoin (↑ caffeine clearance), quinolones (↑ caffeine effects), riluzole (↑ risk of adverse effects of riluzole), terbinafine (↑ caffeine effects), theophylline (↑ theophylline levels), TCAs (precipitation of TCA solutions), verapamil (↑ caffeine concentrations), warfarin (↓ effects of warfarin), yohimbine (↑ risk of hypertensive crisis); | **Dose:** Dry extract: doses should not exceed 3 g daily; | **Monitor:** The laboratory interactions associated with guarana are based on the adverse effect profile of caffeine. Blood pressure, blood glucose, ferritin, heart rate, plasma homocysteine, LFTs, renal function tests, theophylline levels, uric acid level; | **Notes:** Guarana has one of the highest caffeine contents of all plants; the seed contains 2.5%–7% caffeine, compared with 1%–2% in coffee.

guayule *(Parthenium argentatum)* | **Uses:** Insufficient clinical evidence; | **Preg:** Not recommended due to insufficient evidence; | **CIs:** Allergy/hypersensitivity; | **ADRs:** insufficient evidence; | **Interactions:** CYP450 substrates (may alter drug levels), may interact with agents with similar effects (cytotoxic); | **Dose:** Insufficient evidence; | **Monitor:** Insufficient evidence; | **Notes:** There is insufficient evidence in humans to support the use of guayule for any indication. It is primarily used as a source of latex.

guggul *(Commifora mukul)* | **Uses:** Acne, hyperlipidemia, obesity, osteoarthritis, rheumatoid arthritis; | **Preg:**

Not recommended due to insufficient evidence and possible abortifacient effects; **CIs:** Allergy/hypersensitivity; **ADRs:** abdominal upset, altered thyroid function, anorexia, apprehension, bleeding, diarrhea, headache, hiccough, infertility, intestinal gas, nausea, nervousness, rash, restlessness, vomiting; **Interactions:** Anticoagulants/antiplatelets (↑ risk of bleeding), antilipemic agents (additive effects), CYP450 3A4 substrates (induce CYP3A4), diltiazem (↓ bioavailability), ESTROGENS/CONTRACEPTIVES/HORMONE REPLACEMENT THERAPY (additive estrogenic effects/↑ adverse effects), propranolol (↓ bioavailability), SERMS (interfere with effects), thyroid hormones (altered effects); **Dose:** Oral: guggulipid: 500–1,000 mg 3 times daily; guggulsterone: 25 mg 3 times daily, or 50 mg twice daily; **Monitor:** Coagulation panel, estrogens, lipid profile, thyroid function panel; **Notes:** Guggul (gum guggul) is a resin produced by the mukul mirth tree. Guggulipid is extracted from guggul, and contains plant sterols (guggulsterones E and Z), which are believed to be its bioactive compounds.

gumweed *(Grindelia camporum)* **Uses:** Insufficient clinical evidence; **Preg:** Not recommended due to insufficient evidence; **CIs:** Allergy/hypersensitivity, Emetic use, Topical use on open wounds; **ADRs:** bradycardia, depressed nervous system, eye irritation, hypertension, kidney irritation, lung irritation, polyuria, vagus nerve irritation, water loss; **Interactions:** May interact with agents with similar effects or related mechanisms of action (emetic, diuretic, hypotensive); **Dose:** Insufficient evidence; **Monitor:** Insufficient evidence; **Notes:** Gumweed has been used traditionally to treat a number of conditions; however, its clinical use was discontinued in 1960, when a law was passed requiring that all medicines had to have proven efficacy in clinical trials. No company was willing to do clinical trials of gumweed owing to concerns that the plant preparation would not be patentable.

gymnema *(Gymnema sylvestre)* **Uses:** Diabetes (types 1 and 2), hyperlipidemia, obesity; **Preg:** Not recommended due to insufficient evidence; **CIs:** Allergy/hypersensitivity; **ADRs:** dysgeusia, hypoglycemia; **Interactions:** Antidiabetic agents (↑ risk of hypoglycemia), antilipemic agents (additive effects), antiobesity agents (additive effects); **Dose:** Extract: 200 mg twice daily PO. Recommended dose of Proβeta (GS4): 500 mg twice daily at mealtimes (for adults weighing > 100 pounds), or 250 mg twice daily at mealtimes (for adults weighing < 100 pounds); **Monitor:** Blood glucose, lipid profile, weight; | **Notes:** May be standardized to 25% gymnemic acid.

haritaki | **Uses:** Insufficient evidence; | **Preg:** Not recommended due to insufficient evidence; | **CIs:** Allergy/hypersensitivity; | **ADRs:** insufficient evidence; | **Interactions:** Antibiotics (additive effects), antidiabetic agents (↑ risk of hypoglycemia), antifungal agents (additive effects), anti-inflammatory agents (additive effects), antilipemic agents (additive effects), antineoplastic agents (additive effects), antiviral agents (additive effects), isoproterenol (↓ effects of isoproterenol), immunosuppressants (altered effects), sertraline (↓ effects of sertraline); | **Dose:** Dried powder: 2 g PO bid. 4:1 concentrated powder extract: 1 g PO bid. Tablets (500 mg): 1–2 tablets, 1–2 times/day PO; | **Monitor:** Blood glucose, lipid profile; | **Notes:** Haritaki is a common herbaceous plant used extensively in Ayurvedic medicine. Haritaki is used for a variety of conditions, the most common being constipation, digestive conditions, and infection.

H

hawthorn (*Crataegus* spp.) | **Uses:** Angina, anxiety, CHF, CAD, functional cardiovascular disorders, hypertension (in diabetes), orthostatic hypotension; | **Preg:** Not recommended due to insufficient evidence; | **CIs:** Allergy/hypersensitivity, CONCOMITANT USE WITH VASODILATORS; | **ADRs:** abdominal discomfort, agitation, arrhythmia, diaphoresis, dizziness, dyspnea, fatigue, headache, insomnia, nausea, palpitations, rash, sleepiness, sleeplessness, tachycardia; | **Interactions:** Alpha agonists (antagonistic effects), anticoagulants/antiplatelets (↑ risk of bleeding), ANTIHYPERTENSIVES (↑ risk of hypotension), antilipemic agents (additive effects), antineoplastic agents (additive effects), BETA BLOCKERS (↑ risk of hypotension), CALCIUM CHANNEL BLOCKERS (additive vasodilation), CARDIAC GLYCOSIDES (e.g., digoxin; potentiate effects of digoxin); VASODILATORS (e.g., nitrates, phosphodiesterase inhibitors; additive vasodilation); | **Dose:** Oral: 160–900 mg dried extract daily in divided doses; | **Monitor:** Blood pressure, coagulation panel, heart rate, lipid profile; | **Notes:** Hawthorn is widely used in Europe to treat congestive heart failure, with preparations based on flavonoid content. Overall, hawthorn appears to be safe and well tolerated; it is best used under medical supervision.

Heartsease (*Viola tricolor*) | **Uses:** Insufficient clinical evidence; | **Preg:** Not recommended due to insufficient evidence; | **CIs:** Allergy/hypersensitivity; | **ADRs:** insufficient clinical evidence; may cause adverse effects related to salicylate content, including gastrointestinal upset and ↑ bleeding risk; | **Interactions:** May interact with agents with similar effects or related mechanisms of action (antibiotic, antineoplastic, anticoagulant, expectorant, anti-inflammatory, salicylates); | **Dose:** Infusion or tea: 1–4 g dried herb 3 times daily. Tincture: 2–4 mL 3 times daily. Topical: tea or poultice applied 3 times daily; | **Monitor:** Coagulation panel; | **Notes:** Heartsease has been used as a homeopathic remedy.

hemlock | **Uses:** Insufficient evidence; | **Preg:** Avoid use; | **CIs:** Allergy/hypersensitivity, Oral use; | **ADRs:** symptoms of poisoning: coma, convulsions, DEATH, movement problems, nausea/vomiting, polyuria, salivation, tachycardia followed by bradycardia, tachypnea; | **Interactions:** Insufficient evidence; | **Dose:** UNSAFE when used orally; | **Monitor:** Toxic symptoms; | **Notes:** Hemlock is UNSAFE when used orally and can be lethal; may be safe in homeopathic preparations.

H

hemp seed oil | **Uses:** Atopic dermatitis, cachexia, chronic pain, epilepsy, glaucoma, Huntington's disease, insomnia, multiple sclerosis, schizophrenia (treatment resistant); | **Preg:** Avoid use; | **CIs:** Allergy/hypersensitivity, Emphysema (inhalation), Lung cancer (inhalation); | **ADRs:** anxiety, bullous emphysema, cannabis arteritis (peripheral vascular disease), diarrhea, dizziness, fatigue, hepatotoxicity, hyper/hypotension, immunosuppression, nausea, psychotic-like feelings, renal failure, ↑ risk of lung cancer, seizures, sleepiness, tachycardia, weight gain; | **Interactions:** Alcohol (additive effects), anticoagulants/antiplatelets (↑ risk of bleeding), BARBITURATES (↑ drug levels), CNS DEPRESSANTS (additive sedation), disulfiram (↑ risk of hypomania), CNS stimulants (altered effects), cyclosporine (↑ levels of cyclosporine), fluoxetine (↑ risk of hypomania), P-glycoprotein substrates (altered drug levels), THEOPHYLLINE (↑ metabolism of theophylline), vasodilators (additive effects), warfarin (↑ effects of warfarin); | **Dose:** Fluid extract: 1–3 gtt PO qd. Tincture: 5–15 gtt PO qd. Prescription dronabinol (Marinol): 2.5–10 mg PO bid. Inhalation: 65–195 mg of cannabis for smoking; | **Monitor:** Blood pressure, coagulation panel; | **Notes:** The cannabinoid constituent, dronabinol, is an FDA-approved drug (Marinol).

hesperidin | **Uses:** Blood vessel disorders, chronic venous insufficiency, diabetes, hemorrhoids, lymphedema, venous leg ulcers; | **Preg:** Not recommended due to insufficient evidence; | **CIs:** Allergy/hypersensitivity; | **ADRs:** abdominal pain, asthenia, diarrhea, dyspepsia, gastritis, headache, nausea; | **Interactions:** Analgesics (additive effects), anticoagulants/antiplatelets (↑ risk of bleeding), ↑ antidiabetic agents (↑ risk of hypoglycemia), anti-inflammatory agents (additive effects), antilipemic agents (additive effects), calcium (altered effects), CYP450 2C9/2D6/3A4 substrates (inhibits 2C9/2D6/3A4), sedatives (additive effects); | **Dose:** 450 mg of diosmin plus 50 mg of flavonoids expressed as hesperidin (Daflon): 500 mg PO bid; | **Monitor:** Blood glucose, calcium levels, lipid profile; | **Notes:** Hesperidin is a flavone diglycoside that principally is derived from unripe citrus fruit.

H

hibiscus (*Hibiscus* spp.) | **Uses:** Hypertension, *Pediculus humanus* capitis (head lice); | **Preg:** Not recommended due to insufficient evidence and traditional use as a labor stimulant; may suppress fertility and implantation; | **CIs:** Allergy/hypersensitivity; | **ADRs:** birth defects, cancer, dermatitis, infertility; | **Interactions:** Acetaminophen (↓ in half-life), chloroquine (↓ bioavailability), may interact with agents with similar effects or related mechanisms of action (anticancer, antihypertensive, anti-inflammatory, antimalarial, hormonal); | **Dose:** Infusion: 10 g dry calyx with 0.5 L of water (9.6 mg anthocyanin content) daily by mouth for 4 weeks; | **Monitor:** Blood pressure, drug levels (acetaminophen and quinines), urinalysis (creatinine, uric acid, citrate, tartrate, calcium, sodium, potassium, phosphate); | **Notes:** Not to be confused with okra (*Abelmoschus esculentus*), formerly classified as *Hibiscus esculentus*, or Norfolk Island hibiscus (*Lagunaria patersonii*).

hochu-ekki-to | **Uses:** Immune enhancement; | **Preg:** Not recommended due to insufficient evidence; | **CIs:** Allergy/hypersensitivity; | **ADRs:** insufficient evidence; | **Interactions:** Insufficient evidence; | **Dose:** Insufficient evidence; | **Monitor:** Immune parameters; | **Notes:** The herbs in this formula include astragalus root, ginseng root, *Atractylodes lancea* rhizome, Japanese angelica root, bupleurum root, jujube fruit, citrus unshiu peel, glycyrrhiza root (licorice), cimicifuga rhizome, and ginger rhizome. Adverse effects and interactions may be related to those of the individual constituents.

holy basil (*Ocimum sanctum*) | **Uses:** Diabetes; | **Preg:** Not recommended due to insufficient evidence and traditional use to stimulate contraction; | **CIs:** Allergy/hypersensitivity, Pregnancy; | **ADRs:** bleeding, hypoglycemia, infertility, skin irritations; | **Interactions:** Anticoagulants/antiplatelets

(↑ risk of bleeding), antidiabetic agents (↑ risk of hypoglycemia), antilipemic agents (additive effects), CYP 450 substrates (altered drug levels), diltiazem (↑ effects of holy basil), pentobarbital (additive sedation), scopolamine (↑ effects of holy basil); may interact with agents with similar effects or related mechanisms of action (anticoagulant, hypoglycemic, hypolipidemic); **Dose:** Dried leaf: up to 2.5 g dried leaf by mouth as a single dose, or up to 1 oz infused in tea. Juice: 10–20 mL 3 times daily PO; **Monitor:** Blood glucose, blood pressure, coagulation panel, lipid profile; **Notes:** Generally Recognized as Safe (GRAS) status in the United States and is generally safe at low to moderate levels, although clinical supportive evidence is lacking. Related to (but distinct from) sweet basil (*Ocimum basilicum*).

H

honey **Uses:** Burns, dandruff, diabetes mellitus (type 2), Fournier's gangrene, gastroenteritis in infants (inflammation of the stomach and intestine), herpes, hypertension, hyperlipidemia, leg ulcers, plaque/gingivitis, radiation mucositis, rhinoconjunctivitis, skin graft healing, wound healing; **Preg:** Not recommended due to potentially harmful contaminants, such as *Clostridium botulinum* and grayanotoxins, found in some types of honey; **CIs:** Allergy/hypersensitivity, in infants <12 months of age; **ADRs:** honey intoxication: arrhythmia, atrioventricular or intraventricular block, blurred vision, bradycardia, convulsions, diaphoresis, diarrhea, dizziness, dyspnea, hypotension, ↑ maggot infestation of wounds, infant botulism, leukocytosis, nausea, paralysis (mild), ulcers, vomiting, weakness, Wolff-Parkinson-White syndrome; **Interactions:** Antidiabetic agents (↑ blood glucose), phenytoin (↑ absorption), carbamazepine (↓ plasma levels), alcohol (↓ peak blood alcohol levels), may interact with agents with similar effects or related mechanisms of action (antibiotic, antidiabetic, antifungal, anti-inflammatory); **Dose:** Oral: 5 mL as an oral rinse or ingested. Topical: applied as needed. Inhalation: 60% honey solution; **Monitor:** Blood glucose; **Notes:** Honeys from the nectar of flowering plants in the genus *Rhododendron* have been known to cause honey intoxication.

honeysuckle (*Lonicera* spp.) **Uses:** Insufficient clinical evidence; **Preg:** Not recommended due to insufficient evidence; **CIs:** Allergy/hypersensitivity, Pediatric use; **ADRs:** contact dermatitis, cramping, gastrointestinal symptoms, linear itchy raised blisters, muscle cramps; **Interactions:** Insufficient evidence; **Dose:** Insufficient evidence; **Monitor:** Insufficient evidence; **Notes:** There are at least 180 species of honeysuckle, with most species found in Asia and a few in

Europe and the Americas. Used in homeopathy for a number of conditions, but supportive evidence is lacking.

hoodia *(Hoodia gordonii)* | **Uses:** Insufficient clinical evidence; | **Preg:** Not recommended due to insufficient evidence; | **CIs:** Allergy/hypersensitivity; | **ADRs:** insufficient evidence; | **Interactions:** Insufficient evidence; | **Dose:** Dried extract (20:1): up to 800 mg daily PO; | **Monitor:** Insufficient evidence; | **Notes:** Used traditionally to elevate energy while suppressing hunger; currently marketed as a weight-loss supplement.

hop *(Humulus lupulus)* | **Uses:** Insomnia/sleep quality, menopausal symptoms, rheumatic diseases, sedation; | **Preg:** Not recommended due to insufficient evidence and possible hormonal effects; some hop preparations contain alcohol, which is contraindicated in pregnancy; | **CIs:** Allergy/hypersensitivity; | **ADRs:** abdominal pain, ↑/↓ blood sugar, chronic bronchitis, chronic respiratory symptoms, contact dermatitis, drowsiness, dry cough, dyspnea, estrogenic effects, hyperthermia, occupational respiratory diseases, restlessness, sedation, seizures, syncope, vomiting; | **Interactions:** CNS depressants (additive sedation), CYP450 substrates (altered drug levels), may interact with agents with similar effects or related mechanisms of action (antibiotic, antidepressant, antidiabetic, antifungal, anti-inflammatory, antilipemic, antineoplastic, antipsychotic, hormonal, neurological); | **Dose:** Oral: doses increasing to 880 mg twice daily for 4 weeks. Parenteral: not recommended due to soporific effects, weight loss, and death. Topical: gel containing hop phytoestrogens applied daily to the vagina for 1 week, then twice daily for 11 weeks; | **Monitor:** Blood glucose, hormone levels, lipid profile; | **Notes:** Hop extracts may be standardized to the phytoestrogen 8-prenylnaringenin.

horny goat weed *(Epimedium grandiflorum)* | **Uses:** Atherosclerosis, osteoporosis, sexual dysfunction; | **Preg:** Not recommended due to insufficient evidence and possible hormonal effects; | **CIs:** Allergy/hypersensitivity, Hormone-sensitive conditions; | **ADRs:** aggressiveness, delayed-type hypersensitivity responses, dizziness, epistaxis, fever, gastrointestinal disturbances, hypomania, hypotension, irritability, nausea, respiratory arrest, tachyarrhythmia, tendon spasm, vomiting, xerostomia; | **Interactions:** Anticoagulant/antiplatelet (↑ risk of bleeding), antihypertensive agents (↑ risk of hypotension); may interact with agents with similar effects or related mechanisms of action (antilipidemic, estrogenic, immunomodulatory, monoamine oxidase inhibitory, thyroid suppressant); | **Dose:** Up to 15 g raw herb (or equivalent) daily PO; | **Monitor:** Blood pressure, BUN, coagulation panel, hormone levels (serum and excretion), immune parameters, lipid profile, thyroid hormones; | **Notes:** Despite its traditional and popular use, few clinical trials exist in support of horny goat weed. Small controlled trials suggest a potential benefit for the treatment of atherosclerosis symptoms and quality of life associated with hemodialysis. Other promising areas include sexual function.

horse chestnut | **Uses:** Chronic venous insufficiency (CVI); | **Preg:** Not recommended due to insufficient evidence; | **CIs:** Allergy/hypersensitivity, Inflammatory or infectious gastrointestinal disorders, Hepatic impairment, Latex allergy, Renal impairment; | **ADRs:** bleeding, calf spasm, contact dermatitis, dizziness, gastrointestinal tract upset, headache, hepatitis, hypoglycemia, indigestion, kidney damage, liver damage, nausea, pruritus, pseudolupus; | **Interactions:** Anticoagulant/antiplatelet (↑ risk of bleeding), antidiabetic agents (↑ risk of hypoglycemia), antihypertensive agents (↑ risk of hypotension), diuretics (additive effects), hepatotoxic agents (↑ risk of liver damage), nephrotoxic agents (↑ risk of kidney damage); may interact with agents with similar effects or related mechanisms of action (antiangiogenic, anti-inflammatory, neurologic, protein bound); | **Dose:** Oral: 300 mg extract twice daily, containing 50–75 mg escin per dose. Topical: 2% escin gel 3–4 times daily. Parenteral administration is not recommended due to anaphylactic reactions; | **Monitor:** Blood glucose, blood pressure, coagulation panel, LFTs, renal function tests; | **Notes:** Standardized horse chestnut seed extract (HCSE) is generally safe in adults at recommended doses for short periods of time. Horse chestnut flower, branch bark, and leaves should be avoided owing to known toxicity. Horse chestnut contains esculin, which may be lethal.

horseradish *(Armoracia rusticana,* syn. *Cochlearia armoracia)* | **Uses:** Bronchitis, sinusitis, urinary tract infection; | **Preg:** Not recommended due to insufficient evidence and traditional use as an abortifacient; | **CIs:** Allergy/hypersensitivity; | **ADRs:** abortion, allergic reactions, blistering, bloody vomiting, depressed thyroid function, diarrhea, diuresis, gastrointestinal upset, mouth irritation, mucous membrane irritation, nausea, peptic ulcers, ↑ salivation, sinus and eye irritation, skin irritation, urge incontinence, violent sneezing, vomiting, worsened kidney conditions; | **Interactions:** Anticoagulant/

antiplatelet (↑ risk of bleeding), antihypertensive agents (↑ risk of hypotension), antioxidants (↓ effects), diuretics (additive effects), levothyroxine (interfere with therapy); may interact with agents with similar effects or related mechanisms of action (antibiotic, anti-inflammatory, antineoplastic, oxidative, antithyroid); **Dose:** Juice: 15–20 drops between meals. Rheumatism: 3–4 tbsp of horseradish with apple cider vinegar and honey daily. Sinus congestion: ½ tsp grated horseradish, flavored with lemon juice, twice daily; **Monitor:** Blood pressure, coagulation panel, thyroid hormones; **Notes:** The U.S. Food and Drug Administration (FDA) has approved horseradish as Generally Regarded as Safe (GRAS) as a seasoning, spice, and flavoring.

H

horsetail *(Equisetum arvense)* **Uses:** Diuresis, osteoporosis; **Preg:** Not recommended due to insufficient evidence; **CIs:** Allergy/hypersensitivity, Alcoholism, Malnutrition, Pediatric use, Thiamine deficiency; **ADRs:** abdominal distention, asthenia, ataxia, dermatitis, diarrhea, hypokalemia, irreversible neurologic damage, nausea, nervousness, polyuria, thiamine deficiency, Wernicke-Korsakoff syndrome; **Interactions:** Antidiabetic agents (↑ risk of hypoglycemia), chromium (↑ risk of chromium toxicity), diuretics (additive effects), laxatives (additive effects), potassium-depleting agents (↑ risk of hypokalemia), thiamine (↓ effects); may interact with agents with similar constituents (e.g., nicotine), effects, or related mechanisms of action (antigout, cardiac, CNS stimulant, antiosteoporotic, neurological, thiamine depleting); **Dose:** Oral: 300 mg (or equivalent as tea or tincture) 3 times daily; maximum dose 6 g daily; **Monitor:** Blood glucose, potassium levels, renal function tests; **Notes:** *Equisetum arvense* should not be confused with members of the genus *Laminaria*, kelp, or brown alga, for which "horsetail" has been used as a synonym.

Hoxsey formula **Uses:** Cancer; **Preg:** Not recommended due to insufficient evidence; **CIs:** Allergy/hypersensitivity to any of the constituents; **ADRs:** insufficient evidence; **Interactions:** May interact with antineoplastic based on proposed mechanisms of action; **Dose:** Insufficient evidence; **Monitor:** Insufficient evidence; **Notes:** The Hoxsey formula is a therapeutic regimen consisting of an individualized oral tonic, topical preparations, and supportive therapy. Potassium iodide is generally found in the oral tonic, although other ingredients may be added (licorice, red clover, burdock, stillingia root, berberis root, pokeroot, cascara, aromatic USP 14, prickly ash bark, and buckthorn bark). Topical preparations may contain antimony trisulfide, zinc chloride, bloodroot (red paste), arsenic sulfide, talc, sulfur, and a "yellow precipitate" (yellow powder) or trichloroacetic acid (clear solution).

5-HTP **Uses:** Cerebellar ataxia, depression, fibromyalgia, headache, obesity, alcoholism withdrawal symptoms, anxiety, Down's syndrome, Lesch-Nyhan syndrome, psychiatric disorders, sleep disorders; **Preg:** Avoid use; **CIs:** Allergy/hypersensitivity; **ADRs:** abdominal pain, aggressiveness, agitation, amenorrhea, anxiety, bradycardia, depressed mood, diarrhea, dizziness, drowsiness, dyspepsia, EOSINOPHILIA MYALGIA SYNDROME (EMS), euphoria, flatulence, headache, hypomania symptoms, insomnia, irritability, itching, mania, myalgia, nausea, palpitations, pseudobullous morphea, rapid speech, rash, restlessness, rhabdomyolysis, sclerodermatous changes, SEIZURES, shortness of breath, sodium retention, somnolence, taste alteration, transient diastolic hypotension, transient disinhibition and euphoria, urticaria, vertigo, vomiting, weakness, weight gain; **Interactions:** Angiotensin II receptor antagonists (losartan may ↓ serotonin levels), ANTIDEPRESSANTS (↑ risk of serotonergic adverse effects with antidepressants), buspirone (↑ risk of serotonergic adverse effects), carbidopa (↑ risk of developing scleroderma-like illness), CNS depressants (↑ risk of adverse effects), CNS stimulants (↑ risk of adverse effects), decarboxylase inhibitors (↑ risk of serotonergic adverse effects), dextromethorphan (↑ risk of serotonergic adverse effects), lithium (↑ risk of serotonergic adverse effects), meperidine (↑ risk of serotonergic adverse effects), pentazocine (↑ risk of serotonergic adverse effects), phenobarbital (↑ risk of toxicity), reserpine (↑ risk of hypertension), thyroid hormones (altered effects), tramadol (↑ risk of serotonergic adverse effects), trazodone (↑ risk of serotonergic adverse effects), chromium (↑ risk of adverse effects), magnesium (↑ risk of serotonergic adverse effects), melatonin (↑ risk of adverse effects), niacin (↑ risk of serotonergic adverse effects), SAMe (additive effects), herbs or supplements with serotonergic effects; **Dose:** 100–1,600 mg PO daily. **Monitor:** Blood glucose, S/S of hypoglycemia, blood pressure, CBC, urinalysis; **Notes:** Serotonergic effects may interfere with surgery; patient should discontinue 5-HTP therapy a few weeks before surgery; may alter insulin requirements.

huperzine A **Uses:** Alzheimer's disease, cognitive disorders, dementia, learning ability, memory, myasthenia gravis, neuroprotection, organophosphate poisoning, schizophrenia, vascular dementia; **Preg:** Not recommended due to insufficient evidence. Teratogenicity has not been observed in animal

H

studies; | **CIs:** Allergy/hypersensitivity, Renal disorders; | **ADRs:** abdominal cramps, ankle edema, bradycardia, diaphoresis, diarrhea, dizziness (transient), excitability (transient), hyperactivity, insomnia, nasal obstruction, pruritus, slurred speech, syncope, urticaria, visual blurring, vomiting. Huperzine A appears generally safe at doses of up to 400 mcg daily; | **Interactions:** Acetylcholinesterase inhibitors (additive effects), anticholinergic agents (↓ effects), cholinergic agents (additive effects), CYP450 substrates (altered drug levels); may interact with agents with similar effects or related mechanisms of action (anticonvulsant, beta-adrenergic, beta-blocking, cardiovascular, GABAergic, NMDA antagonist); | **Dose:** Oral: up to 200 mcg twice daily. Intravenous/intramuscular: up to 0.3 mg/2 mL 20 minutes prior to completion of surgery; | **Monitor:** Heart rate, LFTs; | **Notes:** Huperzine is derived from Chinese club moss (*Huperzia serrata*). It is currently in phase II clinical trials in the United States and in phase III trials in China for the treatment of Alzheimer's disease. Use cautiously in patients with cardiovascular disease, epilepsy, gastrointestinal obstruction, urogenital tract obstruction, peptic ulcer disease, and pulmonary disorders.

H

hyaluronic acid | **Uses:** Osteoarthritis, skin aging, xerophthalmia; | **Preg:** Not recommended due to insufficient evidence; | **CIs:** Allergy/hypersensitivity; | **ADRs:** bleeding, contusion, hematoma, infection, redness at injection site; | **Interactions:** Anticoagulants/antiplatelets (↑ risk of bleeding); | **Dose:** Dry eyes: 0.2% Hyalist applied 3–4 times/day × 90 days. Osteoarthritis, oral: 80-mg capsules (Hyal-Joint, a natural extract of chicken combs containing 60%–70% hyaluronic acid) PO qd × 8 wk. Osteoarthritis, intra-articular: 20 mg injected weekly into knee × 3 wk; | **Monitor:** Coagulation panel; | **Notes:** Hyaluronic acid is often found in combination with glucosamine, chondroitin, and MSM. There is controversy as to whether the oral form of hyaluronic acid is effective.

hydrangea *(Hydrangea arborescens)* | **Uses:** Insufficient clinical evidence; | **Preg:** Not recommended due to insufficient evidence; | **CIs:** Allergy/hypersensitivity; | **ADRs:** angina, dizziness, gastrointestinal upset, hypoglycemia; | **Interactions:** Diuretics (additive effects); may interact with agents with similar effects or related mechanisms of action (hypoglycemic, antifungal, antihistamine, antilipemic, antimalarial, antibaldness); | **Dose:** Oral: 2–4 g powdered root, 2–4 mL liquid extract, 1 tsp syrup, or 2–10 mL tincture 3 times daily; | **Monitor:** Blood glucose, lipid profile; | **Notes:** Hydrangea may be moderately toxic due to cyanogenic glycosides such as hydrangin, which have been identified in the flowers, leaves, and root.

hydrazine sulfate (HS) | **Uses:** Cachexia (cancer related), cancer, Hodgkin's disease; | **Preg:** Not recommended due to insufficient evidence and potential toxicity; | **CIs:** Allergy/hypersensitivity, Pregnancy, Lactation; | **ADRs:** abnormal heartbeat, anorexia, blurred vision, bronchitis, burns, cancer, coma, confusion, constipation, cough, DEATH, depression, diaphoresis, diarrhea, dizziness, drowsiness, dyspnea, edema, excitability, fever, headache, hepatotoxicity, hypoglycemia, hypotension, hunger, irregular breathing, jaundice, lethargy, malaise, nausea, nephrotoxicity, neuropathy, palpitations, photosensitivity, pneumonia, rash, restlessness, rhinitis, seizures, septic shock, skin irritation, systemic lupus erythematosus, tremors, vein inflammation, violent behavior, vomiting, weakness; | **Interactions:** Alcohol (↑ flushing reaction), antidiabetic agents (↑ risk of hypoglycemia), bleomycin (↑ effects), CNS DEPRESSANTS (↑ toxicity/↓ effectiveness of hydrazine), cyclophosphamide (↑ effects), isoniazid (↑ risk of hepatotoxicity), methotrexate (↑ effects), mitomycin C (↑ effects), MAOIs (↑ effects); | **Dose:** Oral: 60 mg 3 times daily for up to 29 months. Parenteral: 5.4–8.1 g at intervals of 2–6 weeks; | **Monitor:** Blood glucose, CBC, LFTs; | **Notes:** Hydrazine sulfate is approved for use under medical supervision in certain countries (such as Canada), but it is not FDA approved in the United States. Avoid tyramine-containing foods, including anchovies, avocados, bananas, bean curd, beer (alcohol-free/reduced), caffeine (large amounts), caviar, champagne, cheese (particularly aged, processed, or strong varieties such as Camembert, cheddar, and Stilton), chocolate, dry sausage/salami/bologna, fava beans, figs, herring (pickled), liver (particularly chicken), meat tenderizers, papaya, protein extracts/powder, raisins, shrimp paste, sour cream, soy sauce, wine (particularly chianti), yeast extracts, and yogurt.

hydroxycitric acid | **Uses:** Exercise performance, weight loss; | **Preg:** Not recommended due to insufficient evidence; | **CIs:** Allergy/hypersensitivity; | **ADRs:** abdominal pain, headache, nausea; | **Interactions:** antiarrhythmics (altered effects), anticoagulants/antiplatelets (↑ risk of bleeding), antidiabetic agents (↑ risk of hypoglycemia), antilipemic agents (↑ risk of adverse effects), antiobesity agents (additive effects), beta blockers (altered effects), calcium channel blockers (altered effects), cardiac glycosides (potentiation of effects), depolarizing muscle relaxants (↑ risk of arrhythmias), niacin-bound chromium (added weight loss effects), nitrates (altered effects), terfenadine (↑ risk of arrhythmias); | **Dose:** 250–500 mg PO 1–3 times/day; | **Monitor:** Blood glucose, lipid profile, weight; | **Notes:** Hydroxycitric acid is the main constituent of garcinia. Garcinia is an inhibitor of adenosine triphosphate citrate lyase (ATP-citrate-lyase), an important enzymatic step in the conversion of carbohydrate to fat.

hydroxymethylbutyrate (HMB) | **Uses:** Cachexia, exercise capacity, hyperlipidemia, hypertension, immune function, ↑ muscle mass, wound healing; | **Preg:** Not recommended due to insufficient evidence; | **CIs:** Insufficient evidence; | **ADRs:** insufficient evidence; | **Interactions:** May interact with agents with similar effects or related mechanisms of action (hypotensive, hypolipidemic, exercise enhancement, immunostimulatory, antiobesity); | **Dose:** Oral: 3 g daily for up to 8 weeks. Up to 12 g daily has been used for muscle building; | **Monitor:** Blood pressure, BUN, lipid profile, cortisol, immune parameters, CPK; | **Notes:** HMB is a byproduct of metabolism of the amino acid leucine and its keto acid, alpha-ketoisocaproate. HMB is also a precursor to cholesterol.

H

hyoscyamine | **Uses:** Acute rhinitis, antispasmodic, colonoscopy preparation, diagnostic procedures, enema, functional gastrointestinal disorders, infant colic, inflammation, IBS, neurogenic bladder, neurogenic bowel disturbances, nocturnal enuresis, partial heart block, peptic ulcer, surgery preparation, urinary incontinence, ulcers, ureteral colic pain; | **Preg:** Not recommended due to insufficient evidence; | **CIs:** Allergy/hypersensitivity, Glaucoma, Intestinal atony (elderly, debilitated), Myasthenia gravis, Obstructive uropathy, Obstructive disease of GI tract, Paralytic ileus, Toxic megacolon (complicated ulcerative colitis), Ulcerative colitis (severe), Unstable cardiovascular status in acute hemorrhage; | **ADRs:** allergic reactions, ataxia, bloating, blurred vision, constipation, cyclopegia, dizziness, drowsiness, headache, hypohydrosis, impotence, loss of taste, mental confusion, mydriasis, nausea/vomiting, palpitations, psychosis, speech disturbances, suppression of lactation, tachycardia, urticaria, weakness, xerostomia; | **Interactions:** Additive adverse effects from cholingergic blockade: amantadine, antihistamines, haloperidol, MAOIs, phenothiazines, other antimuscarinics, tricyclic antidepressants; antacids (interfere with absorption of hyoscyamine); | **Dose:** Tablets (0.125 mg): 1–2 tablets PO q4h as needed; | **Monitor:** Blood pressure, heart rate; | **Notes:** Caution is warranted in patients with autonomic neuropathy, hyperthyroidism, coronary heart disease, congestive heart failure, cardiac arrhythmias, hypertension, and renal failure. Drowsiness may occur. Caution is warranted when engaging in activities that require mental alertness.

hyssop *(Hyssopus officinalis)* | **Uses:** Crescentic nephritis (rapidly progressive glomerulonephritis [RPGN]); | **Preg:** Not recommended due to insufficient evidence and ↑ risk of seizures; | **CIs:** Allergy/hypersensitivity, Lactation, Seizure disorders; | **ADRs:** convulsions, gastrointestinal discomfort, generalized tonic status, seizures, tonic-clonic seizures, vomiting; | **Interactions:** Drugs that lower seizure threshold (↑ risk of seizures); may interact with agents with similar effects or related mechanisms of action (anticonvulsant, hypoglycemic, antihyperlipidemic, antiviral, glucocorticoid, immunosuppressant, convulsant); | **Dose:** Oral: 2 g dried herb as infusion, 3 times daily; | **Monitor:** Blood glucose, lipid panel; | **Notes:** Medicinal hyssop is mentioned in the Bible but may refer to other species also known as hyssop (*Origanum aegypticum* or *Origanum syriacum*) rather than *Hyssopus officinalis*.

ignatia *(Strychnos ignatii)* | **Uses:** Emotional disorders (emergency use); | **Preg:** Not recommended due to insufficient evidence and possible toxic effects; | **CIs:** Allergy/hypersensitivity, Liver disease (due to potential toxicity); | **ADRs:** agitation, anxiety, back and neck stiffness, convulsions, DEATH, dyspnea, equilibrium disorders, fasciculation, hyperthermia, hyperreflexia, jaw and neck spasms, metabolic acidosis, muscle tension, nephrotoxicity, respiratory spasms, restlessness, rhabdomyolysis, seizures, ↑ sense perception; | **Interactions:** Analeptics/phenothiazines (may ↑ risk of ignatia poisoning); | **Dose:** Dry plant tincture (45% ethanol): 1 drop (10% w/v) 3 times daily PO; | **Monitor:** LFTs; | **Notes:** Although ignatia contains the highly poisonous strychnine, homeopathic remedies containing the extract are diluted enough to be considered safe for use. However, efficacy for any condition is questionable.

Indian gooseberry *(Emblica officinalis)* | **Uses:** Diabetes, eye diseases, hyperlipidemia; | **Preg:** Not recommended due to insufficient evidence; | **CIs:** Allergy/hypersensitivity; | **ADRs:** insufficient evidence; | **Interactions:** Anticoagulants/antiplatelets (↑ risk of bleeding), antidiabetic agents (↑ risk of hypoglycemia), antilipemic agents (additive effects), calcium (↑ calcium levels), doxorubicin (protective effects against doxorubicin toxicity), iron (↓ absorption); | **Dose:** Capsules: 1–2 capsules PO 3 times/day after meals;

| **Monitor:** Blood glucose, lipid profile; | **Notes:** Indian gooseberry (amalaki) juice contains high vitamin C content.

Indian tobacco (lobelia) | **Uses:** Insufficient evidence; | **Preg:** Avoid use; | **CIs:** Allergy/hypersensitivity, High doses (due to TOXIC effects); | **ADRs:** toxic symptoms: convulsions, DEATH, diaphoresis, diarrhea, nausea/vomiting; | **Interactions:** CNS depressants (additive effects), antiasthma drugs (altered effects), antidepressants (additive effects), antihypertensives (↑ risk of hypotension), anti-inflammatory agents (additive effects), diuretics (antagonistic effects), nicotine (↑ risk of adverse effects); | **Dose:** Dried herb (infusion or decoction): ¼–½ tsp of lobelia in 8 oz of water, typically in a mixture with other herbs, steep for 30–40 minutes, take 2 oz PO qid. Liquid extract (1:1 in 50% alcohol): 0.2–0.6 mL PO tid. Smoking cessation: lobeline, a constituent of lobelia, 5 mg PO bid or 0.5 mg PO bid as lozenges. Tincture: 0.6–2 mL PO qd. Vinegar tincture (1:5 in dilute acetic acid): 1–4 mL PO tid; | **Monitor:** Blood pressure; | **Notes:** Indian tobacco (or lobelia) may have an unpleasant, acidic taste. Lobelia is a potentially toxic herb. According to the FDA, lobeline, a constituent of lobelia, can bind to nicotinic receptors and cause adverse effects, including tachycardia, sweating, nausea, vomiting, diarrhea, convulsions, and even death.

inositol nicotinate | **Uses:** Claudication, cerebrovascular insufficiency, hypercholesterolemia, hypertension, necrobiosis lipoidica (skin disorders); | **Preg:** Not recommended due to insufficient evidence; | **CIs:** Allergy/hypersensitivity, Bipolar disorder, Liver disease, Peptic ulcer disease; | **ADRs:** abdominal upset, anaphylactic shock, anxiety, arrhythmia, ascites, bleeding, blurred vision, ↑ creatinine kinase (indicator of muscle damage), dental pain, diarrhea, dizziness, dyspnea, ↑ eosinophils, fatigue, <u>flushing</u>, headache, hepatotoxicity, hyperglycemia, hyperhomocysteinemia, hyper/hypoinsulinemia, hyperuricemia, hypotension, hypothyroidism, jaundice, leukopenia, ↑ liver function tests, macular swelling, nausea, niacin-induced myopathy, palpitations, panic attacks, pruritus, rash, stomach ulcers, thrombosis, tingling, toxic amblyopia, vomiting, xeroderma, xerophthalmia; | **Interactions:** Alcohol (↑ niacin-induced flushing, ↑ hepatotoxicity), allopurinol (↑ risk of hyperuricemia), anticoagulants/antiplatelets (↑ risk of bleeding), antidiabetes drugs (impairs glucose tolerance, ↑ plasma glucose), antihistamines (↓ niacin-induced flushing), antihypertensive agents (additive effects), aspirin (↓ niacin-induced flushing), azathioprine (↑ risk of niacin deficiency), benzodiazepine (↑ benzodiazepine solubility), bile acid sequestrants (↓ niacin absorption), carbamazepine (↑ carbamazepine levels, ↓ inositol levels), chloramphenicol (↑ risk of niacin deficiency), clonidine (↓ niacin-induced flushing), cycloserine (↑ risk of niacin deficiency), CYP450 substrates (inhibits enzyme activity), epinephrine (↓ niacin-induced anaphylactic shock, ↓ epinephrine-induced fatty acid release), estrogen (↑ estradiol solubility), ethionamide (interfere with effects, structural similarities), fluorouracil (↑ risk of niacin deficiency), fibrates (↑ risk of myopathy), griseofulvin (↑ griseofulvin solubility and toxicity), HMG-CoA reductase inhibitiors (↑ risk of myopathy), levodopa/carbidopa (↑ risk of niacin deficiency), lithium (↓ inositol levels), mercaptopurine (↑ risk of niacin deficiency), minerals (may interfere with absorption of minerals), neomycin (↑ effects), nicotine (↑ niacin-induced flushing and dizziness), NSAIDs (↓ niacin-induced flushing and burning), phenytoin (↑ risk of niacin deficiency), primidone (↓ clearance of primidone), probucol (↑ effects), procetofene (↑ effects), progesterone (↑ progesterone solubility), pyrazinamide (↑ risk of pellagra, structural similarities, interfere with activity), testosterone (↑ effects), theophylline (↓ theophylline-induced fatty acid release), thyroid hormones (altered effects), valproic acid (↓ niacin levels, ↓ inositol levels); may interact with agents with similar effects or related mechanisms of action (calcium channel blocking, ganglionic, vasodilatory); **Dose:** Oral: 1,500–4,000 mg qd in 2–4 divided doses for hyperlipoproteinemia and peripheral vascular disorders; **Monitor:** Blood pressure, coagulation panel, lipid profile, cortisol, creatine kinase, homocysteine levels, hormone panel, LFTs, thyroid function tests, uric acid; **Notes:** Potential adverse effects and interactions are based on niacin, the metabolic breakdown product of inositol nicotinate. However, the adverse effects of inositol nicotinate may be less severe because it is slowly broken down into free niacin and inositol.

iodine

Uses: Goiter prevention, bacterial conjunctivitis (pink eye), bladder/bowel irrigation, bleeding, cancer, cognitive function, corpus vitreous degeneration, antisepsis, filarial lymphoedema, goiter treatment, Graves' disease (adjunct iodine/iodides), hearing loss (iodine deficiency), iodine deficiency, molluscum contagiosum, ophthalmia neonatorum (pink eye during delivery of infant) prevention, oral mucositis, pelvic infection, periodontitis/gingivitis, pneumonia, postcesarean endometritis, radiation emergency (potassium iodide thyroid protection), renal pelvic instillation sclerotherapy (RPIS), septicemia, thyrotoxicosis/thyroid storm (adjunct iodides), water purification, wound healing; **Preg:** The U.S. Recommended Dietary Allowance (RDA): 220 mcg daily for pregnant women,

290 mcg daily for breastfeeding women. Iodine deficiency in pregnant or nursing mothers can lead to significant developmental defects in infants; | **Cls:** Allergy/hypersensitivity, Concomitant use with antithyroid drugs; | **ADRs:** abnormal blood counts, acne-like skin lesions, acute iodine poisoning, angioedema, anorexia, arthralgia, bleeding, blepharitis, blistering/crusting/irritation/itching of skin, burning of the mouth/throat/stomach, cardiovascular compromise, chronic iodism, confusion, cough, depression, diarrhea, dysgeusia, easy bruising, eye irritation, fatigue, fever, flu-like symptoms, gastrointestinal upset, headache, ↓/↑ heartbeat, loss of consciousness/coma, myalgia, nausea, numbness, pulmonary edema, ↑ risk of hyperkalemia, ↑ risk of urinary tract infection, ↑ salivation, sneezing, soreness of the gums/teeth, thrombotic thrombocytopenic purpura, thyroid gland dysfunction, tingling pain, urticaria, vasculitis, vomiting, weakness; | **Interactions:** Amiodarone (↑ iodide levels), angiotensin-converting enzyme inhibitors (↑ risk of hyperkalemia), angiotensin receptor blockers (↑ risk of hyperkalemia), ANTITHYROID DRUGS (e.g., methimazole or propylthiouracil; additive effects; ↑ risk of hypothyroidism), lithium, potassium-sparing diuretics (↑ risk of hyperkalemia), herbs and supplements with similar effects; | **Dose:** RDA: 150 mcg daily for adults; 220 mcg daily during pregnancy; 290 mcg daily during lactation. Upper intake level (UL), adults: 1,100 mcg/day; UL children 1–3 years: 200 mcg/day; UL children 4–8 years: 300 mcg/day; UL children 9–13 years: 600 mcg/day; UL children >13 years: 900 mcg/day; | **Monitor:** Potassium levels, thyroid function panel; | **Notes:** Iodine is an element that the human body needs to make thyroid hormone; deficiency can result in numerous health problems such as goiter.

I

ipecac | **Uses:** Poisoning; | **Preg:** Avoid use due to uterine stimulant effects; | **Cls:** Allergy/hypersensitivity, Certain poisonings (corrosives, petroleum distillates, strychnine), Depressed gag reflex, Inflammatory GI conditions, Heart disease, Unconsciousness; | **ADRs:** arrhythmias, aspiration pneumonia, cardiomyopathies, DEATH, diarrhea, dizziness, dyspnea, esophageal rupture, GI irritation, heart failure, hypotension, myopathy, nausea/vomiting, sedation, skin irritation (topical), stomach rupture, tachycardia; | **Interactions:** ACTIVATED CHARCOAL (charcoal adsorbs/inactivates ipecac), bismuth subsalicylate (reduced vomiting following ipecac), CNS depressants (additive effects), THC (altered effects); | **Dose:** Emetic, adults: 15–30 mL, followed by 200–300 mL of water; repeat dose one time if vomiting does not occur within 20 min; children, 6–12 months: 5–10 mL followed by 10–20 mL/kg of water; repeat dose one time if vomiting does not occur within

20 minutes; children, 1–12 years: 15 mL, followed by 10–20 mL/kg of water; repeat dose one time if vomiting does not occur within 20 minutes; | **Monitor:** Blood pressure, electrolytes, heart rate, symptoms of poisoning; | **Notes:** Ipecac is used in an emergency setting for certain types of poisonings. It causes the patient to vomit. The American Academy of Pediatrics recommends that ipecac syrup NOT be stocked at home. The emesis produced by ipecac administration can reduce the effects of many drugs if administered within 1 hour of ingestion.

iron | **Uses:** Anemia of chronic disease, ACE inhibitor–associated cough, attention-deficit hyperactivity disorder (ADHD), cognitive function, fatigue (in women with low ferritin levels), iron deficiency anemia, lead toxicity, preventing iron deficiency anemia (after blood donation, due to gastrointestinal bleeding, exercising women, pregnancy, preterm/low birth weight infants, menstruating women, treatment of predialysis anemia); | **Preg:** Pregnant or breastfeeding women should seek medical advice before taking dietary supplements. FDA Pregnancy Category B: Usually safe, but benefits must outweigh the risks. FDA Pregnancy Category C: Safety for use during pregnancy has not been established for replenishing depleted iron stores in the bone marrow where it is incorporated into hemoglobin; | **CIs:** Allergy/hypersensitivity, Anemia not caused by iron deficiency, High doses, Iron overload; | **ADRs:** abdominal pain, anorexia, arthralgia, arthritis, black teeth, cardiovascular disease, constipation, dark stool, DEATH, diarrhea, dyspnea, fatigue, <u>gastrointestinal irritation</u>, gonadal failure (early menopause, impotence, loss of libido), hemosiderosis, hyperhydrosis, ↑ iron accumulation, nausea, vomiting, weakness; | **Interactions:** Acacia (forms insoluble gel with ferric iron), acetohydroxamic acid (↓ acetohydroxamic acid), allopurinol (↑ iron storage), aminosalicylic acid (↓ iron levels), antacids (↓ iron levels), aspirin (↑ iron deficiency), bile acid sequestrants (↓ iron levels), bisphosphonates (↓ absorption of bisphosphonates), calcium (↓ absorption of heme and nonheme iron), chloramphenicol (↓ response to iron therapy), coffee/tea (↓ iron levels), dairy (↓ iron levels), desferrioxamine (↓ iron levels), dimercaprol (produces harmful chemical when combined with iron), EPO-R (↓ iron levels in bone), acidic agents (↑ iron absorption), H2 blockers (↓ iron levels), levodopa (chelates with levodopa; ↓ levodopa absorption), levothyroxine (↓ levothyroxine absorption), methyldopa (↓ methyldopa absorption), mycophenolate mofetil (↓ mycophenolate mofetil absorption), pancreatic enzyme supplements (↓ iron levels), penicillamine (↓ iron levels), quinolones (↓ absorption of quinolones; ↓ iron levels), riboflavin (improves hematological response to iron supplements), soy (↓ absorption of nonheme iron), tetracycline (↓ absorption of tetracyclines; ↓ iron levels), zinc (interferes with each absorption); | **Dose:** The Recommended Dietary Allowance (RDA) for men (19–50 years) is 8 mg daily; women (19–50 years) 18 mg daily; adults (51 years and older) 8 mg daily; pregnant women (all ages) 27 mg daily; breastfeeding women (19 years and older) 9 mg daily. Upper intake level (UL), ages 14 years and older: 45 mg/day elemental iron; UL for infants and children: 40 mg/day elemental iron; iron deficiency anemia, adults: 50–100 mg tid elemental iron; | **Monitor:** Iron status of the pregnant woman should be measured early (before the 15th week of gestation), and iron supplements should be given as selective prophylaxis based on the serum ferritin level; | **Notes:** There are two forms of dietary iron: heme and nonheme. Sources of heme iron include meat, fish, and poultry. Sources of nonheme iron, which is not absorbed as well as heme iron, include beans, lentils, flours, cereals, and other plant products. Use cautiously in patients with diabetes, gastroenteritis, peptic ulcer disease, ulcerative cholitis, achlorhydria, hemodialysis, hemoglobin diseases, and malabsorption syndromes, and in premature infants.

isoflavones | **Uses:** Isoflavones are produced only by plants in legumes and beans in the Fabaceae (also known as Leguminosae) family. Foods that contain high amounts of isoflavones include soy, peanuts, chick peas, alfalfa, fava beans, and kudzu. When consumed by humans, isoflavones may behave like estrogen in the body. See individual monographs for specific uses; | **Preg:** Not recommended due to insufficient evidence and possible hormonal effects; | **CIs:** Allergy/hypersensitivity, Hormone-sensitive disorders; | **ADRs:** adverse effects related to estrogenic effects; | **Interactions:** Estrogens (additive effects); | **Dose:** Varies; | **Monitor:** Estrogen levels, hormone panel; | **Notes:** It is unclear whether phytoestrogens (such as isoflavones) exert estrogenic or antiestrogenic effects.

isomaltulose | **Uses:** Diabetes, plaque; | **Preg:** Not recommended due to insufficient evidence; | **CIs:** Allergy/hypersensitivity, Disorders in fructose metabolism, Sucrase-isomaltase deficiency; | **ADRs:** insufficient evidence; | **Interactions:** Antidiabetic agents (altered effects); | **Dose:** Insufficient evidence; | **Monitor:** Blood glucose; | **Notes:** Isomaltulose (Palatinose) is a highly sweet disaccharide that occurs naturally in honey and sugar cane. Commercially, it is produced enzymatically from sucrose and reportedly has a low glycemic index.

ivy gourd *(Coccinia indica)* **Uses:** Diabetes; **Preg:** Not recommended due to insufficient evidence; **CIs:** Allergy/hypersensitivity; **ADRs:** appears well tolerated; studies have reported abdominal distention, constipation, flatulence, gastritis; **Interactions:** Antidiabetic agents (additive effects/↑ risk of hypoglycemia), vitamin E (↓ levels), may interact with agents with similar effects or related mechanisms of action (antilipemic, antioxidant, cardiovascular); **Dose:** Oral: 1 g alcoholic extracts daily for 90 days; freeze-dried leaves may be taken as powder or in capsules; **Monitor:** Lipid panel, liver function tests, renal function tests, blood glucose; **Notes:** According to the United States Preventative Services Task Force Level I, American Diabetes Association Guidelines, Level A, preliminary evidence suggests that *Coccinia indica* in diabetes warrants further study for a potential role in treating diabetes.

jackfruit *(Artocarpus heterophyllus)* **Uses:** Hyperglycemia; **Preg:** Fruit is likely safe in food amounts in pregnant or breastfeeding patients based on traditional use. Other parts are not recommended due to lack of sufficient evidence; **CIs:** Allergy/hypersensitivity; **ADRs:** ↑ coagulation, erectile dysfunction, impaired sexual desire and performance, ↓ libido, ↓ sexual arousal; **Interactions:** Anticoagulants/antiplatelets (↑ risk of bleeding); antidiabetic agents (↑ risk of hypoglycemia), may interact with agents with similar effects or related mechanisms of action (antibiotic, antifungal, antiviral, antifertility, immunostimulant, antilibido); **Dose:** Aqueous leaf extract: 20 g/kg PO; **Monitor:** Blood glucose, coagulation panel; **Notes:** Available research examines the role of jackfruit leaves in increasing glucose tolerance.

J

Japanese knotweed *(Polygonum cuspidatum)* **Uses:** Insufficient evidence; **Preg:** Not recommended due to insufficient evidence; **CIs:** Allergy/hypersensitivity; **ADRs:** diarrhea, rash; **Interactions:** Anticoagulants/antiplatelets (↑ risk of bleeding), antilipemic agents (additive effects), CYP450 1A/2E1/3A4 substrates (inhibits CYP450 1A/2E1/3A4), estrogens (additive effects), NSAIDs (altered effects); **Dose:** Insufficient evidence; **Monitor:** Coagulation panel, estrogen levels; **Notes:** Japanese knotwood (or hu zhang) is considered a rich source of trans-resveratrol, as well as emodin, resveratrol, emodin-8-O-D-glucoside, physcion, and piceid. Caution is warranted in patients with hormone-sensitive conditions.

jasmine *(Jasminum spp.)* **Uses:** Alertness, lactation suppression, memory improvement, stroke; **Preg:** Traditional medicine cautions against jasmine use during pregnancy; however, it has been used to ease the labor pain; | **Cls:** Allergy/hypersensitivity; Essential oil should not be ingested; | **ADRs:** dermatitis, poor concentration; | **Interactions:** May interact with agents with similar effects or related mechanisms of action (antifungal, antihypertensive, anxiolytic, diurectic); | **Dose:** Oral: Up to 30 g daily as tea or decoction, up to 10 mL tincture daily. Aromatherapy: 2–4 drops essential oil; | **Monitor:** Blood pressure; | **Notes:** The flowers and oil are used in perfumes, essential oils, and food flavorings such as that in jasmine-scented green tea.

jequirity *(Abrus precatorius)* | **Uses:** Insufficient clinical evidence; | **Preg:** Not recommended due to insufficient evidence and traditional use as an abortifacient; | **Cls:** Allergy/hypersensitivity, Pediatric use, Seeds (ORAL USE); | **ADRs:** abdominal cramps, ↓ appetite, cerebral edema, circulatory collapse, coma, DEATH, dehydration, dermatitis, diarrhea, dyspnea, edema, emphysema, endothelial cell damage, erosions of the abomasal and intestinal epithelium, GASTROENTERITIS (SEVERE), hepatic necrosis, hypertension, nausea, necrotizing conjunctivitis, pulmonary edema, pulmonary hemorrhage, renal necrosis, tachycardia, vascular leak syndrome, vomiting; | **Interactions:** May interact with agents with similar effects or related mechanisms of action (anticoagulant, antihypertensive, hepatotoxic, nephrotoxic); | **Dose:** Insufficient evidence; | **Monitor:** Coagulation panel, liver function tests, renal function tests, vital signs; | **Notes:** Abrin, a constituent of *Abrus precatorius*, is toxic at 5 mg, and ingestion of one bean by a child may be fatal. Severe gastroenteritis may occur; symptoms may not appear for several days.

J

jewelweed *(Impatiens biflora, Impatiens pallida)* | **Uses:** Contact dermatitis (topical); | **Preg:** Not recommended due to insufficient evidence; | **Cls:** Allergy/hypersensitivity, Large consumption; | **ADRs:** jewelweed contains high mineral content, particularly calcium oxalate, which can lead to adverse reactions and toxicity; ↑ risk of renal calculi; | **Interactions:** Diuretics (additive effects); | **Dose:** Insufficient evidence; | **Monitor:** Calcium oxalate levels; | **Notes:** Jewelweed is used as a natural poison ivy treatment. Traditionally used as a food source as well as medicinally to treat a variety of ailments; however, owing to a potential high mineral content, it is considered dangerous when consumed in excess amounts.

jianpi wenshen recipe | **Uses:** Hepatitis B; | **Preg:** Not recommended due to insufficient evidence; | **Cls:** Allergy/

hypersensitivity; **ADRs:** insufficient evidence; **Interactions:** Insufficient evidence; **Dose:** Administered as tea or in pill form; **Monitor:** Insufficient evidence; **Notes:** Jianpi wenshen recipe is a mixture of herbs used in traditional Chinese medicine to treat a number of conditions, including hepatitis B. However, the available evidence does not support efficacy.

jiaogulan *(Gynostemma pentaphyllum)* **Uses:** Cancer, hypercholesterolemia, steatosis; **Preg:** Avoid use due to possible teratogenic effects; **CIs:** Allergy/hypersensitivity, Pregnancy/lactation; **ADRs:** insufficient evidence; **Interactions:** Anticoagulants/antiplatelets (↑ risk of bleeding), antilipemic agents (additive effects), immunosuppressants (interfere with effects); may interact with agents with similar effects or related mechanisms of action (anticancer, anti-inflammatory, hepatotoxic, antidiabetic); **Dose:** Oral: extract, 80 mL daily for 4 months; **Monitor:** Blood glucose, coagulation panel, lipid profile, LFTs; **Notes:** Jiaogulan is best known as a traditional Chinese medicine herb; it is commonly used to counteract aging.

J

jimson weed *(Datura stramonium)* **Uses:** Insufficient clinical evidence; **Preg:** Contraindicated due to extreme toxicity; **CIs:** Allergy/hypersensitivity, Oral or inhaled use, Constipation, Down syndrome, Esophageal Reflux, Fever, Gastric ulcer, GI infection, Hiatal hernia, Narrow-angle glaucoma, Obstructive GI tract conditions, Tachyarrhythmias, Toxic megacolon, Ulcerative colitis, Urinary retention; **ADRs:** abnormal behavior, amnesia, arrhythmia, bleeding, blurred vision, coma, DEATH, delirium, dipsia, disorientation, dry mucous membranes, dysuria, fever, hallucinations, hepatotoxicity, hypertension, mydriasis, nephrotoxicity, respiratory arrest, restlessness, seizures, tachycardia, xerostomia; **Interactions:** Alcohol (↑ effects), anticholinergic agents (↑ anticholinergic effects), CNS depressants (additive effects), digoxin (↑ effects), may interact with agents with similar effects or related mechanisms of action (alkaloid, analgesic, cardiac, antiasthmatic, anticoagulant, antidepressant, antihypertensive, antimicrobial, antipsychotic, antiepileptic, antitumor, beta-adrenergic, diuretic, hepatotoxic, immunomodulatory, muscarinic, narcotic, sedative, stimulant, hallucinatory); **Dose:** Insufficient evidence; **Monitor:** Blood pressure, coagulation panel, EEG, heart rate, iron levels, lactate dehydrogenase, LFTs, WBC count; **Notes:** Not to be confused with *Datura wrightii*, also known as Jimson weed. Jimson weed contains hyoscyamine and scopolamine, which are responsible for its anticholinergic effects.

jointed flatsedge *(Cyperus articulatus)* | **Uses:** Insufficient clinical evidence; | **Preg:** Not recommended due to insufficient evidence; | **CIs:** Allergy/hypersensitivity; | **ADRs:** none; | **Interactions:** May interact with agents with similar effects or related mechanisms of action (antiepileptic, sedative); | **Dose:** Insufficient clinical evidence; | **Monitor:** Insufficient clinical evidence; | **Notes:** Adrue is the "medicine" from the rhizome of jointed flatsedge and is the plant's active ingredient.

jojoba *(Simmondsia chinensis)* | **Uses:** Dementia, mosquito repellent; | **Preg:** Not recommended due to insufficient evidence and possible adverse effects to the fetus; | **CIs:** Allergy/hypersensitivity, Oral consumption; | **ADRs:** contact dermatitis, distention of the small intestine, gastrointestinal upset, ↑ growth hormone, leukocytosis, ↑ thyroxine; | **Interactions:** May interact with agents with similar effects or related mechanisms of action (anti-inflammatory, appetite suppressant, antilipemic, mosquito repellant); | **Dose:** Insufficient evidence; | **Monitor:** Lipid profile, hormone panel, WBC counts; | **Notes:** Jojoba oil is used most commonly as a carrier oil for topical application or aromatherapy.

J

juniper *(Juniperus communis)* | **Uses:** Insufficient clinical evidence; | **Preg:** Not recommended due to insufficient evidence and traditional use as an abortifacient; | **CIs:** Allergy/hypersensitivity, Pregnancy; | **ADRs:** abortion, albuminuria, burns, convulsions, dysmenorrhea, hematuria, hepatotoxicity, hyper-/hypoglycemia, hyper-/hypotension, irritation, nephrotoxicity, purple urine, skin damage, tachycardia; | **Interactions:** Anticoagulants/antiplatelets (↑ risk of bleeding), antidiabetes agents (↑ risk of hypoglycemia), antihypertensive agents (altered effects), diuretics (interfere with therapy); | **Dose:** Oral: essential oil, up to 100 mg daily; dried berries, 2–3 g 3–4 times daily as infusion; tincture, 1–2 mL 3 times daily; | **Monitor:** Blood glucose, coagulation panel, renal function panel; | **Notes:** Juniper berries or berry extracts are used as a fragrance, flavoring, and spice in small amounts. Juniper has been used as a berry tea to treat indigestion, eczema, and other skin diseases.

kamut | **Uses:** Insufficient clinical evidence; | **Preg:** Not recommended due to insufficient evidence; | **CIs:** Allergy/hypersensitivity; | **ADRs:** allergic reactions; | **Interactions:** Insufficient evidence; | **Dose:** Insufficient evidence; | **Monitor:** N/A; | **Notes:** Kamut is a high-protein grain and sometimes used as replacement for wheat flour.

katuka *(Picrorhiza kurroa)* | **Uses:** Insufficient clinical evidence; | **Preg:** Not recommended due to insufficient evidence; | **CIs:** Allergy/hypersensitivity, Autoimmune diseases; | **ADRs:** anorexia, diarrhea, giddiness, immunosuppression, pruritus, rash, vomiting; | **Interactions:** Immunosuppressants (interfere with therapy); may interact with agents with similar effects or related mechanisms of action (antidiabetic, antilipemic, antineoplastic, hepatotoxic); | **Dose:** Insufficient evidence; | **Monitor:** Insufficient evidence; | **Notes:** Usually the root or rhizome of the plant is used traditionally for treating diabetes.

kava *(Piper methysticum)* | **Uses:** Anxiety, benzodiazepine withdrawal, cancer, insomnia, menopausal anxiety, stress; | **Preg:** Discouraged due to possible decreases in uterine tone; | **CIs:** Allergy/hypersensitivity, Concomitant use with CNS depressants, Long-term use, Hepatic dysfunction, Pregnancy/lactation, Parkinson's disease; | **ADRs:** allergic reactions, anorexia, apathy, cirrhosis, DEATH, dizziness, drowsiness, dyspnea, electrocardiogram abnormalities, erythrocytosis, extrapyrmidal side effects (torticollis, oculogyric crisis, and oral dyskinesias), eye irritation, fatigue, fulminant liver failure, gastrointestinal upset, GI distress, headache, hematuria, hepatitis, HEPATOTOXICITY, hypertension, jaundice, ↓ lymphocyte counts, malcoordination, meningismus, mood changes, palpitations, paresthesias, reduced platelet volume, reduced serum albumin, rhabdomyolysis, sedation, sleeplessness, tachycardia, tremor, urticaria, vivid dreams, xerosis; | **Interactions:** Anesthesia (↑ effects), anticancer drugs (may alter pharmacokinetics), CNS DEPRESSANTS (↑ of sedation), CYP450 1A2/2C9/2C19/2D6/2E1/3A4 substrates (inhibits CYP 1A2/2C9/2C19/2D6/2E1/3A4), dopamine (antagonistic effects), HEPATOTOXIC AGENTS (↑ risk of liver damage), levodopa (↓ effectiveness of levodopa), P-glycoprotein substrates (inhibits p-glycoprotein efflux; ↑ drug levels of P-gp substrates); drugs that cause extrapyramidal symptoms (additive effects); may interact with agents with similar effects or related mechanisms of action (ACE inhibitors, diuretic, analgesic, anesthetic, antineoplastic, antidepressant, anticoagulants, hormonal, dopaminergic, neurologic); | **Dose:** Oral: 50–280 mg kava lactones daily at bedtime; 60–120 mg kavapyrones daily at bedtime; | **Monitor:** Albumin, bilirubin, LFTs, RBC count, WBC count; | **Notes:** Sales of kava have been banned in several countries owing to concerns of hepatotoxicity; however, it is still legal in the Unites States. It should be used cautiously as it may cause hepatotoxicity.

K

kefir | **Uses:** Bacterial infections, hyperlipidemia, lactose intolerance; | **Preg:** Not recommended due to insufficient evidence; | **CIs:** Allergy/hypersensitivity; | **ADRs:** abdominal cramping, constipation, diarrhea; | **Interactions:** Antilipemic agents (additive effects), immunosuppressants (altered effects); | **Dose:** 125–500 mL PO qd; | **Monitor:** Lipid profile; | **Notes:** Kefir contains bacteria that may alter the immune system and should be used with caution in immunocompromised patients.

khat *(Catha edulis)* | **Uses:** Cognitive function; | **Preg:** Contraindicated due to birth defects and ↓ birth weight; | **CIs:** Allergy/hypersensitivity, Pregnancy, Psychotic disorders, Glaucoma, Lactation, Prolonged use, Driving; | **ADRs:** aggressiveness, ↑ alertness, anorexia, ↓ appetite, ↑ breathing rate, constipation, delusions, dependency, depression, hallucinations, ↑ heartbeat (tachycardia), hemorrhoidal disease, hyperactivity, hyper-/hypotension, hyper-/hypothermia, inflamed stomach (gastritis), insomnia, irritability, malnutrition, mood swings, mouth cancer, mouth infections, mydriasis, myocardial infarction, nervousness, nightmares, paranoia, parasite infection, straining, talkativeness; | **Interactions:** Antibiotics (↓ ampicillin and amoxicillin availability), bromocriptine (↓ khat addiction), MAO INHIBITORS (↑ risk of hypertensive crisis), may interact with agents with similar effects or related mechanisms of action (adrenergic, antihypertensive, beta-adrenergic, CNS stimulant, antidepressants); | **Dose:** Oral: 100–200 g fresh leaves (chewed and juice swallowed); | **Monitor:** Insufficient evidence; | **Notes:** It is unknown whether khat is physically addictive, yet it has been associated with psychological dependence. It is illegal in the United States. It contains cathine and cathinone, powerful stimulants.

khella *(Ammi visnaga)* | **Uses:** Psoriasis, vitiligo; | **Preg:** Contraindicated due to uterine stimulation effects; | **CIs:** Allergy/hypersensitivity, Pregnancy; | **ADRs:** angina, anorexia, constipation, dizziness, dyspnea, headaches, hepatotoxicity, itchy or swollen skin, ↑ liver enzymes, nausea, permanent jaundice, photosensitivity, skin cancer, skin rashes, sleep disturbances, tightness in throat or chest, urticaria; | **Interactions:** Digoxin (↓ effectiveness), hepatotoxic drugs (↑ risk of liver damage), photosensitizers (↑ photosensitivity); | **Dose:** Oral: extract, 30–60 drops 3–5 times daily; 1 tsp crushed seeds as an infusion. Topical: 2% khellin 3 times weekly; | **Monitor:** Lipid profile, LFTs; | **Notes:** The active constituents are khellin, visnagin, and visnadin. High doses may cause liver damage.

kinetin | **Uses:** Cataract, Ménière's disease, ocular disorders; | **Preg:** Not recommended due to insufficient evidence; | **CIs:** Allergy/hypersensitivity; | **ADRs:** bleeding; | **Interactions:** Anticoagulants/antiplatelets (↑ risk of bleeding), may interact with agents with similar effects or related mechanisms of action (antioxidant, antineoplastic); | **Dose:** Insufficient evidence; | **Monitor:** Coagulation panel; | **Notes:** Kinetin is a chemical analogue of cytokinins, a class of plant hormones that promotes cell division.

kiwi *(Actinidia deliciosa, Actinidia chinensis)* | **Uses:** Asthma (prevention), energy enhancement, respiratory problems (prevention); | **Preg:** Likely safe in food amounts in pregnant or breastfeeding patients based on traditional use. Other uses are not recommended due to lack of sufficient evidence; | **CIs:** Allergy/hypersensitivity, Cross-sensitivity with avocado and latex; | **ADRs:** angioedema, bleeding, collapse, cyanosis, diarrhea, dysphagia, dyspnea, hypertriglyceridemia, hypotension, mouth irritation, nausea, oral allergy syndrome (itching and tingling with or without edema of the lips, mouth and tongue), rhinitis, urticaria, vomiting; | **Interactions:** Avocado (may have cross-sensitivity), may interact with agents with similar effects or related mechanisms of action (antifungal, antioxidant, antiplatelet, serotonergic, hypolipidemic); | **Dose:** Oral: 150–1,200 mL fresh juice, or equivalent as edible fruits; | **Monitor:** Coagulation panel, lipid profile, phosphate test, potassium, urine tests; | **Notes:** The kiwi fruit initially came from China but is now produced in New Zealand, the United States, Italy, South Africa, and Chile.

K

krebiozen | **Uses:** Insufficient clinical evidence; | **Preg:** Not recommended due to insufficient evidence; | **CIs:** Allergy/hypersensitivity, Cancer (not effective); | **ADRs:** mild icterus, pain; | **Interactions:** Insufficient evidence; | **Dose:** Insufficient evidence; | **Monitor:** Insufficient evidence; | **Notes:** Krebiozen, originally called substance X, is derived from horses inoculated with *Actinomyces bovis*. It has been claimed to be useful in the treatment of spontaneous cancer, although the available evidence is insufficient to support this use.

krill (*Euphausia* spp.) | **Uses:** Arthritis, dysmenorrhea, hyperglycemia, hyperlipidemia, premenstrual syndrome; | **Preg:** Insufficient evidence, although krill has been recommended as a nutritional supplement during pregnancy; | **CIs:** Allergy/hypersensitivity; | **ADRs:** diarrhea, dyspepsia, fishy taste, halitosis, nausea, skin oiliness; | **Interactions:** Anticoagulants/antiplatelets (↑ risk of bleeding), antidiabetic agents (↑ risk of hypoglycemia), antilipemic agents (additive effects), orlistat (↓ absorption of fatty acids); | **Dose:** Oral: 500 mg once daily (recommended); up to 3 g daily (in clinical trials); | **Monitor:** Coagulation panel, lipid profile; | **Notes:** Krill oil does not have FDA Generally Regarded as Safe (GRAS) status, although EPA and DHA, which are omega-3 fatty acids found in krill oil, do have FDA, GRAS status. Use cautiously in patients who are allergic to seafood.

kudzu *(Pueraria lobata)* | **Uses:** Alcoholism, cardiovascular disease/angina, deafness, diabetes, diabetic retinopathy, glaucoma, ischemic stroke, menopausal symptoms; | **Preg:** Not recommended due to insufficient evidence; | **CIs:** Allergy/hypersensitivity, Concurrent methotrexate use, Hormone-sensitive conditions; | **ADRs:** hypothermia, rash, weight loss; | **Interactions:** Alcohol (↓ intake), anticoagulants/antiplatelets (↑ risk of bleeding), antidiabetic agents (↑ risk of hypoglycemia), antihypertensive agents (↑ risk of hypotension), benzodiazepines (↓ effects), estrogens (additive or antagonistic effects), mecamylamine (↓ effects), methotrexate (↑ risk of toxicity of MTX), tamoxifen (interfere with effects), vasodilators (additive effects); | **Dose:** Oral: root extract, 50 mg–1.2 g daily by mouth in divided doses; puerarin, 400 mg daily for 10 days. Parenteral: puerarin, 500 mg daily for 2 weeks; | **Monitor:** Alcohol intake, blood glucose, BUN, calcium levels, estrogen levels, hormone profile, LFTs, lipid profile; | **Notes:** Kudzu has been used traditionally to treat a number of ailments.

labrador tea *(Ledum groenlandicum)* | **Uses:** Insufficient clinical evidence; | **Preg:** Avoid due to abortifacient effects; | **CIs:** Allergy/hypersensitivity, Orally in large amounts, Pregnancy; | **ADRs:** abdominal pain, DEATH (large amounts), delirium (large amounts), diarrhea, drowsiness, headache, paralysis (large amounts), symptoms of intoxication; | **Interactions:** CNS depressants (additive sedation); | **Dose:** Insufficient evidence; | **Monitor:** Insufficient evidence; | **Notes:** As a folk medicine, the tea was used externally for all kinds of skin problems. Taken internally, the tea was used to stimulate the nerves and stomach. Syrup made from the tea was sometimes used for cough and hoarseness. However, high amounts may be fatal.

Lactobacillus acidophilus | **Uses:** Allergy treatment (Japanese cedar pollen), asthma, bacterial vaginosis, diarrhea (prevention/treatment), hepatic encephalopathy, hyperlipidemia, irritable bowel syndrome (IBS), lactose intolerance, necrotizing enterocolitis, vaginal candidiasis; | **Preg:** Likely safe in food amounts in pregnant or breastfeeding patients based on traditional use. Other uses are cautioned due to lack of sufficient evidence; | **CIs:** Allergy/hypersensitivity (dairy); Intestinal damage or recent surgery, Severe immunocompromise; | **ADRs:** abdominal discomfort, burning or irritation in the vagina when used vaginally, flatulence; | **Interactions:** Antibiotics (↓ effectiveness of *Lactobacillus acidophilus*), benzodiazepines (↑ side effects), birth control (↑ side effects), immunosuppressants (↑ risk of infection), sulfasalazine (↓ effects); | **Dose:** Oral: up to 10 billion viable bacteria (CFU) daily in divided doses. Vaginal: up to 2 tablets (1 billion CFU per tablet) twice daily. Anal suppository: 1.5 g daily; | **Monitor:** Bacterial counts, drug levels; | **Notes:** Considered a probiotic; beneficial because it produces vitamin K, lactase, and antimicrobial substances such as acidolin, acidolphilin, lactocidin, and bacteriocin. Use cautiously in patients with compromised immune systems.

***Lactobacillus* GG** | **Uses:** Antibiotic-associated diarrhea, atopic dermatitis, bacterial vaginosis, chemotherapy-induced diarrhea, *Clostridium difficile* diarrhea, diarrhea (prevention/treatment), *Helicobacter pylori*, improving or maintaining gut function, irritable bowel syndrome (IBS), pouchitis, respiratory infection, rotaviral diarrhea, traveler's diarrhea, ulcerative colitis, urinary tract infections, | **Preg:** Likely safe in food amounts in pregnant or breastfeeding patients based on traditional use. Other uses are cautioned due to lack of sufficient evidence; | **CIs:** Allergy/hypersensitivity; | **ADRs:** abdominal cramps; | **Interactions:** Antibiotics (↓ effectiveness of *Lactobacillus* GG), benzodiazepines (↑ side effects), birth control (↑ side effects), immunosuppressants (↑ risk of infection), sulfasalazine (↓ effects); | **Dose:** Oral: up to 10 billion CFU daily for 8 weeks; | **Monitor:** Bacterial counts, drug levels; | **Notes:** Considered a probiotic; beneficial because it produces vitamin K, lactase, and antimicrobial substances such as acidolin, acidolphilin, lactocidin, and bacteriocin. Use cautiously in patients with compromised immune systems.

ladies mantle *(Alchemilla vulgaris)* | **Uses:** Insufficient clinical evidence; | **Preg:** Not recommended due to insufficient evidence; traditionally used to aid conception and prevent excessive menstruation; | **CIs:** Allergy/hypersensitivity; | **ADRs:** insufficient evidence; | **Interactions:** Anticoagulants (possible procoagulant effects), iron (↓ iron absorption);

L

| **Dose:** Insufficient evidence; | **Monitor:** Coagulation panel, iron; | **Notes:** Fresh root is used traditionally to stop bleeding.

lady's slipper *(Cypripedium acaule, Cypripedium calceolus)* | **Uses:** Insufficient clinical evidence; | **Preg:** Not recommended due to insufficient evidence; | **CIs:** Allergy/hypersensitivity; | **ADRs:** blistering, dermatitis, giddiness, hallucinations, headache, mental excitement, restlessness; | **Interactions:** Antimalarials/quinine (additive effects/lady's slipper contains quinines), cardiac glycosides (↑ risk of adverse effects), digoxin (↑ risk of adverse effects), CNS depressants (additive effects); | **Dose:** Oral: dried root, 2–4 g as tea; liquid extract, 2–4 mL 3 times daily; capsules, one to two 570-mg capsules 3 times daily with meals; | **Monitor:** Insufficient evidence; | **Notes:** Adverse effects of lady's slipper are not well documented in the available literature. Oral use may cause hallucinations.

lathyrus | **Uses:** Insufficient evidence; | **Preg:** Not recommended due to insufficient evidence; | **CIs:** Allergy/hypersensitivity, ORAL USE (HIGH AMOUNTS OR PROLONGED USE; SEEDS ARE NEUROTOXIC); | **ADRs:** alopecia, angiolathyrism (blood vessel changes), convulsions, DEATH, muscle rigidity, neurogenic bladder, neurolathyrism (neurogenerative disease), NEUROTOXICITY, occupational asthma, osteolathyrism (bone pain and skeletal deformities), shallow breathing, spasticity; | **Interactions:** Anticoagulants/antiplatelets (↑ risk of bleeding); | **Dose:** Insufficient evidence; | **Monitor:** Coagulation panel; | **Notes:** *Lathyrus* is a genus in the pea family and contains species such as *Lathyrus sativus* (grass pea) and *Lathyrus odorata* (sweet pea). Grass pea is used as a famine food, especially in India, the Middle East, and parts of Asia, because the plants are extremely hardy and the seeds are high in protein. Large quantities of the seeds (approximately 400 g *Lathyrus sativus* seeds daily or > 30% of the diet) can cause neurolathyrism (neurogenerative disease), osteolathyrism (bone pain and skeletal deformities), or angiolathyrism (blood vessel changes).

lavender *(Lavandula angustifolia)* | **Uses:** Agitation, alopecia, antibacterial (topical), antispasmodic, anxiety, cancer (perillyl alcohol), cognitive performance, dementia, depression, eczema, insomnia (aromatherapy), otalgia, overall well-being, pain (low back, neck, rheumatic), perineal discomfort following childbirth (bathing), postpartum recovery; | **Preg:** Not recommended due to insufficient evidence and traditional use as an emmenagogue; **CIs:** Allergy/hypersensitivity, Children, Pregnancy; **ADRs:** anemia, anorexia, bleeding, chills (after inhalation), constipation, contact dermatitis, fatigue, gastrointestinal upset, gynecomastia, headache, lipid changes, photosensitivity, nausea, skin pigmentation changes, vomiting; **Interactions:** Anticoagulants/antiplatelets (↑ risk of bleeding), CNS depressants (additive sedation), photosensitizers (↑ risk of skin damage); may interact with agents with similar effects or related mechanisms of action (Alzheimer's agents, analgesics, anesthetics, anxiolytics, antibiotics, antidepressants, antiepileptics, antifungals, antihypertensives, antilipemics, antineoplastics, antispasmodics, neurologicals); **Dose:** Oral: 1–2 tsp dried herb as tea; 800–1,200 mg/m^2 of a 50:50 POH:soybean oil preparation 4 times daily. Inhalation (aromatherapy): 2–4 drops oil in 2–3 c boiling water; up to 10% lavender oil. Topical: 60 drops tincture, dried lavender flowers added to bath, or 20% lavender oil applied as needed; **Monitor:** Coagulation panel, lipid profile; **Notes:** Undiluted essential oil of lavender may be poisonous if taken PO.

L-carnitine **Uses:** Angina (chronic stable), ADHD, AIDS, alcoholism, Alzheimer's disease, arrhythmia, asthenospermia, cerebral ischemia, cirrhosis, congestive heart failure, dementia (elderly), depression, diabetes mellitus, diabetic neuropathy, dialysis (CAPD; hemodialysis), diphtheria, end-stage renal disease, erectile dysfunction, exercise performance, fatigue, fragile X syndrome, hepatic encephalopathy, low birth weight, Huntington's chorea/disease, hyperlipoproteinemia, hyperthyroidism, L-carnitine deficiency, lactic acidosis, memory, miscarriage, myocardial infarction, myocarditis, nutritional deficiencies (primary and secondary carnitine deficiency in adults; full-term infants; premature infants), obesity, peripheral neuropathy, peripheral vascular disease, Peyronie's disease, respiratory distress (adults), respiratory distress (infants), Rett's syndrome, sickle cell disease, surgical uses (bypass), tuberculosis; **Preg:** Not recommended due to insufficient evidence; **CIs:** Allergy/hypersensitivity; **ADRs:** abdominal discomfort, aggression, alopecia, body odor, depression, diarrhea, dyspepsia, euphoria, fatigue, fishy odor, gastralgia, gastrointestinal symptoms, insomnia, mania, nausea, nervousness, skin rash, vomiting; **Interactions:** Adefovir dipivoxil (↓ carnitine levels), Adriamycin (↓ Adriamycin-induced arrhythmia), antiarrhythmics (↓ need for antiarrhythmics), anticoagulants/antiplatelets (↑ risk of bleeding), anticonvulsants (phenobarbital, phenytoin, carbamazepine; ↓ carnitine levels), beta blockers (↓ need for beta blockers), calcium channel blockers (↓ need for calcium channel blockers), cefditoren pivoxil (↓ carnitine levels),

L

cephalosporin (↓ carnitine levels), cinnoxicam (↑ effects), cisplastin (↑ carnitine excretion), D-carnitine (compete for transport systems), digoxin (↓ need for digoxin), diuretics (↓ need for diuretics), antilipemic agents (↓ need for hypolipidemic drugs), ifosfamide (↓ carnitine levels), interleukins (↓ side effects associated with interleukin-2), isotretinoin (↓ levels), nortriptyline (↓ side effects associated with nortriptyline), nucleoside analogues (↓ side effects), paclitaxel (↓ paclitaxel-induced neuropathy), penicillin derivatives (↓ carnitine levels), potassium chloride (↓ potassium chloride–induced rhabdomyolysis), propafenone (↑ effects), pyrimethamine (↓ carnitine levels), sildenafil (↑ effects), sulfadiazine (↓ carnitine levels), thyroid hormones (antagonistic effects), valproic acid (↓ carnitine levels), zidovudine (↓ carnitine levels); | **Dose:** Oral: 1.5–6 g daily (adults), up to 3 g daily (younger than 18 years), | **Monitor:** Blood glucose, BUN, carnitine levels, CD4/CD8 counts, coagulation panel, creatinine, glycerol, immune parameters, insulin, ketone bodies, LFTs, lipid profile, phosphorus, myoglobin, thyroid function panel, WBC count; | **Notes:** D-carnitine or DL-carnitine may cause secondary L-carnitine deficiency and should not be used.

L

lecithin | **Uses:** Alzheimer's disease/dementia, athletic performance, dermatitis, dry skin, Friedreich's ataxia, gallstones, hepatic steatosis, hepatitis, hyperlipidemia, mania, memory/cognitive disorders, Parkinson's disease, respiratory distress, sleep disorders, stress-related disorders, tardive dyskinesia, TPN; | **Preg:** Not recommended due to insufficient evidence; | **CIs:** Allergy/hypersensitivity; | **ADRs:** abdominal discomfort, agitation, body odor, halitosis, hepatotoxicity, nausea; | **Interactions:** Antilipemic agents (additive effects), cholinesterase inhibitors (altered effects), diclofenac (synergistic effects), hepatotoxic agents (↑ risk of liver damage); | **Dose:** 30 mg–50 g PO qd; | **Monitor:** LFTs; | **Notes:** Lecithin is a phospholipid found in egg yolks, organ meats, nuts, and spinach. It contains phosphatidylcholine, which contains choline.

lemon balm ***(Melissa officinalis)*** | **Uses:** Agitation in dementia, anxiety, cognitive (mental) performance, colic, colitis, dyspepsia (indigestion), herpes simplex virus infections, sleep quality; | **Preg:** Not recommended due to lack of sufficient data and possible emmenagogue and hormonal effects; | **CIs:** Allergy/hypersensitivity; | **ADRs:** ↓ alertness, diarrhea, dizziness, drowsiness, ↑ intraocular pressure, nausea, palpitations, skin irritation, wheezing; | **Interactions:** Alcohol (additive sedation), CNS depressants (additive sedation), nicotine (↓ effects), scopolamine (↓ effects), may interact with agents with similar effects or related mechanisms of action (glaucoma medications, thyroid agents, SSRIs); | **Dose:** Oral: up to 4.5 g herb as tea, as needed; 2–6 mL tincture, 3 times daily; 60 drops extract daily; up to 10 g leaves or equivalent daily. Topical: 1% cream up to 4 times daily for 10 days; | **Monitor:** Intraocular pressure, prolactin, TSH; | **Notes:** Lemon balm has FDA Generally Recognized as Safe (GRAS) status. No serious side effects have been reported, although there is limited research of long-term effects.

lemongrass (*Cymbopogon* spp.) | **Uses:** Hypercholesterolemia, sedation; | **Preg:** Avoid use due to uterine stimulating effects; | **CIs:** Allergy/hypersensitivity, Pregnancy; | **ADRs:** burning, hypoglycemia, irritation, ↑ liver function tests, ↑ pancreatic tests, rash; | **Interactions:** CYP450 substrates (altered drug levels), may interact with agents with similar effects or related mechanisms of action (antihypertensive, antidiabetic); | **Dose:** Oral: 2 g or 2 tsp as tea; 140 mg oil daily for 90 days; | **Monitor:** Amylase, bilirubin, blood glucose, lipid profile, liver function tests; | **Notes:** General: lemongrass has Generally Regarded as Safe (GRAS) status in the United States. Based on allergy tests, a common side effect of lemongrass oil is rash, which occurs in 0.8%–1.6% of subjects.

L

lesser celandine *(Ranunculus ficaria)* | **Uses:** Insufficient clinical evidence; | **Preg:** Not recommended due to insufficient evidence; | **CIs:** Allergy/hypersensitivity, ORAL USE, Liver dysfunction; | **ADRs:** hepatotoxicity; | **Interactions:** Hepatotoxic agents (↑ risk of liver damage); | **Dose:** Insufficient evidence; | **Monitor:** Liver function tests; | **Notes:** All parts of the plant may be TOXIC.

licorice *(Glycyrrhiza glabra)* and deglycyrrhizinated licorice (DGL) | **Uses:** Adrenal insufficiency (Addison's disease), aphthous ulcer, aplastic anemia, atopic dermatitis, bleeding stomach ulcers caused by aspirin, dental hygiene, dyspepsia (functional), familial Mediterranean fever, hepatitis, herpes simplex virus, hyperkalemia (resulting abnormally low aldosterone), HIV, hyperprolactinemia (neuroleptic induced), idiopathic thrombocytopenic purpura, inflammation, muscle cramps, obesity, peptic ulcer disease, polycystic ovarian syndrome, upper respiratory tract infections (common cold), viral hepatitis, weight loss; | **Preg:** Contraindicated due to effects on hormones and associated with premature birth; | **CIs:** Allergy/hypersensitivity, Cardiovascular disease, Concurrent use with warfarin, Hormone-sensitive conditions, Hypertension, Hypokalemia, Kidney dysfunction, Pregnancy; | **ADRs:** acute pseudoaldosteronism syndrome, arrhythmias, asthenia, ↓ body fat mass, dropped head syndrome, electrolyte disturbances, headache, hyperprolactinemia, hypertension, hypertensive encephalopathy, myocardial infarction, nausea, nephrotoxicity, paralysis, rhabdomyolysis, ↓ testosterone (men), thyrotoxic periodic paralysis, vision loss, vomiting; | **Interactions:** General: ↑ absorption of drugs by glycyrrhetinic acid; antihypertensive agents (↓ effects), aspirin (↓ aspirin-induced fecal blood loss), benzodiazepines (↓ benzodiazepine withdrawal symptoms), cardiac glycosides (↑ risk of toxicity due to hypokalemia), cisplatin (↓ effects), corticosteroids (↑ effects), CYP450 2B6/2C9/3A4 (may inhibit or induce; altered drug levels), diuretics (thiazide; ↑ risk of hypokalemia), estrogens (additive or antagonistic effects), grapefruit (enhance effects of licorice), iron (↑ absorption), loop diuretics (↑ effects of licorice; ↑ risk of hypokalemia), nitrofurantoin (↓ side effects, ↑ bioavailability, ↑ excretion), phosphate (↑ licorice absorption), salt (↑ adverse effects), ursodeoxycholic acid (↑ effects), WARFARIN (induce CYP2C9, ↓ levels of warfarin); may interact with agents with similar effects or related mechanisms of action (agents used for adrenal insufficiency, aldose reductase inhibitory, aldosterone receptor antagonistic, ACE inhibitors, antiarrhythmic agents, antidepressants, antidiabetic, anti-inflammatory, hypolipidemic, antimicrobial, antineoplastic, antiobesity, antiulcer, antiviral, potassium-depleting, diuretic, hormonal, immunomodulatory, laxative, nephrotoxic); | **Dose:** Oral: 1–4 g daily in divided doses. Topical: 2% cream or gel applied 5 times daily for up to 14 days. Note: The expert panel German Commission E recommends limiting use to 4–6 weeks unless under direct medical supervision; | **Monitor:** 17-hydroxyprogesterone concentrations, blood pressure, ECG, electrolytes, LDH, lipid profile, LFTs, plasma renin, potassium, renal function test, testosterone, viral load; | **Notes:** Licorice can be processed to remove the glycyrrhiza, resulting in DGL (deglycyrrhizinated licorice), which does not appear to share the metabolic disadvantages of licorice.

lignans | **Uses:** Antioxidant, breast CA, cardiovascular disease, cervical CA, cognitive performance, colorectal CA, endometrial CA, hyperlipidemia, HTN, prostate CA, RA, thyroid CA; | **Preg:** Not recommended due to insufficient evidence and possible hormonal effects; | **CIs:** Allergy/hypersensitivity, Gastrointestinal obstruction, Hormone-sensitive conditions, Hypertriglyceridemia; | **ADRs:** abdominal pain, constipation, diarrhea, headache, pruritus; | **Interactions:** Alcohol (↑ effects of alcohol), antiandrogens (altered effects), anticoagulants/antiplatelets (↑ risk of bleeding), antidiabetic agents (↑ risk of hypoglycemia), antihypertensives (↑ risk of hypotension), antilipemic agents (additive effects), aromatase inhibitors (additive effects), CNS depressants (added sedation), CYP450 3A4 substrates (altered effects), digoxin (additive effects), estrogens (additive effects), furosemide (↓ absorption of furosemide), immunosuppressants (additive effects); | **Dose:** 300–500 mg PO qd; | **Monitor:** Blood glucose, coagulation panel, lipid profile; | **Notes:** The lignans are a group of chemical compounds found in whole grains, seeds, nuts, fruits, and vegetables, particularly in flaxseed and sesame seed. Caution is warranted in patients with bleeding disorders and diabetes.

lime *(Citrus aurantifolia)* | **Uses:** Cholera (prevention), iron deficiency, scurvy; | **Preg:** Likely safe in food amounts in pregnant or breastfeeding patients based on traditional use. Other uses are not recommended due to lack of sufficient evidence. | **CIs:** Allergy/hypersensitivity; | **ADRs:** diarrhea, headache, photosensitivity, ↓ tooth minerals; | **Interactions:** CYP450 3A4 substrates (inhibits CYP3A4; ↑ drug levels), digoxin (↑ digoxin transport), mannitol (↑ absorption), photosensitizers (↑ risk of phototoxicity); | **Dose:** Insufficient evidence; | **Monitor:** Electrolytes, renal function tests; | **Notes:** Lime oil contains oxypeucedanin, which may cause photosensitization.

L

lingonberry *(Vaccinium vitis-idaea)* | **Uses:** Urinary tract infection (prevention); | **Preg:** Fruit is likely safe in food amounts in pregnant or breastfeeding patients based on traditional use. Other uses are not recommended due to lack of sufficient evidence. | **CIs:** Allergy/hypersensitivity, Liver disease; | **ADRs:** hepatotoxicity, infertility (men; leaf), nausea, vomiting; | **Interactions:** Hepatotoxic agents (↑ risk of liver damage); may interact with agents with similar effects or related mechanisms of action (anthelmintic, antibiotic, anti-inflammatory, antineoplastic, antioxidant, antiviral, expectorant, antifertility, progestongenic); | **Dose:** Insufficient evidence; | **Monitor:** Bacterial counts, hormone panel, inflammatory markers, LFTs, parasite tests, viral titers; | **Notes:** Lingonberry is traditionally used as a food Scandinavia.

liver extract | **Uses:** Chronic fatigue syndrome, chronic hepatitis (hepatitis C), hepatic disorders, pernicious anemia, surgical uses (urological operation adjunct), | **Preg:** Not recommended due to insufficient evidence; | **CIs:** Allergy/hypersensitivity, Iron metabolism disorders; | **ADRs:** anaphylactic shock, asthmatic reaction, bronchospasm, collapse, cough, DEATH, dyspepsia, fluke infestation, hemochromatosis, hemorrhagic lesions, liver flukes, liver lesions, localized to generalized urticaria, nasal and ocular discharges, nausea, profound shock, pruritus, rigor, slight flushing, substernal pain, syncope, tachycardia, thrombosis, *Vibrio fetus*, vomiting, weakness; | **Interactions:** Human growth hormone (normalizes clearance rate in patients with liver dysfunction), may interact with agents with similar effects or related mechanisms of action (acid-producing, anticoagulant, antihyperlipidemic, antioxidant, antiviral, antineoplastic, immunomodulatory); | **Dose:** Oral: 500 mg extract 1–3 times daily; | **Monitor:** Coagulation panel, hemoglobin, iron, lipid profile, RBC counts; | **Notes:** Liver extract may have a high content of heme iron (3–4 mg/g). Some concern has been raised about the safety of liver extract, because it is made of animal liver, which may be infected with parasites, bacteria, or prion diseases; however, there is insufficient evidence to support these concerns.

liverwort (*Hepatica* ssp.) | **Uses:** Insufficient clinical evidence; | **Preg:** Not recommended due to insufficient evidence; | **CIs:** Allergy/hypersensitivity; | **ADRs:** altered lipid levels, contact dermatitis; | **Interactions:** May interact with agents that alter lipid levels; | **Dose:** Insufficient evidence; | **Monitor:** Lipid profile; | **Notes:** The allergenic component of a liverwort may be a sesquiterpene lactone.

L

lotus *(Nelumbo nucifera)* | **Uses:** Insufficient clinical evidence; | **Preg:** Not recommended due to insufficient evidence and possible antifertility effects; | **CIs:** Allergy/hypersensitivity; | **ADRs:** arrhythmias, bleeding, constipation, flatulence, GI irritation, hyper-/hypotension, hypoglycemia, infertility; | **Interactions:** Pentobarbitone (↑ sleeping time); may interact with agents with similar effects or related mechanisms of action (anticoagulant, antiarrhythmic, hypotensive, hypoglycemic, sedative); | **Dose:** Insufficient evidence; | **Monitor:** Blood glucose, coagulation panel; | **Notes:** Not to be confused with plants from the *Lotus* or *Nymphaea* genera, which are distantly related plants from other botanical families.

lousewort (*Pedicularis* spp.) | **Uses:** Insufficient clinical evidence; | **Preg:** Not recommended due to insufficient evidence; | **CIs:** Allergy/hypersensitivity; | **ADRs:** there are very few reports available or adverse effects associated with *Pedicularis*; | **Interactions:** May chelate iron, may interact with agents with similar effects or related mechanisms of action (anticancer, antioxidant); | **Dose:** Insufficient clinical evidence; | **Monitor:** Iron levels; | **Notes:** The genus *Pedicularis* contains several species referred to as louseworts. The common name was derived from the idea that livestock would get lice from eating the plant.

lovage *(Levisticum officinale)* | **Uses:** Insufficient clinical evidence; | **Preg:** Not recommended due to insufficient evidence and traditional use as an abortifacient; | **CIs:** Allergy/hypersensitivity, Edema, Pregnancy, Lactation, Renal disease; | **ADRs:** abortion, ↑ menstruation, photosensitivity, sodium retention; | **Interactions:** Anticoagulants/antiplatelets (↑ risk of bleeding), diuretics (additive effects), photosensitivity (↑ risk of phototoxicity); | **Dose:** Insufficient evidence; | **Monitor:** Coagulation panel, electrolytes; | **Notes:** Lovage is Generally Recognized as Safe for human consumption as a natural seasoning and flavoring agent by the FDA.

lutein | **Uses:** Antioxidant, atherosclerosis, cancer, cataracts, diabetes mellitus, lens opacities, lung function, macular degeneration, muscle soreness, obesity, pre-eclampsia, retinal degeneration, UV-induced erythema prevention/sunburn; | **Preg:** Likely safe in food amounts in pregnant or breastfeeding patients based on traditional use. Other uses are not recommended due to lack of sufficient evidence; | **CIs:** Allergy/hypersensitivity; | **ADRs:** ↑ cardiovascular disease risk, carotenodermia; | **Interactions:** Alcohol (↓ plasma lutein), beta-carotene (↑ bioavailability of beta-carotene), bile acid sequestrants (↓ lutein absorption), CYP450 substrates (altered drug levels), mineral oil (↓ lutein absorption), nicotine (↓ plasma lutein), orlistat (↓ lutein absorption), retinol (↑ plasma lutein), vitamin E (↓ vitamin E levels); may interact with agents with similar effects or related mechanisms of action (antidiabetic, antilipemic, antioxidant, antineoplastic); | **Dose:** Oral: up to 40 mg daily for 6 months; | **Monitor:** Blood glucose, erythrocyte parameters, lipid profile, markers of oxidative stress, serum tocopherols and carotenoids; | **Notes:** In general, there are no known side effects or precautions with regard to lutein. Strong data support the safety of up to 20 mL daily. Purified crystalline lutein is Generally Recognized as Safe (GRAS) based on animal toxicity studies.

lychee *(Litchi chinensis)* | **Uses:** Insufficient clinical evidence; | **Preg:** Likely safe in food amounts in pregnant or breastfeeding patients based on traditional use. Other uses are not recommended due to lack of sufficient evidence; | **CIs:** Allergy/hypersensitivity; | **ADRs:** rare allergic reactions (anaphylaxis, dermatitis, pruritus, urticaria, flushing, edema,

L

swelling of lips and tongue), dyspnea, epistaxis (excessive use), fever, restlessness; | **Interactions:** May interact with agents with similar effects or related mechanisms of action (analgesic, antidiabetic, anti-inflammatory, antilipemic, antineoplastic, antiviral, cardiovascular, immunomodulatory); | **Dose:** Insufficient evidence; | **Monitor:** Blood glucose, lipid profile; | **Notes:** Lychee fruit consumption is thought to help with gastrointestinal discomfort. According to secondary sources, Chinese people believe that excessive consumption (exact amounts unclear) of raw lychee causes fever and nosebleed.

lycopene | **Uses:** Age-related macular degeneration prevention, antioxidant, asthma (caused by exercise), atherosclerosis (coronary artery disease), benign prostatic hyperplasia (BPH), cancer prevention, cataracts, gingivitis, human papillomavirus, hypertension, infertility, lung cancer prevention, oral mucositis, pre-eclampsia, renal disease, sun protection; | **Preg:** Likely safe in food amounts in pregnant or breastfeeding patients based on traditional use. Other uses are not recommended due to lack of sufficient evidence; | **CIs:** Allergy/ hypersensitivity; | **ADRs:** abdominal pain or cramps, anorexia, diarrhea, flatulence, nausea, vomiting; | **Interactions:** Alcohol (↓ lycopene), androgen (↑ or ↓ androgen), antilipemic agents and bile sequestrants (↓ serum lycopene), beta-carotene (↑ lycopene absorption), nicotine (↓ lycopene levels), probucol (↓ serum carotenoids), UV light (↓ lycopene levels), may interact with agents with similar effects or related mechanisms of action (anticoagulant, antihypertensive, anti-inflammatory, antilipemic, antineoplastic, immunomodulatory); | **Dose:** Oral: 2–30 mg daily; | **Monitor:** Androgen, lipid profile, PSA; | **Notes:** The FDA lists tomato lycopene on its Generally Recognized as Safe (GRAS) list.

lysine | **Uses:** Aphthous ulcers, childhood development, diabetes mellitus, herpes simplex virus, lysine deficiency, metabolic disorders, ocular disorders, osteoporosis, stress; | **Preg:** Not recommended due to insufficient evidence; | **CIs:** Allergy/ hypersensitivity, Renal failure; | **ADRs:** abdominal cramps, ↑ cholesterol levels, diarrhea, dyspepsia, Fanconi's syndrome, gallstones, renal failure; | **Interactions:** Amphetamines (altered effects), anticoagulants/antiplatelets (↑ risk of bleeding), antidiabetic agents (↑ risk of hypoglycemia), antilipemic agents (additive effects), calcium (↑ calcium absorption/↓ urine calcium loss), CNS depressants (added sedation), nephrotoxic agents (↑ risk of kidney damage); | **Dose:** 500–9,000 mg PO qd. RDA: Adults and children 13 years and older: 12 mg/kg/day;

children 2–12 years: 23 mg/kg/day; **Monitor:** Blood glucose, coagulation panel, lipid profile; **Notes:** Sources of lysine include meat, fish, dairy, eggs, and some plants, such as soy and other legumes.

maca ***(Lepidium meyenii)*** **Uses:** Aphrodisiac (male), male hormone regulation, spermatogenesis; **Preg:** Not recommended due to insufficient evidence and possible hormonal effects; **CIs:** Allergy/hypersensitivity, Pregnancy, Lactation; **ADRs:** abdominal pain and bloating, CNS stimulation, leukocytosis, ↓ PT/INR values, ↑ or ↓ sex hormones; **Interactions:** Anticoagulants/antiplatelets (due to high vitamin K content), may interact with agents with similar effects or related mechanisms of action (hormonal, antihypertensive, stimulant); **Dose:** Oral: up to 3 g daily in divided doses for up to 4 months; **Monitor:** Coagulation panel, hormone levels; **Notes:** The long history of this root vegetable as a staple of the Peruvian highland diet suggests a low potential for toxicity.

mace **Uses:** Gingivitis; **Preg:** Not recommended due to insufficient evidence and traditional use as an abortifacient; **CIs:** Allergy/hypersensitivity; **ADRs:** agitation, anxiety, arrhythmia, asthenia, asthma, ataxia, contact dermatitis, dizziness, drowsiness, dysuria, euphoria, headache, hyperactivity, hypotension, ↑ LFTs, nausea/vomiting, tachycardia; **Interactions:** Analgesics (additive effects), anesthetics (additive effects), anticholinergics (additive effects), antilipemic agents (additive effects), antihypertensives (↑ risk of hypotension), antineoplastic agents (altered effects), anxiolytics (additive effects), calcium channel blockers (altered effects), CYP450 1A1/1A2/2B1/2B2 substrates (altered effects), phenobarbital (↓ effects of phenobarbital), hepatotoxic agents (↑ risk of liver damage); **Dose:** Diarrhea: 4–6 tablespoons of powder PO qd. Gingivitis: chew gum after each meal. Nausea: 3–5 gtt essential oil on a sugar lump or in honey; **Monitor:** Blood pressure, LFTs; **Notes:** Nutmeg and mace are two spices originating from the same plant, *Myristica fragrans*. Nutmeg is the seed of the tree and mace is the covering of the seed. Nutmeg has a history of abuse as a replacement for a recreational drug owing to its ability to result in symptoms similar to cannabis intoxication.

M

magnesium (Mg) **Uses:** Arrhythmia, asthma, acute myocardial infarction, anxiety, attention-deficit hyperactivity disorder (ADHD), cancer-associated neuropathic pain, chronic obstructive pulmonary disease (COPD), coronary artery disease

(CAD), constipation, diabetes (type 2), dyspepsia, fibromyalgia, hearing loss, hypercholesterolemia, hypertension, hypomagnesemia, leg cramps, metabolic syndrome, migraine headache, mitral valve prolapse, multiple sclerosis, muscle spasms, nephrolithiasis, post-hysterectomy pain, pre-eclampsia, pregnancy nutritional supplement, premenstrual syndrome (PMS), preterm labor, restless leg syndrome. torsades de pointes, vasoplastic angina; | **Preg:** FDA pregnancy Category A and Category B; acceptable during lactation; high intravenous doses in pregnant women for eclampsia or pre-eclampsia or tocolysis (labor-preventive) may ↑ increase infant mortality; | **CIs:** Allergy/hypersensitivity, Atrioventricular heart block, Renal dysfunction, GI disorders, Intravenous use in toxemia and pregnancy; | **ADRs:** areflexia, asthenia, cardiac arrest, cardiac arrhythmias, coma, DEATH, drowsiness, hypermagnesemia, hypotension, loss of tendon reflexes, polydipsia, respiratory paralysis; | **Interactions:** Aldesleukin (↓ magnesium levels), amifostine (↓ magnesium levels), aminoglycosides (↑ risk of muscular weakness and paralysis; ↓ magnesium levels), amphotericin B (↓ magnesium levels), antibiotics (↓ effects; via chelation), antidiabetic agents (↑ absorption), antihypertensive agents (additive effects; ↑ risk of hypotension), beta-2 agonists (↓ magnesium levels), bile acid sequestrants (↓ magnesium levels), bisphosphonates (↓ absorption), calcium channel blockers (additive effects), carboplatin (↓ magnesium levels), cetuximab (↓ magnesium levels), corticosteroids (↓ magnesium levels), cyclosporine (↓ magnesium levels), digoxin (↓ magnesium levels), diuretics (↓ Mg clearance, ↑ Mg levels), estrogens (↓ magnesium levels), foscarnet (↓ serum Mg, ↑ Mg excretion, Mg depletion), insulin (↓ magnesium levels), levomethadyl (↑ risk of QT prolongation), panitumumab (↓ magnesium levels), penicillamine (↓ magnesium levels), pentamidine (↓ magnesium levels), potassium-sparing diuretics (↑ magnesium levels), quinolone (↓ absorption), skeletal muscle relaxants (potentiate effects of skeletal muscle relaxants), sodium phosphates (↓ magnesium levels), tacrolimus (↓ magnesium levels), tetracycline antibiotics (↓ absorption), thyroid hormones (↓ absorption (via chelation); may interact with agents with similar effects or related mechanisms of action (anticoagulant, anticonvulsant, antidiabetic, antineoplastic, CNS depressant, muscle relaxant, laxative); | **Dose:** Oral: Mg orotate, 17 mM twice daily for 4 weeks; Mg oxide, 500 mg daily for 3 weeks; elemental Mg, up to 360 mg daily for up to 2 months; Mg aspartate, 167 mg daily for 8 weeks; Mg carbonate, up to 1,800 mg daily for 5 weeks; Mg hydroxide, 15 mM daily for 1 year; Mg pyrrolidone carboxylic acid, 360 mg daily for 2 months. Topical: Mg chloride gel applied as needed; Mg sulfate paste, added to baths. Intravenous: Mg

M

sulfate ($MgSO_4$), eclampsia: 10–14 g (appropriately diluted); **Monitor:** Alkaline phosphatase, ACE, blood glucose, blood pressure, calcium levels, coagulation panel, cortisol, diagnex blue, ECG, LFTs, parathyroid hormone, testosterone; **Notes:** Magnesium sulfate is the standard treatment for eclampsia (pregnancy-induced seizure) and pre-eclampsia (pregnancy-induced hypertension). Many antacids and laxatives also contain magnesium.

magnolia and pinelliae formula **Uses:** Pain, mood, overall health; **Preg:** Insufficient evidence; **CIs:** Allergy/hypersensitivity; **ADRs:** insufficient evidence; **Interactions:** Insufficient evidence; **Dose:** Insufficient evidence; **Monitor:** Insufficient evidence; **Notes:** Common names include banxia houpo tang (traditional Chinese medicine) and hange koboku-to (Japanese Kampo). A 1978 study found l-ephedrine, a banned substance, in pinellia tuber (a constituent of magnolia and pinelliae formula). It is unclear if amount of l-ephedrine is clinically significant.

mahonia **Uses:** Atopic dermatitis, psoriasis; **Preg:** Not recommended due to insufficient evidence; **CIs:** Allergy/hypersensitivity; **ADRs:** topical: burning sensation, clothing stains, rash; **Interactions:** Antibiotics (altered effects), antineoplastic agents (additive effects), CNS depressants (additive effects), cyclosporine (↑cyclosporine levels), CYP450 3A4 substrates (inhibits CYP3A4), immunosuppressants (altered effects), tetracycline (↓ absorption of tetracycline), vitamin B (altered metabolism of vitamin B); **Dose:** Infusion: 1–3 teaspoonfuls (5–15 g) of chopped roots boiled in 2 cups (500 mL) water for 15 min and with up to 3 cups of infused, strained and cooled liquid used throughout the day for an unknown duration; tincture: 3 mL PO tid; **Monitor:** Bilirubin, cyclosporine levels; **Notes:** Berberine, a constituent of mahonia (or Oregon grape), may interfere with bilirubin metabolism in jaundiced infants.

M

maitake mushroom ***(Grifola frondosa)*** **Uses:** Cancer, diabetes, immune stimulation; **Preg:** Likely safe in food amounts in pregnant or breastfeeding patients based on traditional use. Other uses are not recommended due to lack of sufficient evidence; **CIs:** Allergy/hypersensitivity; **ADRs:** hypoglycemia, hypotension, occupational hypersensitivity pneumonitis (HP); **Interactions:** May interact with agents with similar effects or related mechanisms of action (antidiabetic, antihypertensive, antineoplastic, antiviral, immunomodulatory);

Dose: Oral: maitake beta-glucan, 0.5–1 mg/kg daily in divided doses; **Monitor:** Insufficient evidence; **Notes:** In Asia, maitake is used as a food and extracts are recommended medicinally for a number of health conditions, including arthritis, hepatitis, and HIV.

malic acid | **Uses:** Insufficient clinical evidence; | **Preg:** Not recommended due to insufficient evidence; does not show reproductive toxicity in animals; | **CIs:** Allergy/hypersensitivity; | **ADRs:** contact dermatitis and urticaria (oral use), skin irritation (topical use); | **Interactions:** May interact with agents with similar effects or related mechanisms of action (antihypertensive, antiobesity); | **Dose:** Insufficient evidence; | **Monitor:** Blood pressure; | **Notes:** Malic acid is an organic dicarboxylic acid found in wines, sour apples, and other fruits.

Manchurian thorn tree | **Uses:** Insufficient evidence; | **Preg:** Not recommended due to insufficient evidence; | **CIs:** Allergy/hypersensitivity; | **ADRs:** insufficient evidence; | **Interactions:** Antidiabetic agents (altered glucose levels); | **Dose:** Insufficient evidence; | **Monitor:** Blood glucose; | **Notes:** Manchurian thorn tree is an adaptogen, traditionally used to increased energy and normalize glucose.

M

mangosteen ***(Garcinia mangostana)*** | **Uses:** Insufficient clinical evidence; | **Preg:** Likely safe in food amounts in pregnant or breastfeeding patients based on traditional use. Other uses are not recommended due to lack of sufficient evidence; | **CIs:** Allergy/hypersensitivity; | **ADRs:** CNS depression; | **Interactions:** CNS depression (additive sedation); may interact with agents with similar effects or related mechanisms of action (anticoagulant, antineoplastic, antihistamine, phosphodiesterase inhibition, antidepressant); | **Dose:** Insufficient evidence; | **Monitor:** Coagulation panel, histamine, phosphodiesterase, serotonin; | **Notes:** In traditional medicine, the fruit hulls (pericarp), leaves, bark, and fruit pulp are used.

maral root | **Uses:** Insufficient clinical evidence; | **Preg:** Not recommended due to insufficient evidence; | **CIs:** Allergy/hypersensitivity; | **ADRs:** insufficient evidence; | **Interactions:** Insufficient evidence; | **Dose:** Insufficient evidence; | **Monitor:** Insufficient evidence; | **Notes:** Maral root or Russian leuzea has been used for centuries in eastern parts of Russia for proteosynthesis, work capacity, reproduction, and sexual function. It is also used as an adaptogen.

marjoram *(Origanum majorana)* **Uses:** Atopic eczema; **Preg:** Likely safe in food amounts in pregnant or breastfeeding patients based on traditional use. Large amounts not recommended due to insufficient evidence and traditional use as an emmenagogue; **CIs:** Allergy/hypersensitivity; **ADRs:** allergic contact dermatitis; **Interactions:** Diuretics (additive effects); may interact with agents with similar effects or related mechanisms of action (anticholinergic, anticoagulant, antioxidant, hypoglycemic); **Dose:** Oral: 1–2 tsp as tea. Topical: essential oil diluted in almond oil; **Monitor:** Blood glucose, coagulation panel; **Notes:** Storage in the light produced considerable changes in the composition of the oil due to the chemical transformation of terpenoids.

marshmallow *(Althaea officinalis)* **Uses:** Eczema, psoriasis; **Preg:** Not recommended due to insufficient evidence; **CIs:** Allergy/hypersensitivity; **ADRs:** ↓ blood glucose; **Interactions:** Antidiabetes agents (↑ risk of hypoglycemia), diuretics (additive effects), oral agents (impaired absorption); may interact with agents with similar effects or related mechanisms of action (antibiotic, anti-inflammatory, antitussive, steroidal); **Dose:** Topical: 5% cream or powder applied three times daily. Oral: 5 g leaf or 6 g root daily; **Monitor:** Blood glucose; **Notes:** The fiber in marshmallow may ↓ absorption of oral agents.

mastic *(Pistacia lentiscus)* **Uses:** Dental plaque, duodenal ulcer, gastric ulcer; **Preg:** Not recommended due to insufficient evidence and possible adverse effects on blood pressure; **CIs:** Allergy/hypersensitivity; **ADRs:** ↓ blood pressure; **Interactions:** Antihypertensives (↑ risk of hypotension); **Dose:** Oral: 1 g mastic powder once or twice daily for up to 4 weeks; **Monitor:** Blood pressure; **Notes:** Mastic is the resin of *Pistacia lentiscus,* a shrub of the sumac family (Anacardiaceae) found in the Mediterranean region.

meadowsweet *(Filipendula ulmaria,* formerly *Spirea ulmaria)* **Uses:** Insufficient clinical evidence; **Preg:** Contraindicated due to salicylic acid content; **CIs:** Allergy/hypersensitivity, Pregnancy, Lactation, Pediatric use, Bleeding disorders, Gastric ulcers; **ADRs:** asthma, bleeding, bleeding risk, blood in stool, bronchospasm, gastric irritation, gastrointestinal bleeding, hypersensitivity, nausea/vomiting, tinnitus; **Interactions:** Anticoagulants/antiplatelets (↑ risk of bleeding), aspirin (additive effects), salicylates (additive effects due to salicylate content in meadowsweet), narcotics (additive effects); | **Dose:** Oral: two to three 570-mg capsules twice daily; infusion/tea: 1 cup of tea (2.5–3.5g [1–2 tsp]) dried flowers or 4–5 g of above-ground parts steeped in 150 mL boiling water for 10 minutes, then strained and ingested several times per day; liquid extract (1:1 in 25% alcohol): 1.5–6 mL 3 times per day; tincture (1:5 in 45% alcohol): 2–4 mL 3 times per day; | **Monitor:** Coagulation panel, blood glucose, hormone panel; | **Notes:** Aspirin (acetylsalicylic acid) is named after spiric acid, another name for salicylic acid derived from the former Latin name for meadowsweet (*Spirea ulmaria*).

melatonin | **Uses:** Alzheimer's disease (sleep disorders), antioxidant, asthma (sleep disturbances), attention-deficit hyperactivity disorder (ADHD), benzodiazepine tapering, bipolar disorder (sleep disturbances), cancer treatment, chemotherapy side effects, circadian rhythm entraining (in blind persons), delayed sleep phase syndrome (DSPS), depression (sleep disturbances), glaucoma, headache (prevention), HIV/AIDS, hypertension, irritable bowel syndrome (IBS), jet lag, insomnia/sleep disorders (idiopathic), insomnia (elderly), Parkinson's disease, periodic limb movement disorder, REM sleep behavior disorder, Rett's syndrome, schizophrenia (sleep disorders), seasonal affective disorder (SAD), sedation (preoperative/antianxiety), seizure disorder (children), sleep disturbances (due to pineal region brain damage), smoking, stroke, tardive dyskinesia, thrombocytopenia, ultraviolet light skin damage protection, work shift sleep disorder; | **Preg:** Contraindicated due to possible hormonal effects, altered pituitary-ovarian function, ↓ ovulation, ↑ uterine contractions, ↑ risk of developmental disorders (high doses); | **CIs:** Allergy/hypersensitivity, Concomitant use with CNS depressants, Pregnancy, Lactation; | **ADRs:** abdominal cramping, angina, arrhythmias, bleeding, ↑ breast size in men, confusion, ↑ Crohn's disease symptoms, disorientation, dizziness, fatigue, hallucinations, headache, hepatomegaly, hormonal changes, hyperglycemia, hyperlipidemia, hyper-/hypotension, irritability, mood changes, nausea, paranoia, sleepiness, sleepwalking, ↓ sperm motility, vivid dreams and nightmares, vomiting; | **Interactions:** Anticoagulants/antiplatelets (↑ risk of bleeding), antidiabetic agents (↑ of hypoglycemia), benzodiazepines (↓ melatonin levels), caffeine (↓ melatonin levels), clonidine (↓ effects), CNS DEPRESSANTS (additive sedation), CYP450 inhibitors (↑ melatonin levels), CYP450 inducers (↓ melatonin levels), estrogens (↑ melatonin levels), flumazenil (inhibit melatonin effects), fluoxetine (↑ psychotic symptoms), fluvoxamine (↑ melatonin levels), haloperidol (↓ haloperidol-induced tardive dyskinesia),

M

immunosuppressants (interfere with effects), isoniazid (↑ effects), methamphetamine (↑ adverse effects), methoxamine (↓ effects), nifedipine (↓ effectiveness of nifedipine), succinylcholine (↑ effects), verapamil (↑ melatonin excretion); **Dose:** Oral, insomnia: 0.1–5 mg in the evening. Dosages for various conditions range from 1 to 75 mg in the evening for various duration. Intramuscular: 20 mg; **Monitor:** Blood glucose, coagulation panel, hormone panel, lipid profile; **Notes:** Melatonin is a neurohormone produced in the brain by the pineal gland, from the amino acid tryptophan.

methione **Uses:** Acetaminophen toxicity, cobalamin deficiency, colorectal cancer, insomnia, neural tube defect prevention, Parkinson's disease; **Preg:** Not recommended due to insufficient evidence; **CIs:** Allergy/hypersensitivity, Acidosis, Hyperhomocysteinemia, Liver disease, Methylenetetrahydrofolate reductase (MTHFR) deficiency, Schizophrenia; **ADRs:** dizziness, drowsiness, ↑ homocysteine levels, hypotension, irritability, nausea, vomiting; **Interactions:** Hepatotoxic agents (↑ risk of liver damage); **Dose:** Acetaminophen toxicity: 2.5 g PO q4h × 4 doses. Insomnia: 500 mg PO qhs. Parkinson's disease: 5 g PO qd; **Monitor:** Homocysteine levels, LFTs; **Notes:** Methionine is one of nine essential amino acids. Sources of methionine include sunflower seeds, beef, eggs, cottage cheese, chicken, fish, pork, liver, sardines, yogurt, pumpkin seeds, sesame seeds, and lentils.

M

methylsulfonylmethane (MSM) **Uses:** Allergic rhinitis, osteoarthritis; **Preg:** Not recommended due to insufficient evidence; **CIs:** Allergy/hypersensitivity; **ADRs:** bloating, diarrhea, difficulty concentrating, fatigue, gastrointestinal discomfort, insomnia; **Interactions:** May interact with agents with similar effects or related mechanisms of action (anti-inflammatory, antioxidant); **Dose:** Oral: 500–8,000 mg daily for up to 12 weeks; **Monitor:** Not applicable; **Notes:** MSM is a naturally occurring form of organic sulfur in a variety of food sources; generally well tolerated, but long-term safety has not been established.

milk thistle ***(Silybum marianum)*** **Uses:** Acute viral hepatitis, *Amanita phalloides*, cancer (prevention), chronic hepatitis, cirrhosis, diabetes (in patients with cirrhosis), dyspepsia, hyperlipidemia, hepatomegaly, liver damage (from drugs and toxins), menopausal symptoms; **Preg:** Not recommended due to insufficient evidence, though pregnant women have taken silymarin 400 mg daily for up to 60 days with no serious adverse effects; | **CIs:** Allergy/hypersensitivity, Estrogen-sensitive disorders; | **ADRs:** abdominal upset, anaphylactic shock, anorexia, arthralgia, diarrhea, dyspepsia, estrogenic effects, flatulence, headache, ↑ hemochromatosis, hepatotoxicity, hyperbilirubinemia, hypoglycemia, irritability/fatigue, impotence, pruritus; | **Interactions:** Alcohol (↓ alcohol-induced hepatotoxicity), amiodarone (↓ amiodarone-induced toxicity), antineoplastic agents (cisplatin, carboplatin, doxorubicin; ↑ effects), antiretroviral agents (CYP450 inhibition/↑ drug concentrations), CYP450 2C9 (inhibits CYP2C9; ↑ levels), glucuronidated agents (↑ levels of glucoronidated agents), estrogen (↑ estrogen clearance), HMG-CoA reductase inhibitors (inhibits effects), P-glycoprotein–modulated agents (altered drug levels); may interact with agents with similar effects or related mechanisms of action (antidiabetic, antilipemic); | **Dose:** Oral: silymarin 230–800 mg daily in 2–3 divided doses; silybin 160–480 mg daily; | **Monitor:** Blood glucose, lipid profile, LFTs; | **Notes:** Products are often standardized to silymarin. Milk thistle is generally considered to be safe. Adverse reactions appear to be mild when used within the recommended dosage parameters, with occasional gastrointestinal symptoms and rare cases of anaphylaxis.

mistletoe ***(Viscum album)*** | **Uses:** Arthritis, cancer, common cold, hepatitis, HIV, recurrent respiratory disease; | **Preg:** Not recommended due to insufficient evidence and possible uterine stimulant effects; | **CIs:** Allergy/hypersensitivity, Autoimmune disease, Immunosuppressed patients, Pregnancy; | **ADRs:** altered blood cell counts, anorexia, bradycardia, burning sensation, coma, congested intestine, dehydration, delirium, depressive moods, diarrhea, edema, eye and muscle problems, eye irritation, fatigue, fever, flu-like symptoms, gastroenteritis, general malaise, gingivitis, hallucinations, headache, hepatotoxicity, hyperemia, hypotension, myocardial infarction, nausea, nephrotoxicity, nocturia, pain (generalized, bone, joint), pancreatic hemorrhage, rash, seizures, skin inflammation at injection site, sleeplessness, vomiting; | **Interactions:** Antihypertensives (↑ risk of hypotension), immunosuppressants (↓ effectiveness; ↑ risk of organ failure and death), tyramine (↑ risk of hypertensive crisis), may interact with agents with similar effects or related mechanisms of action (abortifacient, antidiabetic, anti-inflammatory, antineoplastic, cardiovascular, cholinergic, agents that lower seizure threshold, diuretic, hepatotoxic, neurological, thyroid agents); | **Dose:** Oral: 2.5 g as tea, up to 2 cups daily; up to 4 mL tincture or extract daily; Iscador 0.05 mg–0.1 mg 3 times daily, increased over several weeks to 5–10 mg 3 times daily. Parenteral: Iscador 20–40 mg, or Helixor

(5% levulose) 300–500 mg/250 mL infused for 2 hours twice weekly, for 6–9 infusions over 6 weeks; **Monitor:** Blood glucose, blood pressure, BUN, creatinine, complete blood count, serum protein, LFTs; **Notes:** American mistletoe has caused toxic effects in humans; however, in 1,754 cases of exposure reported in the literature from 1985 to 1992, there is a lack of fatalities associated with American mistletoe.

modified citrus pectin **Uses:** Detoxification, prostate cancer; **Preg:** Likely safe when consumed in amounts found in food; **CIs:** Allergy/hypersensitivity; **ADRs:** constipation, electrolyte loss, fecal impaction; **Interactions:** May ↓ absorption of oral agents, may interact with agents with similar effects or related mechanisms of action (antilipemic, antineoplastic, chelating); **Dose:** Oral: 6–30 g daily in divided doses, dissolved in water and diluted with lemon or powdered form; 800-mg capsules 3 times daily; **Monitor:** Lipid profile, PSA, urinalysis; **Notes:** Modified citrus pectin is Generally Regarded as Safe (GRAS) by the FDA; few adverse effects have been reported.

mugwort ***(Artemisia vulgaris)*** **Uses:** Scars; **Preg:** Not recommended due to insufficient evidence and traditional use as an abortifacient; **CIs:** Allergy/hypersensitivity, Pregnancy, Lactation; **ADRs:** abortion, anaphylaxis, asthma, atopic eczema, conjunctivitis, contact dermatitis, CNS damage, nausea, pollinosis, respiratory and dermatological allergic responses, seasonal allergic rhinitis, upper and lower respiratory tract sensitization, urticaria, vomiting; **Interactions:** Anticoagulants/antiplatelets (↑ risk of bleeding), potassium (↑ potassium excretion); **Dose:** Oral: 2 cups of mugwort tea daily for 6 days, prepared with 1 oz of mugwort leaf infused in 1 pint of boiling water for 5–10 minutes; **Monitor:** Coagulation panel, potassium levels; **Notes:** Mugwort is on the Commission E (Germany's regulatory agency for herbs) list of unapproved herbs with insufficient evidence of safety and effectiveness.

muira puama ***(Ptychopetalum olacoides)*** **Uses:** Erectile dysfunction, sexual dysfunction (females); **Preg:** Not recommended due to insufficient evidence and possible hormonal effects; **CIs:** Allergy/hypersensitivity; **ADRs:** altered blood pressure, altered heart function, anabolic side effects (↑ energy, ↑ aggression, ↑ appetite, changes in voice or enlargement of genitalia), central nervous system (CNS) stimulation; **Interactions:** Anticoagulants/antiplatelets (↑ risk of bleeding), antihypertensive agents (interfere with effects); may

M

interact with agents with similar effects or related mechanisms of action (analgesic, antidepressant, hormonal, sympathomimetic, opioid cross-tolerance); | **Dose:** Oral: up to 2.6 g daily. Topical: up to 16 drops tincture; | **Monitor:** Coagulation panel, blood pressure, heart rate, hormone panel; | **Notes:** *Liriosma ovata* and *Acanthea virilis* are commonly incorrectly sold as muira puama.

mullein (*Verbascum* spp.) | **Uses:** Earache, otitis media; | **Preg:** Not recommended due to insufficient evidence; | **CIs:** Allergy/hypersensitivity; | **ADRs:** insufficient evidence; | **Interactions:** Anticoagulants/antiplatelets (↑ risk of bleeding); | **Dose:** Insufficient evidence; | **Monitor:** Coagulation panel; | **Notes:** As of 2005, the FDA reported that mullein flowers are likely safe for use as natural flavoring and in small amounts.

myrcia (*Myrcia* spp.) | **Uses:** Diabetes (type 2); | **Preg:** Not recommended due to insufficient evidence and possible adverse effects; | **CIs:** Allergy/hypersensitivity; | **ADRs:** abdominal discomfort, agranulocytosis, bloating, ↓ blood glucose, ↑ blood pressure, chills, diarrhea, dizziness, drowsiness, fever, flatulence, nausea, ↓ taste, ↓ thyroid hormone; | **Interactions:** May interact with agents with similar effects or related mechanisms of action (hypoglycemic, antihypertensive, thyroid agents); | **Dose:** Oral: 1–2 g leaf powder in tablet or capsule form; 1 cup of leaf infusion, 2–3 times daily; | **Monitor:** Blood glucose, blood pressure, thyroid hormones; | **Notes:** Traditionally used to treat diabetes.

M

N-acetyl cysteine (NAC) | **Uses:** Acetaminophen toxicity, ARDS, angina, asthma, atelectasis, bronchitis, cancer, cerebral adrenoleukodystrophy, chemotherapy adverse effects (including cardiotoxicity), COPD, cystic fibrosis, endotracheal crusting, epilepsy, fatigue, fibrosing alveolitis, glutathione production, heavy metal detoxification, HIV/AIDS, hyperhomocysteinemia, ifosfamide toxicity, influenza (prevention), MI, nephropathy (prevention), ovulation (induction), PCOS, pulmonary disorders, renal impairment, sepsis, Sjögren's syndrome, trichotillomania; | **Preg:** Likely safe when used appropriately; | **CIs:** Allergy/hypersensitivity; | **ADRs:** abdominal pain, allergic reactions, angina, chills, clamminess, constipation, diarrhea (large doses), drowsiness, fever, headache, hepatotoxicity, hypotension, nausea/vomiting, rash, rhinorrhea, unpleasant odor; | **Interactions:** Activated charcoal (↓ charcoal effects), anticoagulants/antiplatelets (↑ risk of bleeding), antihypertensives, cephalosporins (e.g., cefuroxime), NITROGLYCERIN (↑ risk of severe hypotension), thyroid hormones (altered effects); | **Dose:** Inhalation: 3–5 mL of the 20% solution or 6–10 mL of the 10% solution 3–4 times/day. Intravenous: loading dose 140 mg/kg, followed by 12 maintenance doses of 70 mg/kg every 4 hours. Oral: 200–500 mg PO up to 3 times/day; | **Monitor:** Blood pressure, coagulation panel, creatinine, cysteine (free), ketones, LFTs; | **Notes:** NAC is an FDA-approved drug used mostly commonly for the management of acetaminophen overdose. NAC breaks down mucus, helps the body synthesize glutathione, and protects the body from acetaminophen toxicity.

nattokinase | **Uses:** HTN, deep vein thrombosis (DVT); | **Preg:** Not recommended due to insufficient evidence; | **CIs:** Allergy/hypersensitivity; | **ADRs:** ↑ risk of bleeding; | **Interactions:** Anticoagulants/antiplatelets (↑ risk of bleeding), antihypertensives (↑ risk of hypotension); | **Dose:** General: 100 mg 3 times daily or 2,000–6,000 fibrinolytic units (FU) daily. DVT: 2 capsules of Flite Tabs (150-mg blend of nattokinase plus pycnogenol) PO taken 2 hours before flight and 2 capsules taken 6 hours later. HTN: 1–2 capsules PO qd (NSK-II, each containing 2,000 FU of nattokinase per milligram); | **Monitor:** Blood pressure, coagulation panel; | **Notes:** Nattokinase is an enzyme extracted and purified from the popular traditional Japanese food natto. The cheese-like natto is made by fermenting soybeans with a bacteria called *Bacillus subtilis natto*.

N

neem ***(Azadirachta indica)*** | **Uses:** Dental plaque (oral bacteria), gastroduodenal ulcers, mosquito repellent, psoriasis; | **Preg:** Not safe due to abortifacient and teratogenic effects observed in animal studies; | **CIs:** Allergy/hypersensitivity, Lactation, Pregnancy, Pediatric use; | **ADRs:** altered sensations, anemia, arrhythmia, ↓ blood sugar, changes in blood cell count, coma, DEATH (in children), diarrhea, drowsiness, ↑ liver enzyme, myocardial infarction, ↑ risk of birth defects, seizures, starvation, toxic encephalopathy, uterine damage, vomiting; | **Interactions:** Acetaminophen (↑ hepatotoxicity), diuretics (additive effects), immunosuppressants (↓ effectiveness), mitomycin C (↓ effectiveness), morphine (↑ analgesia); | **Dose:** Oral: 30–60 mg bark extract twice daily for 10 weeks. Topical: gel formula twice daily before meals (in the mouth for dental plaque); 2%–5% oil as insect repellant; | **Monitor:** Ammonia levels, bilirubin, blood glucose, CBC, potassium, testosterone, thyroid function tests; | **Notes:** Commonly used to treat infections and as a pesticide.

niacin (vitamin B_3, nicotinic acid), niacinamide

Uses: Age-related macular degeneration, Alzheimer's disease, atherosclerosis, cognitive function, diabetes (type 1 and type 2), headaches, hyperlipidemia, pellagra, myocardial infarction (prevention of reoccurrence), osteoarthritis (niacinamide), ↑ phosphorus level, skin conditions; **Preg:** Niacin (Niaspan): Pregnancy category C. If a woman with primary hypercholesterolemia (types IIa or IIb) becomes pregnant, niacin should be discontinued. If a woman being treated for hypertriglyceridemia (types IV or V) becomes pregnant, the drug may be continued only if the benefits outweigh the risks. The need for niacin is said to increase by 3 mg daily of niacin equivalents, particularly in the second and third trimesters, to cover increased energy utilization and maternal and fetal growth. The recommended dietary allowance (RDA) for niacin in pregnant women is 18 mg daily. The tolerable upper intake level of niacin in pregnant women is 35 mg daily. However, supplementation during pregnancy is usually not required; the catabolism of tryptophan is accelerated during pregnancy, resulting in increased niacin production; **CIs:** Allergy/hypersensitivity, Active peptic ulcer, Arterial bleeding, Active liver disease; **ADRs:** anaphylactic shock, anxiety, arrhythmia, ascites, ↑ blood clotting, blurred vision, ↑ creatine kinase (indicator of muscle damage), dental pain, diarrhea, dizziness, dry skin, ↑ eosinophils, <u>flushing</u>, gout, headache, hepatotoxicity, ↑ homocysteine levels (may ↑ risk of heart disease), hyperglycemia, hypotension, hypothyroidism, jaundice, keratoconjunctivitis sicca (dry eye), leukopenia, macular swelling, mild stomach upset, nausea, niacin-induced myopathy, palpitations, panic attacks, ↓ platelet count, pruritus, rash, ↑ stomach ulcers, toxic amblyopia, ↑ uric acid levels, vomiting, warm sensation; **Interactions:** Alcohol (↑ niacin-induced flushing, ↑ risk hepatotoxicity), testosterone (↑ effects), anticoagulants/antiplatelets (↑ risk of bleeding/ ↓ platelet count/↑ PT), antihistamines (↓ niacin-induced flushing), antihypertensive agents (↑ risk of hypotension), aspirin (↓ niacin-induced flushing and burning), bile acid sequestrants (↑ hypolipidemic effects, ↓ niacin absorption, ↑ adverse effects, ↑ myopathy risk), fibrates (↑ adverse effects, ↑ myopathy risk), HMG-CoA reductase inhibitors (↑ adverse effects, ↑ myopathy, ↑ rhabdomyolysis, ↑ hepatotoxicity, ↑ hypolipidemic effects), ↑ benzodiazepine solubility, ↑ estradiol solubility, CYP450 substrates (altered drug levels), epinephrine (↓ niacin-induced anaphylactic shock; ↓ epinephrine-induced fatty acid release), griseofulvin (↑ griseofulvin solubility and toxicity), insulin (↓ insulin requirements, may ↑ blood glucose), neomycin (↑ effects), nicotine (↑ niacin-induced flushing and dizziness), NSAIDs (↓ niacin-induced flushing and burning), primadone

N

(↑ half-life, ↓ conversion to phenobarbital and phenylethylmalonamide), probucol (↑ effects), procetofene (↑ effects), progesterone (↑ progesterone solubility), pyrazinamide (↑ risk of pellagra, ↓ niacin production), theophylline (↓ theophylline-induced fatty acid release), thyroid hormones (↓ serum thyroxine), may interact with agents with similar effects or related mechanisms of action (calcium channel blocking, ganglionic, vasodilatory); | **Dose:** Dietary reference intake (1 mg niacin = 60 mg tryptophan) is from 14–18 mg daily for adults; upper intake level is 35 mg daily. Doses as high as 6,000 mg daily have been used under medical supervision; | **Monitor:** Blood pressure, coagulation panel, lipid panel, cortisol, creatine kinase, fibrinogen, glucagon, homocysteine levels, hormone panel, LFTs, thyroid function tests, uric acid; signs and symptoms of muscle pain or weakness; | **Notes:** Niacin (not niacinamide) appears to be a relatively safe, inexpensive, and effective treatment for hyperlipidemia; niacinamide (not niacin) may have a preventative role in type 1 diabetes mellitus.

nicotinamide | **Uses:** Acne, diabetes (type 1), high phosphorus (during dialysis), maculopathy, osteoarthritis, pellagra, pemphigus foliaceus, radiotherapy side effects, skin care; | **Preg:** Safe; RDA: 17–18 mg/day for females above the age of 14; | **CIs:** Allergy/hypersensitivity; | **ADRs:** dry hair, fatigue, flushing, GI upset, headache, hypotension (at high doses, above 600 mg), liver damage (high doses), nausea/vomiting, rash, sedation; | **Interactions:** Anti-inflammatory agents (additive effects), antihypertensives (↑ risk of hypotension), CNS depressants (additive effects), CYP450 substrates (altered effects), hepatotoxic agents (↑ risk of liver damage), immunosuppressants (altered effects); | **Dose:** Oral, general: 500 mg–3 g PO qd; topical, acne: 4% nicotinamide gel applied to skin twice daily; | **Monitor:** Blood glucose, phosphorus levels; | **Notes:** Nicotinamide is the amide of nicotinic acid (vitamin B_3). Nicotinamide does not have the same effects as niacin.

nitrilosides | **Uses:** Cancer; | **Preg:** Avoid use; | **CIs:** Allergy/hypersensitivity, Pregnancy; | **ADRs:** CYANIDE TOXICITY (symptoms: ataxia, blindness, coma, cyanosis, DEATH, dizziness, dyspnea, fever, headache, liver damage, low blood pressure, mental confusion, nausea/vomiting, optic nerve lesions, shortness of breath), goiter, urticaria, skin rash; | **Interactions:** Insufficient evidence; | **Dose:** 250–1,000 mg amygdalin PO qd; | **Monitor:** Cyanide levels; | **Notes:** Nitriloside is a generic term for beta-cyanophoric glycosides, a large group of water-soluble, sugary compounds found in a number of plants. Amygdalin (Laetrile), one of the most common nitrilosides, occurs in the kernels of the seeds many fruits, particularly apricots. The terms Laetrile and amygdalin are often used nterchangeably. The American Cancer Society states that Laetrile, or amygdalin, is effective in treating cancer. Amygdalin can cause cyanide poisoning.

nomame herba | **Uses:** Insufficient evidence; | **Preg:** Not recommended due to insufficient evidence; | **CIs:** Allergy/hypersensitivity; | **ADRs:** diarrhea; | **Interactions:** Antineoplastic agents (altered effects), antiobesity agents (additive effects); | **Dose:** 100–900 mg PO 2–3 times/day before meals; | **Monitor:** Weight; | **Notes:** Nomame herba (*Cassia nomame*) is a Chinese medicinal herb that is being marketed in weight loss formulations. Taking *Cassia nomame* is thought to reduce fat breakdown in the intestinal tract, resulting in less fat absorption. It is thought that absorption of fat-soluble vitamins is not affected.

noni *(Morinda citrifolia)* | **Uses:** Antioxidant, hearing loss; | **Preg:** Not recommended due to insufficient evidence and traditional use as an abortifacient; | **CIs:** Allergy/hypersensitivity, Liver dysfunction, Renal dysfunction, Hyperkalemia; | **ADRs:** ↓ blood pressure, hepatotoxicity; | **Interactions:** Anticoagulants/antiplatelets (Coumadin resistance, case report; noni contains vitamin K in some preparations), may interact with oral agents due to ↓ gastric transit time, may interact with agents with similar effects or related mechanisms of action (agents that ↑ potassium, analgesic, ACE inhibitors, antihelminthic, antiangiogenic, procoagulant, antidiabetic, antihypertensive, anti-inflammatory, antineoplastic, antiviral, diuretic, hepatotoxic, immunomodulatory, metabolic); | **Dose:** Oral: Up to 2 oz twice daily for 3 months; | **Monitor:** Blood glucose, blood pressure, coagulation panel, CRP, LDH, LFTs, potassium, viral titers, WBC counts; | **Notes:** Noni juice and/or fruit itself is not a source for vitamin K; therefore, it would be unsubstantiated to draw any conclusions concerning a potential warfarin/coumarin interaction with a case report.

N

nopal (*Opuntia* spp.) | **Uses:** Alcohol-induced hangover, benign prostatic hypertrophy (BPH), diabetes, hyperlipidemia; | **Preg:** Likely safe in food amounts in pregnant or breastfeeding patients based on traditional use. Other uses are not recommended due to lack of sufficient evidence; | **CIs:** Allergy/hypersensitivity, Autoimmune disorders, Immunocompromised patients, Liver dysfunction; | **ADRs:** abdominal fullness, acute monoarthritis, ↓ blood pressure, colonic obstruction, dermatitis, esophageal blockage, headache, intestinal blockage, keratoconjunctivitis, mild diarrhea, nausea, osmylogenic asthma, rectal perforation, rhinitis, ↑ stool frequency, ↑ stool volume, synovitis; | **Interactions:** Acidic agents (↓ effects), antidiabetic agents (additive effects; ↑ risk of hypoglycemia), antihypertensive agents (↑ risk of hypotension), antilipemic agents (additive effects), antiulcer agents (interfere with effects), hepatotoxic agents (↑ risk of liver damage), oral agents (↓ absorption), thyroid hormones (↓ thyroxin levels); | **Dose:** Oral: 500 g broiled stems as single dose; 10.1 g stem extract as a single dose; 10 capsules nopal powder 3 times daily for 1 week; up to 1 mL flower extract; up to 1 g flowers; | **Monitor:** Blood glucose, lipid profile, thyroid function panel, uric acid; | **Notes:** Nopal is the most commonly used herbal hypoglycemic agent among persons of Mexican descent.

nux vomica *(Strychnos nux-vomica)* | **Uses:** Insufficient clinical evidence; | **Preg:** Contraindicated due to known toxicity; | **CIs:** ORAL USE (seeds, toxic amount of strychnine), Pediatrics; Pregnant women; | **ADRs:** abdominal cramps, bilateral horizontal nystagmus, carpopedal spasm, chest discomfort, confusion, dizziness, dyspnea, hyperreflexia, hyperthermia, hyperventilation, knee jerks with several beats of clonus, leg pain, metabolic and respiratory acidosis, myalgias, myoglobinuric renal failure, painful seizures, partial seizure, perioral numbness, rhabdomyolysis, spasms, and tonic contractions of all limb muscles; | **Interactions:** Antipsychotic agents (↑ effects), hepatotoxic agents (↑ risk of liver damage); | **Dose:** Oral: Homeopathic strengths include 6X, 12X, 30X, and 30C; traditionally, sublingual doses are taken one-half hour before or after eating, brushing teeth, or drinking anything but water; | **Monitor:** Urine tests, vital signs; | **Notes:** In *The Complete German Commission E Monographs: Therapeutic Guide to Herbal Medicines*, nux vomica preparations were not deemed as justifiable therapies, given the risks of use and lack of evidence supporting therapeutic effectiveness.

oat *(Avena sativa)* | **Uses:** Cardiovascular disease, constipation, diabetes, fat redistribution syndrome, gastric cancer, hyperlipidemia, obesity; | **Preg:** Likely safe in food amounts in pregnant or breastfeeding patients based on traditional use. Other uses are not recommended due to lack of sufficient evidence; | **CIs:** Allergy/hypersensitivity; | **ADRs:** allergic reaction, contact dermatitis, gastrointestinal upset; | **Interactions:** Antidiabetic agents (↑ risk of hypoglycemia), antilipemic agents

O

(additive effects), morphine (↓ morphine-induced antinociceptive effects), oral agents (↓ absorption due to fiber content), sodium lauryl sulfate (↓ SLS-induced skin irritation), nicotine (↓ nicotine-induced cytotoxicity); | **Dose:** Oral 4 g oat beta-glucans daily for 5 weeks. Topical: insufficient clinical evidence; | **Monitor:** Blood glucose, lipid profile, weight; | **Notes:** Oats are likely safe for those with celiac disease requiring a gluten-free diet; immune responses in gluten-sensitive individuals are likely due to contamination with other grains. Use cautiously in patients with gastrointestinal dysfunction.

octacosanol | **Uses:** Amyotrophic lateral sclerosis (ALS), Parkinson's disease; | **Preg:** Not recommended due to insufficient evidence; | **CIs:** Allergy/hypersensitivity; | **ADRs:** ↓ blood pressure, ↑ glucose, gum bleeding, ↑ LFTs, skin rash; | **Interactions:** ANTICOAGULANTS/ANTIPLATELETS (↑ risk of bleeding), antidiabetic agents (altered effects), antihypertensives (↑ risk of hypotension), antilipemic agents (additive effects), levodopa/carbidopa (may worsen dyskinesias), nitroprusside (additive effects); | **Dose:** Oral, ALS: 40 mg PO qd; Parkinson's disease: 5 mg PO tid with meals; | **Monitor:** Blood glucose, blood pressure, coagulation panel, lipid profile, serum creatinine, LFTs; | **Notes:** Octacosanol is the main component of policosanol. Octacosanol inhibits platelet aggregation and may cause excessive bleeding if used before surgery. Patients should discontinue octacosanol 2 weeks before surgery. Use cautiously in patients with Parkinson's disease as octacosanol may worsen carbidopa/levodopa-related dyskinesias.

oleander | **Uses:** Cancer, CHF; | **Preg:** Avoid use; | **CIs:** Allergy/hypersensitivity, Oral use, Arrhythmias, Pregnancy; | **ADRs:** abdominal pain, altered mental status, buccal erythema, cardiovascular toxicity, DEATH, diaphoresis, diarrhea, headache, hypotension, jaundice, mydriasis, nausea/vomiting, renal failure, visual disturbances; | **Interactions:** Antiarrhythmics (altered effects), antihypertensives (↑ risk of hypotension), calcium (enhance the effects of oleander), DIGOXIN (cardiac glycoside toxicity), DIURETICS (↑ risk of potassium depletion), laxatives (↑ risk of potassium depletion), MACROLIDE ANTIBIOTICS (↑ risk of cardiac toxicity), TETRACYCLINE ANTIBIOTICS (↑ risk of cardiac toxicity); | **Dose:** Oral use should be avoided; | **Monitor:** Electrolytes, heart rate; | **Notes:** The term "oleander" refers to two common plant species, *Nerium oleander* (common oleander) and *Thevetia peruviana* (yellow oleander), which grow in temperate climates throughout the world. Both species contain cardiac glycosides with digoxin-like effects, and both species are TOXIC with well-described reports of FATAL ingestion. Anvirzel (Ozelle Pharmaceuticals, Inc.), an aqueous extract of *Nerium oleander*, is currently being studied in phase I trials for its antitumor effects. As of November 2006, the manufacturer's website (www.ozelle.com) accurately reflects the status of this investigational drug, including the lack of safety and efficacy data. However, before this, in March 2000, the FDA issued a warning to Ozelle Pharmaceuticals because claims were made on the Ozelle Web site that Anvirzel was safe and effective based on preliminary and inconclusive data.

olive leaf | **Uses:** Insufficient evidence; | **Preg:** Not recommended due to insufficient evidence; | **CIs:** Allergy/hypersensitivity; | **ADRs:** insufficient evidence; | **Interactions:** Antiviral agents (altered effects); | **Dose:** Insufficient evidence; | **Monitor:** Viral load; | **Notes:** Olive leaves come from the olive tree, a native of the Mediterranean. Although olives and olive oil are used as foods, olive leaf is primarily used medicinally or as a tea. Olive leaf has displayed antifungal and antiviral properties in laboratory study.

omega-3 fatty acids, fish oil, alpha-linolenic acid | **Uses:** Angina pectoris, arrhythmias, asthma, atherosclerosis, cancer prevention, cardiovascular disorders, CHD prevention, Crohn's disease, cyclosporine nephrotoxicity, cystic fibrosis, depression, dysmenorrhea, eczema, GI disorders, HTN, hypertriglyeridemia, infant development, lupus erythematosus, nephrotic syndrome, pneumonia, pre-eclampsia, psoriasis, prostate cancer, psychiatric disorders, Raynaud's syndrome, schizophrenia, skin disorders, respiratory disorders, rheumatoid arthritis, stroke prevention, ulcerative colitis; | **Preg:** Considered safe in therapeutic doses; supplementation increased gestation; DHA preferred omega-3 fatty acid for brain/eye development; FDA recommends pregnant/nursing women avoid eating types of fish with higher levels of methylmercury; | **CIs:** Allergy/hypersensitivity, Diabetes (doses > 3 g/day), immunodeficiency (doses > 3 g/day); | **ADRs:** abdominal bloating/pain, bleeding (large doses), fishy aftertaste, halitosis, heartburn, hemorrhagic stroke (large doses), hyperglycemia (large doses), hypotension, immunosuppression (large doses), intestinal gas, ↑ LDL cholesterol, loose stools (large doses), nausea (large doses), skin rash, weight gain; | **Interactions:** Anticoagulants/antiplatelets (↑ risk of bleeding), antidiabetic agents (↑ risk of hypoglycemia), antihypertensives (↑ risk of hypotension), contraceptives (altered effects), orlistat (↓ absorption of fish oil), vitamins A and D (↑ risk of vitamin A or D toxicity; with cod liver oil), vitamins E (↓ vitamin E levels); | **Dose:** Oral: bipolar disorder, adjunct: 6.2 g EPA/3.4 g DHA PO qd (hypomania may develop); cyclosporine nephrotoxicity: 2.2 g EPA and 1.4 g DHA PO qd; depression: 9.6 g PO qd (use w/ antidepressants); dysmenorrhea: 1.08 g EPA/0.72 g DHA PO qd; hyperlipidemia: 1–6 g PO qd; hypertriglyceridemia: 1–4 g PO qd; HTN: 2.04 g EPA and 1.4 g DHA qd; infant development: 200–250 mg algal DHA PO qd; post–cardiac intervention: 3–6 g PO qd; post-MI: 0.85–1.08 g EPA PO qd: Raynaud's syndrome: 3.96 g EPA/2.64 g DHA PO qd; rheumatoid arthritis: 3.8 g EPA/2 g DHA PO qd; | **Monitor:** Blood pressure, coagulation panel, lipid profile; | **Notes:** Caution is warranted in patients with fish allergies.

onion | **Uses:** Allergies, alopecia areata, diabetes, HTN, scar prevention; | **Preg:** Not recommended due to insufficient evidence; | **CIs:** Allergy/hypersensitivity; | **ADRs:** asthma, ↓ blood pressure, contact dermatitis, dyspepsia, gastroesophageal reflux, hypoglycemia, "tulip finger" (painful tingling and erythema of the fingertips); | **Interactions:** Anticoagulants/antiplatelets (↑ risk of bleeding), antidiabetic agents, (↑ risk of hypoglycemia), antihypertensives (↑ risk of hypotension), aspirin (altered allergy effects), diuretics (additive effects); | **Dose:** Oral: 50 g PO qd. Topical: apply gel tid × 1 mo; | **Monitor:** Blood glucose, blood pressure, coagulation panel; | **Notes:** The primary adverse effects associated with onion are dermatological and gastrointestinal.

O

oregano | **Uses:** Parasitic infection; | **Preg:** Safe when used in amounts found in food; insufficient evidence regarding medicinal use; | **CIs:** Allergy/hypersensitivity; | **ADRs:** insufficient evidence; | **Interactions:** Anticoagulants/antiplatelets (↑ risk of bleeding), antidiabetic agents (↑ risk of hypoglycemia), diuretics (additive effects); estrogens (additive effects); | **Dose:** Oral, parasitic infections: 200 mg emulsified oil PO tid with meals × 6 wk. Topical, bath: 100 g dried leaf steeped in 1 L water × 10 min, strained and added to full bath; topical, oil: apply twice daily to affected area. Tea (as a mouth rinse): unsweetened oregano tea, gargle, or mouthwash; | **Monitor:** Blood glucose; coagulation panel; | **Notes:** Oregano is a perennial herb that contains phenolic compounds such as carvacrol and thymol. The leaves, stems, and flowers are used medicinally. It is commonly used as a food flavoring and preservative. Traditionally, oregano has been used to treat respiratory and gastrointestinal disorders and menstrual irregularities.

pagoda tree | **Uses:** Insufficient evidence; | **Preg:** Not recommended due to insufficient evidence; | **CIs:** Allergy/hypersensitivity, UNSAFE for oral use; | **ADRs:** DEATH, facial edema; | **Interactions:** Anticoagulants/antiplatelets (↑ risk of bleeding); | **Dose:** Insufficient evidence; | **Monitor:** Coagulation panel; | **Notes:** The seeds of the pagoda tree are not safe to consume. Use may cause facial edema, cystine poisoning, and even death.

palm oil | **Uses:** Malaria, hyperlipiemia, vitamin A deficiency; | **Preg:** Likely safe when used appropriately; | **CIs:** Allergy/hypersensitivity; | **ADRs:** ↓ bone mineral content, carotenoderma (high amounts); | **Interactions:** Anticoagulants/antiplatelets (↓ the effectiveness of anticoagulants/antiplatelets), antilipemic agents (additive effects), beta-carotene (excess beta-carotene), vitamin A (excess vitamin A), vitamin E (excess vitamin E); | **Dose:** Oral: hyperlipidemia, adults: 10 mL/day boiled crude palm oil after lunch or dinner; preventing vitamin A deficiency, children 5 years and older: 3 tbsp (9 g) per day; children younger than 5 years: 2 tbsp (6 g) per day; pregnant women: 4 tbsp (12 g) per day; | **Monitor:** Coagulation panel, lipid profile, vitamin A levels; | **Notes:** Palm oil is a source of beta-carotene and vitamin E. Caution is warranted in patients undergoing surgery due to increased risk of bleeding. Palm oil should be discontinued before surgery.

pancreatin | **Uses:** Cystic fibrosis, diabetes, digestion, gastrectomy, hiatal hernia complex, malnutrition, pancreatic cancer, pancreatic insufficiency, pancreatic surgery recovery, steatorrhea; | **Preg:** Not recommended due to insufficient evidence; | **CIs:** Allergy/hypersensitivity, Fibrosing colonopathy; | **ADRs:** abdominal pain, abnormal feces, altered glucose control, anorexia, asthmatic symptoms, contact dermatitis, cough, dizziness, fibrosing colonopathy, flatulence, gastrointestinal upset, headache, hyperuricosuria, occupational rhinitis, pruritic erythema, xerostomia; | **Interactions:** Acarbose (↓ efficacy of acarbose), analgesics (additive effects), antidiabetic agents (↓ effects), antineoplastic agents (potentiate effects), folic acid (↓ absorption of folic acid), misoprostol (↑ efficacy of pancreatin); | **Dose:** Digestive aid: 500–1,000 mg PO tid at the beginning of meals; 8,000–25,000 USP units of lipase PO qd at the beginning of meals; | **Monitor:** Uric acid; | **Notes:** Extreme caution is warranted in patients at risk for hyperuricemia, including patients with gout, renal impairment, or hyperuricemia. Pancreatic enzyme preparations vary greatly in their contents and properties. Most pancreatic enzyme

P

preparations are prescription medications indicated for supplementation in patients with exocrine pancreatic insufficiency due to conditions such as cystic fibrosis or chronic pancreatitis.

pantethine | **Uses:** Athletic performance, cystinosis, hyperlipidemia, IHD; | **Preg:** Not recommended due to insufficient evidence; | **CIs:** Allergy/hypersensitivity; | **ADRs:** diarrhea, dyspepsia, gastrointestinal discomfort, nausea; | **Interactions:** Anticoagulants/antiplatelets (↑ risk of bleeding), antilipemic agents (additive effects); | **Dose:** 600–1,200 mg PO qd; 400 mg/day IM; | **Monitor:** Coagulation panel, lipid profile; | **Notes:** Discontinue pantethine 2 weeks before surgery due to bleeding risk.

pantothenic acid | **Uses:** Athletic performance, ADHD, burns, hyperlipidemia, osteoarthritis, pantothenic acid deficiency, RA, wound healing; | **Preg:** When used in RDA (6 mg/day); | **CIs:** Allergy/hypersensitivity, GI obstruction (pantothenic acid injection), Hemophilia (dexpanthenol, derivative of pantothenic acid); | **ADRs:** diarrhea, dyspepsia, nausea; | **Interactions:** Anticoagulants/antiplatelets (↑ risk of bleeding), antibiotics (↓ levels of pantothenic acid), cholinesterase inhibitors (additive effects); | **Dose:** Dietary supplement: 5–10 mg PO qd. RDA: Men and women, 14 years and older, 5 mg PO qd; Children 9–13 years, 4 mg PO qd; Children 4–8 years, 3 mg PO qd; Children 1–3 years, 2 mg PO qd; Infants 7–12 months, 1.8 mg PO qd; Infants 0–6 months, 1.7 mg PO qd; Pregnant women, 6 mg PO qd; and Lactating women, 7 mg PO qd; | **Monitor:** Coagulation panel, pantothenic acid levels; | **Notes:** Pantothenic acid (vitamin B_5) is essential to all life and is a component of coenzyme A (CoA), a molecule that is necessary for numerous vital chemical reactions to occur in cells. Dexpanthenol is a derivative of pantothenic acid; the injection form is FDA approved for prophylaxis after abdominal surgery to reduce the risk of paralytic ileus.

pao pereira | **Uses:** Insufficient evidence; | **Preg:** Not recommended due to insufficient evidence; | **CIs:** Allergy/hypersensitivity; | **ADRs:** insufficient evidence; | **Interactions:** Antineoplastic agents (altered effects); | **Dose:** Oral: infusion: 3–5 cups/day; tincture: 2–8 mL/day; | **Monitor:** PSA levels; | **Notes:** Traditionally, pao pereira has been used to suppress the proliferation of HIV, herpesviruses, and cancer. Preliminary research suggests pao pereira may be used for prostate cancer.

papain | **Uses:** Exercise recovery, herpes zoster, jellyfish sting, lung abscess, pharyngitis, prevention of postoperative adhesion formation, radiation adverse effects, rheumatic disorders, sore throat, wound healing, xerotic skin; | **Preg:** Not recommended due to insufficient evidence; | **CIs:** Allergy/hypersensitivity, Clotting disorders; | **ADRs:** abdominal cramps, allergic conjunctivitis, allergic reactions, bleeding, blisters (topical), diaphoresis, diarrhea, esophageal perforation, fatigue, gastritis, irritation (topical), rhinorrhea, sneezing, ulcer; | **Interactions:** Anticoagulants/antiplatelets (↑ risk of bleeding); | **Dose:** 1,500 mg PO qd; | **Monitor:** Coagulation panel; | **Notes:** Cross-sensitivity in individuals allergic to kiwi and fig.

papaya | **Uses:** Antioxidant, burns, cancer (prevention), diabetes, human papillomavirus, skin ulcers, vitamin A deficiency; | **Preg:** Not recommended due to insufficient evidence and possible teratogenic and abortifacient effects; | **CIs:** Allergy/hypersensitivity, Latex allergy; | **ADRs:** airway sensitization, angioedema, burning sensation, gastrointestinal distress; | **Interactions:** Antibiotics (altered effects), anticoagulants/antiplatelets (↑ risk of bleeding; may potentiate the effects of warfarin), antilipemic agents (additive effects), immunosuppressants (altered effects), iron (↑ iron absorption), potassium (↑ potassium levels), vasodilators (altered effects); | **Dose:** Oral: 3–9 g fermented papaya PO qd; chewable enzyme tablets (250 mg of papaya powder, 150 mg of dried pineapple juice powder, and 10 mg of papain): 1 tablet PO tid, after meals. Topical: papaya paste, applied to a gauze pad to burnt skin, 1–2 times/day; | **Monitor:** Coagulation panel (may ↑ INR); | **Notes:** Papaya has traditionally been used for digestive problems. Papaya contains the proteolytic enzymes papain and chymopapain, which have been isolated and studied for their proteolytic effects on injured dermal tissue and for dissolving obstructed meat boluses.

para-aminobenzoic acid (PABA) | **Uses:** Asthma, cancer pain, dermatomyositis, herpes, hair loss, lichen sclerosus, melasma prevention, morphea, pemphigus vulgaris adjuvant, Peyronie's disease, photoprotection, scleroderma, vitiligo; | **Preg:** Likely safe when used topically; oral use not recommended due to insufficient evidence; | **CIs:** Allergy/hypersensitivity; | **ADRs:** allergic reactions, anorexia, contact dermatitis (topical), diarrhea, dyspepsia, fever, ↑ LFTs, rash, vitiligo, ↑ WBC count; | **Interactions:** Anticholinergic agents (↓ levels), anticoagulants/antiplatelets (↑ risk of bleeding), antidiabetic agents (↑ risk of hypoglycemia), cimetidine (↑ PABA absorption), cortisone (↑ effects), DAPSONE (↓ effects), procainamide (altered effects), SULFONAMIDE ANTIBIOTICS (↓ effects), tinidazole (↓ excretion of PABA); | **Dose:** Oral (potassium salt of PABA), adults: 12 g PO qd in 4–6 divided doses; children: 220 mg/kg/day in 4–6 divided doses; take with meals. Topical, sunscreen: apply 1%–15% for sun protection; | **Monitor:** LFTs, WBC count; | **Notes:** Caution is warranted in patients with kidney dysfunction. Adjust dose as needed.

parsley | **Uses:** Antioxidant; | **Preg:** Likely safe in amounts in food; not recommended in medicinal amounts due historical use as an abortifacient; | **CIs:** Allergy/hypersensitivity; | **ADRs:** large amounts: blood dyscrasias, bradycardia, deafness, hallucinations, hepatic dysfunction, hypotension, nephrotoxicity, photodermatitis; | **Interactions:** Anticoagulants/antiplatelets (interfere with anticoagulant effects), antidiabetic agents (↑ risk of hypoglycemia), aspirin (altered parsley allergy), diuretics (interfere with effects), laxatives (additive effects), MAO inhibitors (↑ risk of hypertensive crisis), vasodilators (additive effects); | **Dose:** Oral: Dilute a few drops of oil in a cup of water, gargle, and expectorate; 1–2 pearls 1–3 times/day; | **Monitor:** Blood glucose, coagulation panel; | **Notes:** Traditionally, parsley is used as a spice. Its oils have been used in halitosis and having antibacterial and antifungal activity. Parsley constituents—apiole and myristicin—in large amounts have been associated with hematological, renal, and hepatic toxicity.

parsnip | **Uses:** Insufficient evidence; | **Preg:** Safe in amounts found in food; insufficient evidence regarding medicinal use; | **CIs:** Allergy/hypersensitivity; | **ADRs:** photosensitivity; | **Interactions:** Photosensitizers (↑ risk of phototoxicity); | **Dose:** Insufficient evidence; | **Monitor:** N/A; | **Notes:** Parsnips were historically used as an aphrodisiac.

P

passion flower | **Uses:** Adjustment disorder, anxiety, CHF, opiate withdrawal; | **Preg:** Not recommended due to insufficient evidence and uterine stimulating effects; | **CIs:** Allergy/hypersensitivity; | **ADRs:** altered consciousness, dizziness, drowsiness, nausea/vomiting, sedation, tachycardia, vasculitis; | **Interactions:** Anticoagulants/antiplatelets (↑ risk of bleeding), antihypertensives (↑ risk of hypotension), antitussives (additive effects), caffeine (altered effects), CNS depressants (additive effects), CYP 450 substrates (altered effects), flumazenil (↓ effects of passion flower), naloxone (↓ effects of passion flower); | **Dose:** Anxiety: 45 drops of passiflora liquid extract plus 30 mg oxazepam PO qd × 4 wk. Insomnia: 200 mg PO qhs (standardized to contain 3.5% isovitexin per dose). General: dried herb: 0.5–2 g, 3–4 times/day; tincture (1:8): 1–4 mg 3–4 times/day; tea: 1 cup PO qd, made from 4–8 g dried herb in 150 mL boiling water; | **Monitor:** Blood pressure, coagulation panel; | **Notes:** Passion flower may depress the CNS and may cause additive effects when used with anesthesia. Passion flower should be discontinued 2 weeks before surgery.

pau d'arco | **Uses:** Cancer; | **Preg:** Avoid use due to abortifacient effects, may be toxic to fetus; | **CIs:** Allergy/hypersensitivity; | **ADRs:** bleeding, diarrhea, dizziness, gastrointestinal upset, vomiting; | **Interactions:** Antiangiogenic agents (additive effects); anticoagulants/antiplatelets (↑ risk of bleeding), immunosuppressants (additive effects); | **Dose:** Capsules: 1–4 g PO qd. Tablets: 1–4 g PO qd in 2–3 divided doses. Tea: 1 tsp loose dried bark boiled in 150 mL water × 5–15 min, 2–8 times/day. Tincture: 20–30 gtts, 2–3 times/day; | **Monitor:** Coagulation panel; | **Notes:** Much of the scientific research conducted to date has demonstrated a number of antineoplastic effects attributed to pau d'arco and its constituents, especially beta-lapachone, in vitro and in animals.

PC-SPES | **Uses:** Prostate CA; | **Preg:** Not recommended due to insufficient evidence and possible hormonal effects; | **CIs:** Allergy/hypersensitivity; | **ADRs:** diarrhea, erectile dysfunction, hot flashes, hypertriglyceridemia, indigestion, leg cramps, ↓ libido, mastalgia, pulmonary thrombosis; | **Interactions:** Antacids (↓ effectiveness), antiandrogens (additive effects), anticoagulants/antiplatelets (↑ risk of bleeding), estrogens (additive effects), paclitaxel (altered effects); | **Dose:** Based on known safety concerns associated with PC-SPES, no dosing regimen is recommended; | **Monitor:** PSA levels; | **Notes:** PC-SPES is an herbal combination product that was produced and marketed until early 2002 by BotanicLab, Inc. for the treatment of prostate cancer. The initials PC stand for prostate cancer, and *spes* is Latin for hope. The composition of PC-SPES has been conflicting. Based on a Chinese herbal formula, the ingredients of PC-SPES were officially listed as including *Serenoa repens* (saw palmetto) and seven other herbs: *Chrysanthemum morifolium* (chrysanthemum, mum, Chu-hua); *Ganoderma lucidum* (reishi mushroom, Ling Zhi); *Glycyrrhiza glabra* (licorice); *Isatis indigotica* Fort (Da Qing Ye, dyer's wood); *Panax pseudo-ginseng* (San Qi); *Rabdosia rubescens* (rubescens, Dong Ling Cao); and *Scutellaria baicalensis* (skullcap, Huang-chin). Diethylstilbestrol, indomethacin, and warfarin and several natural products have been found in some PC-SPES preparations.

P

peony | **Uses:** Allergic dermatitis, antioxidant, *Campylobacter pyloridis,* chronic hepatitis, CHD, cor pulmonale, hemolytic disease in newborn, hormone regulation, hyperlipidemia, lung CA, menstrual irregularities, muscle cramps, nephritis, preeclampsia, RA, uterine fibroids, wrinkle prevention; | **Preg:** Avoid during the first trimester of pregnancy and tree peony bark should not be used at all during pregnancy. Traditionally, peony has been used as an abortifacient and emmenagogue; | **CIs:** Allergy/hypersensitivity; | **ADRs:** angina, colic, contact dermatitis, contusion, diarrhea, dyspepsia, epistaxis, gum bleeding, nausea/vomiting; | **Interactions:** Anticoagulants/antiplatelets (↑ risk of bleeding), antilipemic agents (additive effects), antiviral agents (altered effects), CYP450 2C9 (↓ levels), hormonal agents (altered effects), phenytoin (↓ effectiveness), tamoxifen (altered effects), vasodilators (additive effects); | **Dose:** Tea: 1 cup/day PO (prepared using 1 g flowers steeped in 150 mL boiling water for 5–10 min and then strained). Wrinkle prevention, cream: 0.5% partially purified paeoniflorin × 8 wk; | **Monitor:** Heart rate, blood pressure, coagulation panel; | **Notes:** Extreme caution is warranted when using peony during pregnancy in the second and third trimesters. Peony should be avoided during the first trimester.

peppermint oil | **Uses:** Abdominal distention, antispasmodic, asthma, brain injury, cough, cracked nipples (prevention), dyspepsia, functional bowel disorders, IBS, hemiplegic shoulder pain, halitosis, nasal congestion, nausea (postoperative), postherpetic neuralgia, tension headache, tuberculosis, UTI; | **Preg:** Not recommended due to insufficient evidence; | **CIs:** Allergy/hypersensitivity, Achlorhydria; | **ADRs:** abdominal bloating, abdominal pain, acute lung injury, acute renal failure, anal burning, asthma exacerbation, blurry vision, bradycardia, brain lesions, breast infection, burning mouth syndrome, chemical burn, contact dermatitis, drop in respiratory rate, dyspepsia, eye irritation, flatulence, hypersensitivity reactions, interstitial nephritis, lichenoid reaction, mild pancreatitis, minty taste in the mouth, mouth wounds, muscle tremor, nausea, necrosis, neurotoxicity, non-thrombocytopenic purpura, perianal burning, pulmonary edema, skin rash and irritation, symphathovagal response, tachycardia, urticaria, vomiting; | **Interactions:** Antacids/H2 antagonists/PPIs (premature dissolution of enteric-coated peppermint oil), cyclosporine (↑ cyclosporine levels), CYP450 1A2/2C9/2C19/3A4 substrates (inhibits CYP450 1A2/2C9/2C19/3A4); | **Dose:** Digestive disorders: 0.2–0.4 mL PO tid (avg daily amount is 6–12 gtt). Colonic spasm: 8 mL/day PO. Esophageal spasm: 5 gtt in 10 mL water

P

PO qd. IBS, capsules: 1–2 caps PO tid 15–30 min before meals × 1 mo (capsules contain 0.2 mL peppermint oil). Nausea/vomiting, leaf: 3–6 g PO qd, tincture: 5–15 gtt/150 mL PO qd. Sore throat: 1 lozenge PO prn for sore throat (lozenge contains 2–10 mg peppermint oil). Tension headache: 10% peppermint oil in ETOH sol, apply to forehead/temples, repeat after 15 and 30 min. General, other uses, inhaled: 3–4 gtt oil in hot water prn (inhale vapors/aromatic steam); Other uses, topical: apply topically prn; Other uses, oral, tincture (1:5 prep in 45% ethanol): 2–3 mL PO tid; spirits (10% and 1%; leaf extract): 1 mL (20 gtt) in water; dried extract: 2–4 g PO tid; tea (prepared w/dried leaves/250 mL boiling water): 3–4 cups PO qd; infusion (1.5–3 g peppermint oil/150 mL water): 1 cup PO tid; | **Monitor:** N/A; | **Notes:** Although peppermint has been studied for nonulcerative dyspepsia, it should be noted that the most common complaint in trials of oral peppermint oil is heartburn.

perilla | **Uses:** Allergies, aphthous stomatitis, asthma; | **Preg:** Not recommended due to insufficient evidence; | **CIs:** Allergy/hypersensitivity; | **ADRs:** contact dermatitis; | **Interactions:** Barbituates (additive effects), antilipemic agents (additive effects), NSAIDs (↓ effects); | **Dose:** Tea: 500 mL boiling water to ¼ cup dry herb, steep 10 to 15 minutes, consumed throughout the day. Asthma: 10–20 g perilla seed oil PO qd; | **Monitor:** Lipid profile; | **Notes:** Perilla is used to treat asthma and is generally well tolerated.

perillyl alcohol | **Uses:** Cancer; | **Preg:** Not recommended due to insufficient evidence; | **CIs:** Allergy/hypersensitivity; | **ADRs:** abdominal bloating, anorexia, constipation, cramps, diarrhea, dysgeusia, fatigue, gastrointestinal reflux, headache, hot flashes, hypertension, hypokalemia, leukocytosis, mucositis, nausea, pancreatitis, satiety; | **Interactions:** Antilipemic agents (additive effects), cisplatin (↑ effects), imatinib (synergistic effects); | **Dose:** 1.2–11.2 g/m^2 PO 3–4 times daily; | **Monitor:** WBC count; | **Notes:** Animal studies suggest perillyl alcohol can be a regressive agent against pancreatic, mammary, and liver tumors. It may also have an application as a chemopreventive mediator for colon, lung, and skin cancer. Perillyl alcohol is under sponsorship from the National Cancer Institute (NCI), and is undergoing phase II clinical trials.

periwinkle | **Uses:** Cancer, dementia, Hodgkin's disease, idiopathic thrombocytopenic purpura, stroke; | **Preg:** Avoid use; | **CIs:** Allergy/hypersensitivity, Oral use; | **ADRs:** ↓ blood pressure, bone marrow depression, diarrhea, gastrointestinal upset, KIDNEY DAMAGE, LIVER DAMAGE, myelosuppression, nausea/vomiting, NEUROLOGICAL DAMAGE, pancytopenia, rash, skin flushing; | **Interactions:** Anticoagulants/antiplatelets (↑ risk of bleeding), antihypertensives (↑ risk of hypotension), CYP450 substrates (altered effects), hepatotoxic agents (↑ risk of liver damage), immunosuppressants (↑ risk of immunosuppression), MAOIs (↑ risk of hypertensive crisis), nephrotoxic agents (↑ risk of kidney damage), vasodilators (additive effects); | **Dose:** Insufficient available evidence; | **Monitor:** LFTs, kidney function, WBC count; | **Notes:** The use of periwinkle as a dietary supplement is not recommended because it contains vinca alkaloids, which are TOXIC and may cause damage to the liver, kidneys, and nerves as well as death. The vinca alkaloids, including vinblastine and vincristine isolated from Madagascar periwinkle, are FDA-approved chemotherapeutic agents.

peyote | **Uses:** Insufficient available evidence; | **Preg:** Avoid use; | **CIs:** Allergy/hypersensitivity; | **ADRs:** anxiety, DEATH, diaphoresis, fear, gastrointestinal distress, hallucinations, hyper-/hypotension, mydriasis, nausea/vomiting, paranoia, psychosis, sedation, tachycardia; | **Interactions:** Antihypertensives (altered effects), CNS depressants (altered effects), STIMULANTS (↑ risk of adverse CNS effects); | **Dose:** Insufficient evidence; | **Monitor:** N/A; | **Notes:** Peyote is commonly used in rituals and as a hallucinogen. In 1990, the United States Supreme Court ruled that states may prohibit the use of peyote for religious purposes. There are cases of death with peyote ingestion. Mescaline can be extracted from peyote. Peyote and mescaline are Schedule I controlled substance hallucinogens.

P

phenylalanine | **Uses:** ADHD, dental anesthesia, chronic pain, depression, low back pain, multiple sclerosis, phenylalanine deficiency, vitiligo; | **Preg:** Not recommended due to insufficient evidence; | **CIs:** Allergy/hypersensitivity, Hyperphenylalaninemia, Parkinson's disease (particularly DL-phenylalanine); | **ADRs:** anxiety, constipation, dyspepsia, fatigue, headache, hypomania, insomnia, nausea, sedation, TARDIVE DYSKINESIA; | **Interactions:** Antipsychotic drugs (↑ risk of tardive dyskinesia), baclofen (↓ absorption of baclofen), CNS depressants (↑ risk of sedation), LEVODOPA (exacerbate tremor), MAOIs, (↑ risk of hypertensive crisis); | **Dose:** ADHD (adults): 50–400 mg DL-phenylalanine PO tid. Chronic pain: 250 mg D-phenylalanine PO qid. Dental anesthesia: 2 or 4 g D-phenylalanine, 30 minutes before acupuncture. Depression: 500 mg L-phenylalanine PO bid (morning and noon), may titrate up to a maximum of 14 g/day. Low back pain: 1.5 g

D-phenylalanine PO qd in 3 divided doses or 4 g, 30 minutes before acupuncture. Multiple sclerosis: 500 mg L-phenylalanine PO bid plus lofepramine 70 mg PO qd and vitamin B_{12} 1,000 mcg IM qd. Vitiligo: 50, 70, or 100 mg/kg L-phenylalanine PO qd. ADHD (children): 10–20 mg/kg D-phenylalanine PO qd in 4 divided doses. Vitiligo (topical): 50–100 mg/kg L-phenylalanine 15 minutes after daily oral L-phenylalanine 50 or 100 mg/kg, along with UVA exposure; | **Monitor:** N/A; | **Notes:** DL-phenylalanine can exacerbate tremor and "on-off" syndrome in patients with Parkinson's disease. Use cautiously in patients with schizophrenia.

phosphates, phosphorus | **Uses:** Burns, constipation, diabetic ketoacidosis, hypercalcemia, hypercalciuria, hyperparathyroidism, hypophosphatemia, laxative, osteoporosis, refeeding syndrome prevention, renal calculi, TPN, vitamin D–resistant rickets; | **Preg:** Safe when used at RDA; | **CIs:** Allergy/hypersensitivity; | **ADRs:** constipation, diarrhea, electrolyte disturbances, gastrointestinal discomfort, nausea; | **Interactions:** Alcohol (↑ levels of phosphorus), antacids (↓ absorption of phosphate), anticonvulsants (↓ levels of phosphate), bile acid sequestrants (↓ absorption of phosphate), bisphosphonates (↑ risk of hypocalcemia), calcitrol (↑ risk of hyperphosphatemia), calcium (↓ absorption of phosphate and calcium), corticosteroids (↑ levels of phosphorus), iron (↓ absorption of phosphate and iron), magnesium (↓ absorption of phosphate and magnesium), sevelamer (↓ levels of phosphate), sucralfate (↓ levels of phosphate), teriparatide (↓ levels of phosphate); | **Dose:** RDA: adults, older than 18 years: 700 mg/day; children 9–18 years: 1,250 mg/day; children 4–8 years: 500 mg/day; children 1–3 years: 460 mg/day; infants 7–12 mo: 275 mg/day; infants 0–6 mo: 100 mg/day. The Tolerable Upper Intake Level (UL) for adults ages 19–70 years old is 4 g/day; for adults 70 years and older, the UL is 3 g/day. The recommended UL in pregnant women is 3.5 g/day, and in breastfeeding women, it is 4 g/day. Rectal: dibasic sodium phosphate: 6.84–7.56 g as a single dose; monobasic sodium phosphate: 18.24–20.16 g as a single dose. IV: 50 mmoles over 24 hours used during refeeding syndrome; | **Monitor:** Phosphate levels; | **Notes:** Conditions that may be worsened with excessive phosphorus/phosphate supplementation include burns, heart disease, pancreatitis, rickets, osteomalacia, underactive parathyroid glands, underactive adrenal glands, and liver disease.

P

phosphatidyl choline | **Uses:** Alcohol-induced liver damage, Alzheimer's disease, cancer, dialysis, fatty deposits, gallstones, hepatitis, hyperlipidemia, memory, tardive dyskinesia; | **Preg:** Not recommended due to insufficient evidence; | **CIs:** Allergy/hypersensitivity; | **ADRs:** injection: bruising, burning, edema, erythema, pruritus, tenderness; oral: diarrhea, GI upset, hyperhidrosis; | **Interactions:** Anticholinergic agents (↓ effectiveness of anticholinergics), cholinergic agents (excessive acetylcholine levels), cholinesterase inhibitors (↑ acetylcholine levels); | **Dose:** Injection, subcutaneous: 0.2–0.5 mL of a 5% phosphatidyl choline (250 mg/5 mL), in various intervals. Oral: 500–1,000 mg PO 2–3 times/day; Chronic hepatitis: 1.8 g daily; Subacute hepatic failure: 350 mg 3 times daily; Acute viral hepatitis: 300 mg 3 times daily; Chronic active ulcerative colitis: 6 g daily retarded-release phosphatidyl choline–rich phospholipids; Hyperlipoproteinemia: 300 mg daily; | **Monitor:** N/A; | **Notes:** The term "lecithin" refers to 100% phosphatidyl choline in the food industry, which is used as a food emulsifier. It is used as the active ingredient contained in cosmetic injection products.

phosphatidyl serine | **Uses:** ADHD, age-related memory disorders, stress; | **Preg:** Not recommended due to insufficient evidence; | **CIs:** Allergy/hypersensitivity; | **ADRs:** GI distress, insomnia, nausea; | **Interactions** Acetylcholinesterase inhibitors (↑ acetylcholine levels), anticholinergic agents (↓ effectiveness of anticholinergics), anticoagulants/antiplatelets (↑ risk of bleeding), cholinergic agents (↑ acetylcholine levels); | **Dose:** 100 mg PO 2–3 times/day; | **Monitor:** Coagulation panel, cortisol levels; | **Notes:** Phosphatidyl serine is a phospholipid, a fat-soluble compound. Phospholipids are essential components of cell membranes, with very high concentrations found in the brain.

P

Pinus radiata | **Uses:** Antioxidant, cardiovascular health, cognitive performance; | **Preg:** Not recommended due to insufficient evidence; | **CIs:** Allergy/hypersensitivity; | **ADRs:** contact dermatitis, rhinoconjunctivitis; | **Interactions:** Antihypertensives (↑ risk of hypotension), antilipemic agents (additive effects); | **Dose:** 1–2 capsules of Enzogenol (capsule containing 120 mg *Pinus radiata* flavonoid extract and 60 mg vitamin C); | **Monitor:** Blood pressure, lipid profile; | **Notes:** Pollen from *Pinus radiata* may cause seasonal rhinoconjunctivitis.

plant sterols | **Uses:** Androgenetic alopecia, BPH, gallstones, HIV, hyperlipidemia, immune function, RA, tuberculosis (adjunct); | **Preg:** Not recommended due to insufficient evidence; | **CIs:** Allergy/hypersensitivity; | **ADRs:** asthma, constipation, diarrhea, dyspepsia, erectile dysfunction, flatulence, nausea; **Interactions:** Acarbose (↑ absorption), acid-labile antibiotics (improve absorption of antibiotics), activated charcoal (↓ levels of sterols), anticoagulants/antiplatelets (↑ risk of bleeding), antidiabetic agents (↑ risk of hypoglycemia), antilipemic agents (additive effects), beta-carotene (↓ absorption of beta-carotene), estrogens (additive effects), ezetimibe (inhibits absorption of sterols), immunosuppressants (altered effects), laxatives (additive effects), HMG-CoA reductase inhibitors (↓ levels of sterols), vitamin E (↓ absorption of vitamin E); **Dose:** Adults: 60 mg–6 g PO qd; children: 1.5–3 g PO qd; **Monitor:** Blood glucose, coagulation panel, lipid profile; **Notes:** Plant sterols are found in plant-based foods such as fruits, vegetables, soybeans, breads, peanuts, and peanut products. Plant sterols are also present in bourbon and oils, such as olive, flaxseed, and canned tuna. Beta-sitosterol is one of the most common dietary phytosterols (plant sterols) found and synthesized exclusively by plants.

pleurisy *(Asclepias tuberosa)* **Uses:** Insufficient available evidence; **Preg:** Not recommended due to insufficient evidence; **CIs:** Allergy/hypersensitivity, Concurrent use with cardiac glycosides; **ADRs:** Insufficient available evidence; **Interactions:** Antidepressants (altered effects), CARDIAC GLYCOSIDES (e.g., digoxin, additive effects), diuretics (↑ risk of hypokalemia), estrogens (interfere with therapy); **Dose:** Insufficient available evidence; **Monitor:** Heart rate; **Notes:** The roots of the pleurisy plant have been found to contain cardiac glycosides and should be avoided with digoxin.

P

podophyllum *(Podophyllum hexandrum, Podophyllum peltatum)* **Uses:** Leukoplakia, RA, uterine CA, warts; **Preg:** Not recommended due to insufficient evidence and possible teratogenic effects; **CIs:** Allergy/hypersensitivity, Gallbladder disease, Pregnancy; **ADRs:** ataxia, burning sensation (topical), diarrhea, dysgeusia, hypokalemia, leukopenia, nausea/vomiting, neutropenia, pancytopenia, stomach discomfort, tachycardia, thrombocytopenia, urinary retention; **Interactions:** Antihypertensives (↑ risk of hypotension), antipsychotic agents (exacerbate extrapyrimidal symptoms caused by antipsychotic agents), hepatotoxic drugs (↑ risk of liver damage), laxatives (↑ risk of dehydration and electrolyte disturbances); **Dose:** Oral, RA: 300 mg PO qd × 12 wks. Topical, warts: 0.5%–2% applied twice daily to affected area for 3 days a week for 5 weeks; **Monitor:** Blood pressure, WBC count; | **Notes:** Podophyllum can increase liver function tests. Podophyllotoxin is a plant-derived compound used to produce two cytostatic drugs, etoposide and teniposide.

poison ivy *(Toxicodendron radicans)* | **Uses:** Insufficient evidence; | **Preg:** Avoid use; | **CIs:** Allergy/hypersensitivity, Topical or oral use; | **ADRs:** Oral: diarrhea, intestinal colic, mucous membrane irritation, nausea/vomiting; topical: black spot dermatitis, blisters, contact dermatitis, pruritus, skin reddening, swelling; | **Interactions:** *Ginkgo biloba* (cross-reactivity); | **Dose:** Avoid oral or topical use; | **Monitor:** N/A; | **Notes:** Cross-reactivity with cashews and mangos.

pokeweed *(Phytolacca americana)* | **Uses:** Schistosomiasis (prevention), tonsillitis; | **Preg:** Not recommended due to insufficient evidence and traditional use as an abortifacient; | **CIs:** Allergy/hypersensitivity, Oral use; | **ADRs:** toxic effects: abdominal pain, burning sensation of the mouth/throat, convulsions, DEATH, diarrhea, eosinophilia, hepatotoxicity, hypotension, nausea/vomiting, respiratory failure, salivation, tachycardia, thrombocytopenia, transient blindness, urinary incontinence, weakness; | **Interactions:** Antihypertensives (↑ risk of hypotension), diuretics (additive effects); | **Dose:** Emetic or purgative: 1 g of dried pokeweed root, based on unsubstantiated reports. Immune stimulation, rheumatism: 60–100 mg daily of the root and berries, based on unsubstantiated reports. | **Monitor:** Toxic effects; | **Notes:** All parts of the pokeweed plant are considered TOXIC.

P

policosanol | **Uses:** Blood clot prevention, CHD, intermittent claudication, hyperlipidemia, reactivity; | **Preg:** Not recommended due to insufficient evidence; | **CIs:** Allergy/hypersensitivity, Surgery; | **ADRs:** ↓ blood pressure, dyspepsia, ↑/↓ glucose, headache, skin rash, vertigo; | **Interactions:** ANTICOAGULANTS/ANTIPLATELETS (↑ risk of bleeding), antidiabetic agents (altered effects), antihypertensives (↑ risk of hypotension), antilipemic agents (additive effects), nitroprusside (additive effects); | **Dose:** 5–80 mg/day for up to 3 years; | **Monitor:** Coagulation panel, lipid profile; | **Notes:** Policosanol inhibits platelet aggregation and may cause excessive bleeding if used before surgery. Patients should discontinue policosanol 2 weeks before surgery.

polydextrose | **Uses:** Child growth; | **Preg:** Not recommended due to insufficient evidence; | **CIs:** Allergy/

hypersensitivity; **ADRs:** abdominal cramping, bloating, diarrhea, eczema, flatulence, irritability; **Interactions:** Antidiabetic agents (altered effects), antilipemic agents (altered effects), laxatives (additive effects); **Dose:** 16–90 g daily; **Monitor:** Blood glucose, lipid profile; **Notes:** Polydextrose is a dietary fiber that is used as a bulking agent in a variety of foods.

Polypodium leucotomos extract and anapsos

Uses: Atopic dermatitis, dementia, psoriasis, skin damage, sunburn, vitiligo; **Preg:** Not recommended due to insufficient evidence; **CIs:** Allergy/hypersensitivity; **ADRs:** abdominal discomfort, pruritus, sedation; **Interactions:** Anticoagulants/antiplatelets (↑ risk of bleeding), antihypertensives (↑ risk of hypotension), beta blockers (altered effects), cardiac glycosides (altered effects), CNS depressants (↑ sedation), immunosuppressants (altered effects); **Dose:** 120–750 mg PO qd × 4 wk; **Monitor:** Heart rate; **Notes:** The South American species *Polypodium leucotomos* L. is commonly known as "calaguala." Extracts of this species, called "anapsos," have been marketed and used as a treatment for multiple indications. It has positive inotropic and chronotropic effects.

pomegranate *(Punica granatum)*

Uses: Antioxidant, atherosclerosis, COPD, erectile dysfunction, fungal infection, hyperlipidemia, HTN, menopausal symptoms, periodontitis, plaque, prostate CA, stomatitis, sunburn; **Preg:** Safe when consumed in food; not recommended in medicinal amounts due to insufficient evidence; **CIs:** Allergy/hypersensitivity; **ADRs:** allergic reactions, angioedema (topical), contamination, diarrhea, flatulence, hypotension, red itchy eyes (topical), rhinorrhea (topical), urticaria (topical); **Interactions:** ACE inhibitors (additive effects), antidiabetic agents (altered effects), antihypertensives (↑ risk of hypotension), antilipemic agents (additive effects), CYP450 2D6 and 3A4 (inhibits CYP450 2D6 and 3A4), estrogens (additive effects), rosuvastatin (↑ levels of rosuvastatin); **Dose:** 50–400 mL pomegranate juice/day; **Monitor:** Blood glucose, blood pressure; **Notes:** Dried pomegranate peel may contain aflatoxin, which is a potent hepatocarcinogen and toxin. Pomegranate root and stem contain pellertierine, and oral overdoses can cause strychnine-like effects in the form of reflex arousal that can escalate to paralysis. At amounts greater than 80 g, people have experienced vomiting, including bloody emesis, followed by dizziness, chills, vision disorders, collapse, and possibly death due to respiratory failure.

P

populus | **Uses:** Insufficient available evidence; | **Preg:** Not recommended due to insufficient evidence; | **CIs:** Allergy/hypersensitivity; | **ADRs:** allergic reactions, asthma, contact dermatitis, rhinoconjunctivitis; | **Interactions:** Anticoagulants/antiplatelets (↑ risk of bleeding), anti-inflammatory agents (additive effects); | **Dose:** Insufficient available evidence; | **Monitor:** Insufficient available evidence; | **Notes:** Populus pollen, bark, wood, and sawdust are known to cause allergic reactions in sensitive people, including contact dermatitis, rhinoconjunctivitis, and asthma.

probiotics | **Uses:** Allergies, amoebiasis, antibiotic-associated diarrhea, asthma, atopic dermatitis, bacterial vaginosis, cardiovascular disease, cirrhosis, collagenous colitis, colon cancer, Crohn's disease, dental caries, diarrhea (acute), ear infections, fertility, growth, *Helicobacter pylori,* hepatic encephalopathy, immune enhancement, IBS, lactose intolerance, necrotizing enterocolitis (prevention), pancreatitis, pneumonia, pouchitis, radiation sickness, RA, respiratory tract infections, rotaviral diarrhea, sinusitis, supplementation (preterm/low-birth weight infants), traveler's diarrhea, ulcerative colitis, UTI, vaccine adjunct, vaginal candidiasis; | **Preg:** Not recommended due to insufficient evidence; | **CIs:** Allergy/hypersensitivity; | **ADRs:** bloating, diarrhea, flatulence, gastrointestinal distress; | **Interactions:** Antibiotics (↓ effectiveness of probiotics), immunosuppressants (altered effects); | **Dose:** Probiotics are commercially available as capsules, yogurts, powder, and dairy products. The most common probiotics are *Lactobacillus, Saccharomyces,* and *Bifidobacterium*. Various doses have been used but typically range from 1–10 billion cells PO qd (higher doses up to 600 billion bacteria PO qd have been used); children: 2–5 billion colony-forming units of *Lactobacillus acidophilus* and *Bifidobacterium* PO qd; | **Monitor:** N/A; | **Notes:** Use with caution in immunocompromised patients.

P

progesterone | **Uses:** Amenorrhea, abnormal uterine bleeding, Alzheimer's disease, brain injury, breast cancer (prevention), cardiovascular disease, dysmenorrhea, endometrial hyperplasia, HRT, infertility, mastalgia, mastodynia, menopause, osteoporosis, PMS, preterm birth (prevention); | **Preg:** Avoid use; | **CIs:** Allergy/hypersensitivity, Allergy to progesterone or peanut oil (oral), Breast cancer, Cerebral apoplexy (history of), Hepatic dysfunction (severe), Missed abortion, Vaginal bleeding (undiagnosed), Thromboembolic disorders; | **ADRs:** acne, alopecia, amenorrhea, appetite changes, breakthrough bleeding or spotting, cerebrovascular disorders, depression, edema, gastrointestinal disturbances, hepatotoxicity, hirsutism, mastalgia, menstrual irregularities, pain or swelling at injection site, photosensitivity, pruritus, pulmonary embolism, retinal thrombosis, sodium retention, thrombophlebitis, weight gain or loss; | **Interactions:** Antidiabetic agents (↑ risk of hypoglycemia), bromocriptine (interfere with effects of bromocriptine), CYP2C19 inducers (altered effects), CYP3A4 inducers (altered effects), estrogens (↑ risk of breast tenderness), red clover (↓ effectiveness of progesterone); | **Dose:** IM: amenorrhea: 5–10 mg/day for 6–8 days; functional uterine bleeding: 5–10 mg/day for 6 doses. Intravaginal: dosage range for intravaginal progesterone gel varies. Oral: amenorrhea: 400 mg PO qd × 10 days; endometrial hyperplasia (prevention): 200 mg PO qd × 12 days of a 28-day cycle with conjugated estrogens; HRT: 200 mg PO qd × 12 days of 25-day cycle with conjugated estrogens. Topical: dosage range for topical progesterone depends on the strength of the extract; | **Monitor:** Blood glucose, LFTs, LH/FSH, progesterone levels; | **Notes:** Natural progesterone is used in hormone replacement therapies. It is often used for PMS and problems associated with menopause. Intravaginal progesterone gel (Crinone 8%) is FDA-approved for infertility; micronized progesterone (Prometrium) is approved for endometrial hyperplasia and secondary amenorrhea. Caution is warranted in patients with cardiovascular disease, diabetes, fluid retention, or history of depression.

propolis | **Uses:** Aphthous stomatitis, burns, cervicitis, common cold, dental analgesia, *Helicobacter pylori*, infection, HSV-1 and 2, Legg-Calvé-Perthes disease, plaque/gingivitis, postherpetic corneal complications, rheumatic disease, rhinopharyngitis prevention (children), sulcoplasty, URI (children), vaginitis; | **Preg:** Not recommended due to insufficient evidence; | **CIs:** Allergy/hypersensitivity, Asthma; | **ADRs:** allergic reactions, burning, cheilitis, contact dermatitis, edema, erythematous vesicular lesions, hyperkeratotic dermatitis, mucositis, perioral eczema, pruritus, renal failure, stomatitis, vesiculitis; | **Interactions:** Antibacterial agents (additive effects), anticoagulants/antiplatelets (↑ risk of bleeding), antiretroviral agents (additive effects), immunosuppressants (altered effects); | **Dose:** Oral, for infection: 500 mg PO tid × 3 days; mouthwash: 5% aqueous alcohol solution. Topical, cervicitis: 5% ointment or cream applied daily × 10 days; topical, genital herpes: 3% ointment applied 4 times/day. Children, rhinopharyngitis prevention: 0.5 mL nasal spray weekly × 5 months; | **Monitor:** Coagulation panel, WBC count; | **Notes:** Propolis is a natural flavonoid-rich resin created by bees used in the construction of hives.

P

PSK (polysaccharide krestin) | **Uses:** Cancer (adjuvant); | **Preg:** Not recommended due to insufficient evidence; | **CIs:** Allergy/hypersensitivity; | **ADRs:** anorexia, darkening of fingernails, diarrhea, gastrointestinal discomfort/upset, hepatotoxicity, leukopenia, nausea/vomiting; | **Interactions:** Hepatotoxic agents (↑ risk of liver damage), immunosuppressants (altered effects); | **Dose:** 3 g PO qd; | **Monitor:** LFTs, WBC count; | **Notes:** Polysaccharide krestin (PSK), a constituent of coriolus mushroom, is given as a biological response modifier and an adjunct to standard chemotherapy. Leukopenia and hepatotoxicity have been reported, but patients were also using chemotherapy.

psyllium ***(Plantago ovata, Plantago isphagula)*** | **Uses:** Anal fissures, cervical dilator, colon CA, colonoscopy preparation, constipation, diarrhea, fat excretion, flatulence, hemorrhoids, hypercholesterolemia, hyperglycemia, IBD, obesity; | **Preg:** Generally considered safe, but studies are lacking; | **CIs:** Allergy/hypersensitivity, Fecal impaction, GI atony, GI obstruction, Spastic colon, Phenylketonuria (products that contain aspartame), Swallowing disorders; | **ADRs:** abdominal pain, bloating, constipation, diarrhea, dyspepsia, indigestion, rhinitis, wheezing; | **Interactions:** Antidiabetic agents (↑ risk of hypoglycemia), carbamazepine (↓ absorption), digoxin (↓ absorption), iron (↓ absorption), laxatives (additive effects), lithium (↓ levels), oral drugs (↓ absorption), riboflavin (↓ absorption), salicylates (↓ levels), tetracyclines (↓ levels), warfarin (↓ absorption); | **Dose:** 2.2–45 g PO daily in divided doses; | **Monitor:** Blood glucose, lipid profile; | **Notes:** Adequate fluid intake is required when taking psyllium-containing products. Inadequate water may cause psyllium to swell and block the throat or intestines.

pycnogenol | **Uses:** Asthma, ADHD, blood clot prevention, chronic venous insufficiency, coronary artery disease, deep vein thrombosis, diabetes, diabetic microangiopathy, dysmenorrhea, endometriosis, erectile dysfunction, HTN, hyperlipidemia, leg cramps, menopausal symptoms, plaque, pregnancy-related pain and discomfort (back pain, pelvic pain, hip pain); retinopathy, SLE, venous leg ulcers; | **Preg:** Not recommended due to insufficient evidence, has been used safely during third trimester. The manufacturer recommends avoidance during the first trimester due to lack of clinical study in this population; | **CIs:** Allergy/hypersensitivity; | **ADRs:** ↓ blood glucose, gastrointestinal discomfort, headache, nausea, vertigo; | **Interactions:** Anticoagulants/antiplatelets (↑ risk of bleeding), antidiabetic agents (↑ risk of hypoglycemia), antihypertensives (↑ risk of hypotension), antilipemic agents (additive effects), immunosuppressants (altered effects); **Dose:** Adults: 50–450 mg PO qd. Children, for asthma and ADHD: 1 mg/kg PO qd × 4 wk; **Monitor:** Blood glucose; **Notes:** Pycnogenol is the patented trade name for a water extract of the bark of the French maritime pine (*Pinus pinaster* ssp. *atlantica*) and contains oligomeric proanthocyanidins (OPCs).

pygeum ***(Prunus africanum, Pygeum africanum)*** **Uses:** BPH; **Preg:** Not recommended due to insufficient evidence and possible hormonal effects; **CIs:** Allergy/hypersensitivity; **ADRs:** abdominal pain, constipation, diarrhea, nausea; **Interactions:** 5-alpha reductase inhibitors (additive effects), androgens (antagonistic effects), estrogens (additive effects), saw palmetto (additive effects), stinging nettle (additive effects); **Dose:** 75–200 mg (standardized to a 14% content of sterols) PO qd in single or 2 divided doses; **Monitor:** PSA; **Notes:** Pygeum is widely used in Europe for BPH. The demand for pygeum has increased so much that the tree was reported as a threatened species.

pyruvate **Uses:** Aging skin, alcoholic liver disease, athletic performance, cardioprotection, cataracts, CHF, COPD, dialysis, hyperlipidemia, weight loss; **Preg:** Not recommended due to insufficient evidence; **CIs:** Allergy/hypersensitivity; **ADRs:** bloating, borborygmus, burning (topical), diarrhea, flatulence, gastrointestinal distress; **Interactions:** Antidiabetic agents (↓ pyruvate levels), antihypertensive agents (↑ risk of hypotension), antilipemic agents (additive effects), antiobesity agents (additive effects), laxatives (additive effects); **Dose:** Inhalation, COPD: sodium pyruvate 3 times/day. IV infusion, alcoholic liver disease: 10 days infusion of 54–86.4 g pyruvate daily, 150–180 mg/min, 6–8 hr and 15 days of 50–54 g daily, 100 mg/min, 6 hr. Oral: 6–44 g/day PO in conjunction with low-fat, low-cholesterol diet. Topical, cataracts: 5% sodium pyruvate prepared in artificial tears instilled in the eye to be operated upon for cataract extraction, 4 times at 10-min intervals. Topical, aging: 50% pyruvic acid facial peel, applied once weekly × 4 wk; **Monitor:** Lipid profile, weight; **Notes:** Death has been reported in a child with restrictive cardiomyopathy who received pyruvate loading test.

quassia **Uses:** Head lice; **Preg:** Not recommended due to insufficient evidence and possible hormonal effects; **CIs:** Allergy/hypersensitivity, Cardiomyopathy (IV use), Patients trying to become pregnant; **ADRs:** blindness, dysgeusia, infertility, nausea/vomiting, vision changes; **Interactions:** Antacids/H2-blockers/proton pump inhibitors (antagonistic effects), anticoagulants/antiplatelets (↑ risk of bleeding), CNS depressants (sedation), hormonal agents (altered effects), potassium-depleting drugs (↑ risk of hypokalemia); **Dose:** Tea: to make, simmer 1–2 g of wood in 150 mL of boiling water for 10–15 minutes, strain, and drink 1 cup 2–3 times daily. Topical, for lice: apply tincture for 1 week; **Monitor:** Potassium levels; **Notes:** Quassia is used as a natural insecticide. It has cytotoxic and emetic properties.

quercetin **Uses:** Cardiovascular disease, exercise endurance, HTN, immune function, kidney transplant, lung cancer prevention, ovarian cancer prevention, pancreatic CA prevention, prostatis; **Preg:** Not recommended due to insufficient evidence; **CIs:** Allergy/hypersensitivity, Renal dysfunction; **ADRs:** constipation, gastrointestinal upset, hair thinning, headache, hematoma, nephrotoxicity; **Interactions:** Anticoagulants/antiplatelets (↑ risk of bleeding), antineoplastic agents (altered effects), cyclosporine (↑ levels of cyclosporine), CYP450 2C8/2C9/3A4 substrates (quercetin inhibits CYP450 2C8/2C9/3A4), P-glycoprotein (quercetin inhibits gastrointestinal P-glycoprotein efflux pump), quinolones (competitive inhibition); **Dose:** Oral: 500 mg PO bid. IV: 60–1,700 mg/m^2 by IV bolus weekly or in 3-week intervals; **Monitor:** Kidney function; **Notes:** Quercetin is a flavonol, belonging to the class of flavonoids, that occurs ubiquitously in foods of plant origin, such as red wine, onions, green tea, apples, berries, and *Brassica* vegetables (cabbage, broccoli, cauliflower, turnips). Quercetin is also found in *Gingko biloba*, St. John's wort, and American elder.

quinoa ***(Chenopodium quinoa)*** **Uses:** Insufficient available evidence; **Preg:** Not recommended due to insufficient evidence; **CIs:** Allergy/hypersensitivity; **ADRs:** insufficient evidence; **Interactions:** Antilipemic agents (additive effects); **Dose:** Insufficient evidence; **Monitor:** Lipid profile; **Notes:** Quinoa may be eaten by those with celiac disease or those who cannot consume or digest gluten.

raspberry ***(Rubus idaeus)*** **Uses:** Antioxidant, induce labor; **Preg:** Safe when used in amounts in food; possibly unsafe when used in medicinal amounts; **CIs:** Allergy/hypersensitivity; **ADRs:** contamination, sedation; **Interactions:** CNS depressants (↑ sedation), diuretics (additive effects), estrogens (additive effects), salicylates (raspberries may contain salicylates); **Dose:** 2 g dried leaf in 240 mL of boiling water for 5 minutes and then straining. Childbirth: 2.4 g/day from 32 weeks' gestation until labor; **Monitor:** Estrogen levels; **Notes:** Red raspberry leaf has estrogenic effects. It may also contain salicylates.

red clover ***(Trifolium pratense)*** **Uses:** BPH, breast CA (may also increase risk), endometrial CA, hypercholesterolemia, mastalgia, menopause, osteoporosis, prostate CA; **Preg:** Safe when used in foods; unsafe in medicinal amounts; **CIs:** Allergy/hypersensitivity; **ADRs:** headache, mastaglia, menstrual changes, myalgia, nausea, rash, vaginal spotting; **Interactions:** Anticoagulants/antiplatelets (↑ risk of bleeding), CYP450 substrates (red clover inhibits CYP 1A2, 2C19, 2C9, 3A4), estrogens (altered effects), tamoxifen (altered effects); **Dose:** 40–80 mg of red clover isoflavones/day; **Monitor:** Coagulation panel, estrogen level; **Notes:** Red clover is a legume, which like soy contains "phytoestrogens" (plant-based compounds structurally similar to estradiol, which are capable of binding to estrogen receptors as an agonist or antagonist). Use cautiously in patients with hormone-sensitive conditions.

red yeast rice ***(Monascus purpureus)*** **Uses:** CHD, diabetes, hyperlipidemia; **Preg:** Avoid use; **CIs:** Allergy/hypersensitivity, Pregnancy; **ADRs:** bloating, dizziness, flatulence, gastrointestinal discomfort, headache, kidney damage, ↑ LFTs, MYOPATHY, peripheral neuropathy, RHABDOMYOLYSIS; **Interactions:** Alcohol (↑ risk of liver damage), anticoagulants/antiplatelets (↑ risk of bleeding), coenzyme Q10 (↓ CoQ10 levels), cyclosporine (↑ risk of myopathy), CYP450 3A4 (↑ levels of lovastatin in red yeast rice), gemfibrozil (↑ risk of myopathy), grapefruit (↑ levels of lovastatin in red yeast rice), HMG-CoA reductase inhibitors (↑ risk of adverse effects), levothyroxine (↓ efficacy of levothyroxine), protease inhibitors (altered effects), niacin (↑ risk of myopathy), St. John's wort (↓ levels of lovastatin in red yeast rice); **Dose:** 600–1,200 mg PO qd; maximum: 2,400 mg PO qd; **Monitor:** LFTs, kidney function; **Notes:** The active ingredient in red yeast rice is believed to be monacolin K, a compound identical to lovastatin (a "statin"). In 1998, the FDA determined that red yeast rice did not conform to the definition of a dietary supplement under the 1994 Dietary Supplement and Health Education Act (DSHEA). The manufacturers of these products, including Pharmanex Inc., makers of Cholestin, have since recalled and reformulated these products.

R

rehmannia | **Uses:** Aplastic anemia, Sheehan's syndrome; | **Preg:** Not recommended due to insufficient evidence; | **CIs:** Allergy/hypersensitivity; | **ADRs:** ↓ blood glucose, dizziness, edema, fatigue, palpitations; | **Interactions:** Anticoagulants/antiplatelets (↑ risk of bleeding), antidiabetes drugs (↑ risk of hypoglycemia), antihypertensives (↑ risk of hypotension), antilipemic agents (additive effects), antineoplastic agents (↓ toxicity), corticosteroids (synergistic effects), thyroid hormones (altered effects); | **Dose:** Extract (1:2): 30–60 mL PO per week or 4–12 mL PO qd. Sheehan's syndrome: 90 g of cleaned and finely chopped *Rehmannia glutinosa* root added to 900 mL of water and boiled down to 200 mL PO 3-day courses with an intermission of 3, 6, and 14 days; | **Monitor:** Blood glucose, coagulation panel, lipid profile, thyroid panel; | **Notes:** Rehmannia has been used extensively in traditional Chinese medicine (TCM). Use cautiously in patients with diabetes because rehmannia may reduce blood glucose levels.

reishi mushroom | **Uses:** Arthritis, CA, CHD, diabetes mellitus, hepatitis B, HTN, postherpetic neuralgia, proteinuria, *Russula subnigricans* poisoning; | **Preg:** Not recommended due to insufficient evidence; | **CIs:** Allergy/hypersensitivity; | **ADRs:** ↓ blood pressure, dermatitis, dizziness, GI bleeding, headache, hepatotoxicity, insomnia, ↓ libido, mastalgia, nausea/vomiting, pruritus, skin rash; | **Interactions:** Adenosine (↑ levels of adenosine), amphetamines (antagonistic effects), analgesics (additive effects), anesthetics (altered effects), antibiotics (synergistic effects), anticoagulants/antiplatelets (↑ risk of bleeding), antidiabetic agents (↑ risk of hypoglycemia); antihypertensives (↑ risk of hypotension), antineoplastic effects (altered effects), hepatotoxic agents (↑ risk of liver damage), protease inhibitors (altered effects), thyroid hormones (altered effects); | **Dose:** Ganopoly (contains 600 mg extract of *Ganoderma lucidum* per capsule): 1,200–1,800 mg PO 2–3 times/day; | **Monitor:** Blood glucose, blood pressure, LFTs; | **Notes:** Reishi mushrooms may have hepatotoxic effects.

rhodiola | **Uses:** Bladder CA, exercise performance enhancement, fatigue, generalized anxiety disorder (GAD), hypoxia, lung injury, mental performance; | **Preg:** Not recommended due to insufficient evidence; | **CIs:** Allergy/hypersensitivity; | **ADRs:** ↑ blood pressure, dizziness, dry mouth, insomnia, irritability, leukocytosis, restlessness; | **Interactions:** Anxiolytics (additive effects), antidepressants (additive effects), antineoplastic agents (additive effects), antihypertensive agents (additive effects); CNS depressants (additive effects), immunosuppressants (additive effects), opioids (additive effects); **Dose:** 100 mg–4 g daily; **Monitor:** Blood pressure; **Notes:** *Rhodiola rosea* is considered to be an "adaptogen" and extensively studied in the former Soviet Union.

rhubarb **Uses:** Aplastic anemia, constipation, fatty liver, GI disorders, gingivitis, hepatitis, herpes, hypercholesterolemia, memory impairment, nasopharyngeal carcinoma, nephritic syndrome, obesity, pre-eclampsia, renal failure, surgery, systemic inflammation reaction syndrome, upper GI bleed; **Preg:** Not recommended due to insufficient evidence and possible uterine stimulant effects; **CIs:** Allergy/hypersensitivity, Children, Crohn's disease, Diarrhea, History of kidney stones, IBS, Intestinal obstruction, Ulcerative colitis, Use for more than 2 wk; **ADRs:** abdominal pain, arrhythmias, burning of the mouth and throat, contact dermatitis, diarrhea, electrolyte loss, hematuria, hepatotoxicity, hyperkalemia, jaundice (neonatal), kidney stones, nausea/vomiting, seizures, weakness; **Interactions:** Corticosteroids (↑ risk of potassium-depletion/hypokalemia), digoxin (↑ risk of potassium depletion/hypokalemia), diuretics (↑ risk of potassium depletion/hypokalemia), hepatotoxic drugs (↑ risk of liver damage), laxatives (↑ electrolyte loss), minerals (↓ absorption), nephrotoxic drugs (↑ risk of kidney damage), oral drugs (↓ absorption), potassium-depleting drugs (↑ risk of potassium depletion/hypokalemia), warfarin (↑ risk of INR/bleeding); **Dose:** Upper GI bleed: 3 g alcoholic extract tablets or 6 mL of syrup 2–4 times/day × 2 wk. Gingivitis: 5% rhubarb extract injected with micro syringe into gum daily × 20 days. Constipation: 1 tsp (5–6 g) of powdered root boiled in 1 cup of water for 10 minutes and ingested 1 tbsp (15 cc) at a time, up to 1 cup PO qd; dried root: 1–4 PO qd. Obesity: 1 g refined rhubarb extract 2–3 times daily, taken 30 minutes before meals, × 12 wk. Pre-eclampsia: 0.75 g PO qd from the 28th week until delivery. Renal failure: 6–9 g PO qd for 6–22 mo; **Monitor:** Electrolytes; **Notes:** Rhubarb leaves are considered toxic due to their oxalic content and should not be ingested. Anthraquinones found in rhubarb roots are potentially mutagenic and genotoxic. Tannins in rhubarb leaves may also be hepatotoxic. Rhubarb may discolor urine and interfere with laboratory and diagnostic tests.

R

riboflavin **Uses:** AIDS-related lactic acidosis, anemia, cataracts, cervical cancer, cognitive function, depression, eating disorders, esophageal CA, ethylmalonic encephalopathy, malaria, migraine prevention, neonatal jaundice, pre-eclampsia, riboflavin deficiency; **Preg:** Safe when consumed at RDA (1.4 mg/

day); | **CIs:** Allergy/hypersensitivity; | **ADRs:** burning sensation, discolored urine, numbness, photosensitivity, pruritus; | **Interactions:** Antibiotics (↓ levels of riboflavin), anticholinergic agents (↓ absorption of riboflavin), doxorubicin (↓ levels of riboflavin), oral contraceptives (↓ levels of riboflavin), phenobarbital (↑ levels in liver), phenothiazines (↓ levels of riboflavin), probenecid (↑ levels of riboflavin), psyllium (↓ absorption of riboflavin), quinacrine (↓ levels of riboflavin), tamoxifen (altered effects), TCAs (altered effects); | **Dose:** RDA: adults, men (14 years and older): 1.3 mg/day; adults, women (older than 18 years): 1.1 mg/day; children, 14–18 years: 1 mg/day; children 9–13 years: 0.9 mg/day; children 4–8 years: 0.6 mg/day; children 1–3 years: 0.5 mg/day; infants: 7–12 months: 0.4 mg/day; infant 0–6 months: 0.3 mg/day; pregnant women: 1.4 mg/day; lactating women: 1.6 mg/day; | **Monitor:** Riboflavin levels; | **Notes:** Riboflavin (vitamin B_2) is a water-soluble vitamin found in milk (and other dairy products), eggs, enriched cereals/grains, meats, liver, and green vegetables (such as asparagus or broccoli).

ribose | **Uses:** Adenylosuccinase deficiency, athletic performance, cardiovascular disease, chronic fatigue syndrome, congestive heart failure, coronary artery bypass surgery, fibromyalgia, McArdle's disease, mental fatigue, muscle mass; | **Preg:** Not recommended due to insufficient evidence; | **CIs:** Allergy/hypersensitivity; | **ADRs:** headache, hyperuricemia, hyperuricosuria, hypoglycemia; | **Interactions:** Alcohol (↑ risk of hypoglycemia), antidiabetic agents (↑ risk of hypoglycemia), aspirin (↑ risk of hypoglycemia), choline magnesium trisalicylate (↑ risk of hypoglycemia), propranolol (↑ risk of hypoglycemia), salicylates (↑ risk of hypoglycemia); | **Dose:** Oral: 15–60 mg PO qd in divided doses. Intravenous: 3.3 mg/kg/min infusion as a 10% solution (for imaging of coronary arteries using thallium-201); | **Monitor:** Blood glucose, phosphate levels; | **Notes:** Ribose and its related compound, deoxyribose, are the building blocks of the backbone chains in nucleic acids, known as RNA and DNA, respectively. Research has shown that ribose may help speed recovery of the heart muscle after a heart attack, and improve blood flow to the heart in those affected by ischemia. Ribose supplementation has been used to support heart function and rejuvenate cardiac tissue after both heart attack and heart surgery.

R

rooibos | **Uses:** Insufficient available evidence; | **Preg:** Not recommended due to insufficient evidence; | **CIs:** Allergy/hypersensitivity; | **ADRs:** contamination; | **Interactions:** CYP450 substrates; | **Dose:** 1 tsp in hot water PO qd;

Monitor: N/A; **Notes:** Rooibos (or red bush tea) tea contains a large amount of flavonoids and acts as a potent antioxidant.

rose hips **Uses:** Antioxidant, dermatoses, dysmenorrhea, immune system enhancement, ophthalmological disorders, osteoarthritis, wound healing; **Preg:** Amounts higher than those found in foods are not recommended due to insufficient evidence; **CIs:** Allergy/hypersensitivity, History of kidney stones; **ADRs:** allergic reactions, asthma, constipation, diarrhea, fatigue, flushing, headache, insomnia, keratitis, nausea/vomiting, renal calculi, rhinitis, rhinoconjunctivitis, urticaria, wheezing; **Interactions:** Aluminum (↑ absorption of aluminum), anticoagulants/antiplatelets (interfere with anticoagulant effects), antilipemic agents (additive effects), antineoplastic agents (additive or synergistic effects), antiretroviral agents (additive or synergistic effects), diuretics (additive effects), estrogens (↑ absorption and effects of estrogen), fluphenazine (↓ blood levels), immunosuppressants (altered effects), iron (↑ absorption of iron), laxatives (additive effects), salicylates (↑ excretion of ascorbic acid/↓ excretion of salicylates), warfarin (↓ warfarin response); **Dose:** Decoction: steep 2–2.5 g of the crushed rose hips in 150 mL boiling water for 10–15 minutes and then strain; osteoarthritis: 5 g of Hyben Vital PO qd × 3 mo; **Monitor:** Coagulation panel, lipid profile; **Notes:** Large amounts of vitamin C found in rose hips may increase the risk of kidney stones. Vitamin C may cause false negative results in amine-dependent tests for occult blood in stool, urine glucose determinations, and acetaminophen tests. It can cause false increases in aspartate aminotransferase (AST, SGOT), bilirubin, and carbamazepine laboratory tests.

rosemary **Uses:** Alopecia areata, anxiety, stress; **Preg:** Not recommended in medicinal amounts due to insufficient evidence and traditional use as an abortifacient; **CIs:** Allergy/hypersensitivity, Pregnancy, Seizure disorder; **ADRs:** contact dermatitis, diuresis, hypotension, nausea, seizures, vomiting; **Interactions:** ACE inhibitors (additive effects), anticoagulants/antiplatelets (↑ risk of bleeding), antidiabetic agents (altered effects), CYP450 2B/1A1/2E1 substrates (rosemary may induce CYP450 2B/1A1/2E1), diuretics (additive effects), drugs that lower seizure threshold (↑ risk of seizures); **Dose:** 4–6 g PO qd; **Monitor:** Blood sugar, electrolytes; **Notes:** Rosemary essential oil can be toxic if taken orally even in fairly low doses, and the maximum safe dose is not currently available. According to unsubstantiated sources, a rosemary oil

R

overdose may lead to spasms, gastroenteritis, vomiting, irritated kidney, uterine bleeding, coma, and death.

royal jelly | **Uses:** Hyperlipidemia, PMS; | **Preg:** Not recommended due to insufficient evidence; | **CIs:** Allergy/hypersensitivity, Dermatitis; | **ADRs:** allergic reactions, anaphylaxis, asthma, conjunctivitis, contact dermatitis, dyspnea, eczema, edema, hemorrhagic colitis, pruritus, skin irritation, urticaria; | **Interactions:** Anticoagulants/antiplatelets (↑ risk of bleeding), antilipemic agents (additive effects); | **Dose:** Oral, hyperlipidemia: 50–100 mg PO qd; PMS: 2 tablets PO bid (combination product containing royal jelly 6 mg, bee pollen extract 36 mg, and bee pollen plus pistil extract 120 mg [Femal]); | **Monitor:** Coagulation panel, lipid profile; | **Notes:** Use extreme caution in patients with asthma or atopy. Use cautiously in patients with asthma.

rutin | **Uses:** Chronic venous insufficiency, edema, hemorrhoids, HTN, leg ulcers, Ménière's disease, microangiopathy, retinal vein occlusion, retinopathy, schizophrenia, skin conditions, thrombosis; | **Preg:** Rutin supplements have been safely used during pregnancy; | **CIs:** Allergy/hypersensitivity; | **ADRs:** alopecia, constipation, diarrhea, dizziness, gastritis, gastrointestinal disturbances, headache, skin rash, upper respiratory tract infection, vomiting; | **Interactions:** Diuretics (additive effects), iron (chelates iron), quinolones (antagonistic effects); | **Dose:** 500 mg PO qd or bid; 500 mg–1 g PO qd or bid as hydroxyethylrutosides; | **Monitor:** Electrolytes; | **Notes:** Rutin is found in various plants (e.g., rue, tobacco, and buckwheat).

Saccharomyces boulardii | **Uses:** Acne, amebiasis, antibiotic-associated diarrhea, *Clostridium difficile* diarrhea, Crohn's disease, cystic fibrosis, diarrhea, *Helicobacter pylori*, HIV-related diarrhea, nutritional support (premature infants), traveler's diarrhea, ulcerative colitis; | **Preg:** Not recommended due to insufficient evidence; | **CIs:** Allergy/hypersensitivity; | **ADRs:** bloating, constipation, edema, flatulence, fungemia, leukocytosis, polydipsia; | **Interactions:** Antibiotics (altered effects), antidiarrheals (antagonistic effects), antifungals (↓ effects of *Saccharomyces boulardii*), iodoquinol (synergistic effects), mesalamine (synergistic effects), metronidazole (synergistic effects); | **Dose:** Diarrhea: 250 mg–1 g PO bid–qid; | **Monitor:** CBC; | **Notes:** *Saccharomyces boulardii* is classified as a probiotic. Multiple case reports describe fungemia. Some laboratories are unable to differentiate between *Saccharomyces cerevisiae* and *Saccharomyces boulardii* when testing patients with fungemia following use of *Saccharomyces boulardii*.

R

safflower | **Uses:** Angina, CAD, cor pulmonale, cystic fibrosis, familial hyperlipidemia, fatty acid deficiency, Friedreich's ataxia, hepatitis C, hypercholesterolemia, HTN, kidney disease, malnutrition, lithium toxicity, nutritional supplement (infant formula), skin disorders, TPN, type 2 diabetes; | **Preg:** Not recommended due to insufficient evidence and traditional use as an abortifacient; | **CIs:** Allergy/hypersensitivity, Pregnancy; | **ADRs:** acne, anorexia, ↓ blood pressure, contact dermatitis, diarrhea, dysgeusia, fullness, hypertriglyceridemia, ↑ LFTs, stomach cramps; | **Interactions:** Anticoagulants/antiplatelets (↑ risk of bleeding), antidiabetic agents (↑ risk of hypoglycemia), antihypertensives (↑ risk of hypotension), antilipemic agents (additive effects), cimetidine (↑ levels of linoleic acid), immunosuppressants (altered effects); | **Dose:** Cystic fibrosis: 102–132 mg/kg PO qd × 6 wk. Fatty acid deficiency, ethyl ester of safflower oil: 6 g PO qd × 8 wk. HTN, safflower oil: 1–6 g PO qd × 8 wk. Hyperlipidemia: 14 g PO qd × 6 wk; | **Monitor:** Blood glucose, blood pressure, lipid profile, LFTs; | **Notes:** Use parenteral safflower oil emulsions cautiously in newborns, because serum triglycerides and free fatty acids must be monitored to avoid the complications of intolerance.

sage | **Uses:** Alzheimer's disease, cognitive impairment, herpes, lung CA prevention, menopausal symptoms, mood enhancement, pharyngitis; | **Preg:** Not recommended due to insufficient evidence and possible hormonal and abortifacient effects; | **CIs:** Allergy/hypersensitivity, Pregnancy, Seizure disorders; | **ADRs:** ↑ blood pressure, contact dermatitis, sedation, SEIZURES; | **Interactions:** Anticonvulsants (altered effects), antidiabetic drugs (↑ risk of hypoglycemia), CNS depressants (↑ risk of sedation), CYP450 3A4 substrates (sage inhibits CYP3A4), drugs that lower seizure threshold (↑ risk of seizures), estrogens (additive effects), thyroid hormones (altered effects); | **Dose:** Alzheimer's disease and cognitive impairment, essential oil of *Salvia lavandulaefolia*: 25–50 mcL PO qd. Menopausal symptoms, tablets: 120 mg plus 60 mg alfalfa PO qd. Mood enhancement, dried leaf: 300–600 mg PO qd. Pharyngitis, *Salvia officinalis* extract: 15% spray containing 14 mcL of *Salvia* per dose 6–9 times daily × 3 days; | **Monitor:** Blood glucose, blood pressure; | **Notes:** Sage has been noted to cause seizures. Thujone constituent found in some species of sage is considered toxic.

S

saiboku-to | **Uses:** Insufficient available evidence; | **Preg:** Not recommended due to insufficient evidence; | **CIs:** Allergy/hypersensitivity; | **ADRs:** insufficient evidence;

| **Interactions:** Steroids (↑ effects); | **Dose:** Insufficient evidence; | **Monitor:** Insufficient evidence; | **Notes:** Saiboku-to contains bupleurum, hoelen, pinellia, magnolia, Asian ginseng, Asian skullcap, licorice, perilla, ginger, and jujube. The combination of herbs is thought to have significant anti-inflammatory and antihistamine effects. Saiboku-to is a Japanese herbal formula that is commonly used to treat asthma.

saiko-keishi-to | **Uses:** Insufficient evidence; | **Preg:** Not recommended due to insufficient evidence; | **CIs:** Allergy/hypersensitivity; | **ADRs:** insufficient evidence; | **Interactions:** Insufficient evidence; | **Dose:** Insufficient evidence; | **Monitor:** Insufficient evidence; | **Notes:** Saiko-keishi-to is made up of nine herbs: bupleurum root, pinellia tuber, scutellaria root, jujube fruit, ginger rhizome, ginseng root, cinnamon bark, peony root, and glycyrrhiza root. It is commonly used to treat duodenal ulcer, pancreatitis, and chronic liver disease.

salatrim | **Uses:** Appetite suppressant; | **Preg:** Not recommended due to insufficient evidence; | **CIs:** Insufficient evidence; | **ADRs:** mild gastrointestinal symptoms (nausea, diarrhea, cramping); | **Interactions:** Insufficient evidence; | **Dose:** Insufficient evidence; | **Monitor:** Insufficient evidence; | **Notes:** Salatrim is an acronym for short- and long-chain acyl triglyceride molecules, and mainly is composed of short-chain fatty acids (SCFAs) and stearic acid. It is a light tan oil or semisolid. It was developed as a reduced-calorie fat, based on the reduced caloric content of SCFAs and the reduced absorption of stearic acid. Salatrim (Benefat) is a GRAS substance (GRASP 4G0404) under 21 CFR 170.30. Food products containing salatrim were launched commercially in 1995.

salvia divinorum | **Uses:** Insufficient evidence; | **Preg:** Not recommended due to insufficient evidence; | **CIs:** Allergy/hypersensitivity; | **ADRs:** bradycardia, diaphoresis, fever, hallucinations; | **Interactions:** Opioids (additive effects); | **Dose:** Oral: 200–500 mcg (diterpene salvinorin A from salvia) PO qd. Inhalation: 200–750 mcg of leaves, smoked. Buccal: 200 mcg–50 g fresh leaves or 2–10 g of chewed dried leaves (rehydrated); | **Monitor:** Body temperature; | **Notes:** Salvia may have hallucinogenic effects when used orally or by inhalation.

SAMe | **Uses:** ADHD, AIDS-related myelopathy, cholestasis, depression, fibromyalgia, intrahepatic cholestasis, liver disease, osteoarthritis; **Preg:** Not recommended in the first trimester or during breastfeeding owing to lack of sufficient data. SAMe has been used in the third trimester for the treatment of intrahepatic cholestasis; **CIs:** Allergy/hypersensitivity, Bipolar disorder; **ADRs:** anxiety, ↓ blood glucose, diarrhea, dizziness, epigastric pain, erythema, flushing, headache, insomnia, mania, nausea/vomiting, palpitations, pruritus, skin rash, tachycardia; **Interactions:** ANTIDEPRESSANTS (↑ risk of serotonergic effects), antidiabetic agents (↑ risk of hypoglycemia), dextromethorphan (↑ risk of serotonergic effects), levodopa (exacerbate parkisonian symptoms), linezolid (↑ risk of serotonergic effects), MAOIs (additive effects), meperidine (↑ risk of serotonergic effects), pentazocine (↑ risk of serotonergic effects), tramadol (↑ risk of serotonergic effects); **Dose:** Oral: 800–1,600 mg PO qd in 2–3 divided doses. IV/IM: 150–1,600 mg qd IV or IM; **Monitor:** Blood glucose, LFTs; **Notes:** SAMe has been associated with hypomania and mania in patients with or without a history of bipolar disorder. SAMe may worsen parkinsonian symptoms.

sandalwood **Uses:** Alertness, anxiety; **Preg:** Avoid use due to reports of abortifacient effects; **CIs:** Allergy/hypersensitivity, Kidney disease, Pregnancy; **ADRs:** dermatitis; **Interactions:** Anticancer agents (additive effects), antifungal agents (additive effects), anxiolytics (altered effects), diuretics (additive effects); **Dose:** Insufficient available evidence; **Monitor:** Electrolytes; **Notes:** Perfume in sandalwood incense can cause an allergic reaction.

sanghuang **Uses:** Cancer; **Preg:** Not recommended due to insufficient evidence; **CIs:** Allergy/hypersensitivity; **ADRs:** insufficient evidence; **Interactions:** Antiangiogenic agents (altered effects), immunosuppressants (altered effects); **Dose:** Tea: 2–3 pieces of sanghuang mixed with 1,500 mL of water, boiled for 5–10 minutes, from 2–8 times, with barley or corn tea added; **Monitor:** N/A; **Notes:** Sanghuang is a medicinal mushroom that is used for cancer; however, human trials are lacking.

S

sanicle **Uses:** Asthma, atopic eczema, otitis media; **Preg:** Not recommended due to insufficient evidence; **CIs:** Allergy/hypersensitivity, GI mucosal irritation; **ADRs:** gastrointestinal upset, nausea/vomiting, photodermatosis; **Interactions:** Caffeine (↑risk of stimulant effects), diuretics (additive effects); **Dose:** Dried, aerial parts: 4–6 g PO qd; **Monitor:** Electrolytes; **Notes:** Sanicle was once commonly used as a folk herbal remedy for treating wounds and skin conditions and was applied topically for skin inflammation and hemorrhoids. Sanicle has also purportedly been used as a homeopathic remedy for nervous disorders, cough, and bronchitis. In Andean cuisine, sanicle is used as a spice.

sarsaparilla | **Uses:** Insufficient available evidence; | **Preg:** Not recommended due to insufficient evidence; | **CIs:** Allergy/hypersensitivity; | **ADRs:** diuresis, occupational asthma (from inhalation of root dust); | **Interactions:** Digoxin (↑ absorption of digoxin), diuretics (additive effects); | **Dose:** Insufficient available evidence; | **Monitor:** Digoxin levels, electrolytes; | **Notes:** The FDA has approved sarsaparilla as a food additive.

sassafras | **Uses:** Insufficient available evidence; | **Preg:** Not recommended due to insufficient evidence; | **CIs:** Allergy/hypersensitivity, Oral use (contains safrole, a carcinogen), Liver disease; | **ADRs:** diaphoresis, HEPATOTOXICITY, sedation, urinary irritation; | **Interactions:** Anticoagulants/antiplatelets (interfere wih effects), CNS depressants (additive sedation), CYP450 1A2/2A6/2E1/2D6/3A4 substrates (sassafras is an inhibitor), HEPATOTOXIC AGENTS (↑ risk of liver damage); | **Dose:** Insufficient available evidence; | **Monitor:** LFTs, toxic effects; | **Notes:** Sassafras should not be used internally because safrole is carcinogenic. Sassafras oil may cause a false-positive in blood phenytoin laboratory tests.

saw palmetto | **Uses:** Androgenetic alopecia, chronic pelvic pain syndrome, hypotonic neurogenic bladder, prostate CA, prostatitis, transurethral resection of the prostate (TURP); | **Preg:** Avoid due to insufficient evidence and possible hormonal effects; | **CIs:** Allergy/hypersensitivity, Pregnancy; | **ADRs:** abdominal pain, bleeding, ↑ blood pressure, diarrhea, dyspnea, fatigue, myalgia, nausea/vomiting, sexual dysfunction, ulcer; | **Interactions:** Androgens (↓ effectiveness), antibiotics (additive antibacterial effects, specifically with ciprofloxacin and azithromycin), anticoagulants/antiplatelets (↑ risk of bleeding), antihypertensives (antagonistic effects), anti-inflammatory agents (additive effects), estrogens (antagonize effects); | **Dose:** Fluid extract of berry pulp (1:1): 1–2 mL PO tid. Ground, dried, or whole berries: 1–2 g PO qd. Tea: prepare with 2 tsp dried berry and 24 oz water, simmer slowly until liquid is reduced by half, take 4 ounces PO tid. Tincture (1:4): 2–4 mL PO tid. BPH: 320 mg PO qd (80%–90% fatty acid and sterols [liposterolic content]). Topical, alopecia: apply lotion BID to scalp × 50 wk;

S

Monitor: Coagulation panel, PSA; **Notes:** PSA levels may be artificially lowered by saw palmetto.

schisandra **Uses:** Adaptogen, eczema, familial Mediterranean fever (FMF), liver disease, vision; **Preg:** Not recommended due to insufficient evidence and possible hormonal effects; **CIs:** Allergy/hypersensitivity, Epilepsy, GERD, Patients with intracranial pressure, PUD, Surgery; **ADRs:** anorexia, ↓ blood glucose, dyspepsia, skin rash, urticaria; **Interactions:** Anticoagulants/antiplatelets (↑ risk of bleeding), antidiabetic agents (↑ risk of hypoglycemia), antiviral agents (altered effects), calcium channel blockers (altered effects), cholinergic drugs (additive effects); CNS depressants (altered effects), CYP450 2C9 substrates (↓/↑ levels of drugs metabolized by CYP2C9), CYP450 3A4 substrates (↓/↑ levels of drugs metabolized by CYP3A4), tacrolimus (↑ levels of tacrolimus), warfarin (↓ levels of warfarin); **Dose:** General: Fruit, dried: 1.5–15 g PO qd 100 days; tincture 2–4 mL PO tid × 1 mo; powder: 1.5–6 g PO qd; tea: 1–3 cups PO tid prepared by using 1–6 g dried schisandra berries in 1–3 c boiling water; capsules: 1.5 g PO qd; decoction: prepare by boiling 5 g of crushed schisandra berries in 100 mL of water; this is then divided into 3 doses and taken over a 24-hour period. Hepatitis: standardized extract (20 mg lignan [equivalent to 1.5 g crude schisandra]) PO qd. As an adaptogen: 91.1 mg PO bid, standardized to 3.1 mg schisandrin and gamma-schisandrin. Liver disease: 7.5 mg of HpPro (a natural analogue of schisandrin C, a constituent of schisandra) PO tid × 4 wk; **Monitor:** Blood glucose, LFTs; **Notes:** After pretreatment with schisandra, reduced sleeping times induced by pentobarbital were noted. Schisandra should be avoided in patients undergoing surgery.

scopolamine **Uses:** Alzheimer's disease, abdominal pain, ACE inhibitor–associated cough, addiction, airway obstruction, anesthesia (prevention of dreams), antidepressant, arrhythmia, asthma, biliary colic, bowel disorders, emesis (cisplatin-induced), headache (chronic), heart failure (chronic), HTN, IBS, labor/delivery, motion sickness, MI, nausea/vomiting, otitis media (children), postoperative pain, PUD, poisoning, renal colic, sedation/anxiety (preoperative), seizures, syncope, tardive dyskinesia, urinary incontinence, vertigo; **Preg:** FDA Pregnancy Category C (no adequate human or animal studies; or adverse fetal effects in animal studies, but no available human data); **CIs:** Allergy/hypersensitivity, Angle-closure glaucoma, GI/GU obstruction, Myasthenia gravis, Paralytic ileus, Tachycardia, Thyrotoxicosis; **ADRs:** agitation, blurred vision,

S

confusion, constipation, dizziness, drowsiness, dry mouth, dysuria, flushing, hallucinations, headache, ophthalmalgia, palpitations, nervousness, rash, restlessness, tachycardia; | **Interactions:** ANTICHOLINERGICS (↑ risk of adverse effects), antihistamines (↑ risk of adverse effects), CNS depressants (↑ CNS depression), GRAPEFRUIT (↑ levels of scopolamine), tricyclic antidepressants (↑ risk of adverse effects); | **Dose:** IV/IM/SC: 0.6–1 mg in divided doses. Ophthalmic: 1–2 gtt to the eye(s) up to 4 times/day. Oral: 1–2 tablets an hour before travel or 0.3 mg PO tid or 0.6 mg PO q6h. Transdermal (Transderm Scop): 1 system q72 hr (1.5 mg of scopolamine designed to deliver 0.5 mg over 3 days); | **Monitor:** BUN, CBC, LFTs, renal function, serum alkaline phosphatase; | **Notes:** Scopolamine (also called hyoscine) is one of the naturally occurring muscarinic receptor antagonists in belladonna plants. The most common adverse effects associated with scopolamine are dry mouth, dizziness, drowsiness, and blurred vision.

scotch broom | **Uses:** Cardiovascular conditions, diuresis, labor induction; | **Preg:** Avoid due to abortifacient effects; | **CIs:** Allergy/hypersensitivity, Pregnancy, Oral use (amounts greater than in food), Cardiovascular disease; | **ADRs:** blurry vision, CARDIAC TOXICITY, confusion, diaphoresis, diarrhea, dizziness, fatigue, gastrointestinal distress, headache, mydriasis, nausea/vomiting, ocular palsy, skin irritation, tachycardia, weakness; | **Interactions:** ANTIARRHYTHMICS (quinidine; ↑ risk of cardiac toxicity), antihypertensives (altered effects); CYP450 2D6 inhibitors (↑ risk of scotch broom toxicity), CYP450 2D6 inducers (↓ effectiveness of scotch broom), diuretics (additive effects), HALOPERIDOL (↑ risk of cardiac toxicity), MAOIs (↑ risk of hypertensive crisis), nicotine (antagonistic effects), vasodilators (additive effects); | **Dose:** It is not clear what dose(s) of scotch broom are safe or effective for any medical condition, and use should be only under medical supervision. Infusion: add 1 oz of dried tops/flowers to a pint of boiling water (or 1 tsp of dried tops/flowers of scotch broom added to 200 mL boiling water), and take as a cupfull once or twice daily as needed. Juice: make by pressing the bruised, fresh tops/flowers of scotch broom and add one-third volume alcohol, allow to sit for 7 days, followed by filtration and taken daily as needed. Tea: 1–2 g (1 level tsp) of scotch broom herb (above-ground parts) steeped in 150–200 mL of boiling water, then strained after 5–10 min and taken as a cupfull, up to 3 times daily as needed. Tincture: 0.5–2 mL (above ground parts; 1:5 preparation in 45% ethanol [v/v]) daily. Toxicity has been reported with consumption of more than 300 mg of sparteine or 30 g of the above-ground parts. | **Monitor:** Heart rate, blood pressure;

S

Notes: There is particular concern about the potential toxicity of scotch broom owing to the presence of small amounts of the toxic alkaloids sparteine and isosparteine, which are found in both the flowers and herb (above-ground parts of the plant). Spartiene has cardiovascular depressing effects similar to the drug quinidine (a class 1a antiarrhythmic agent).

sea buckthorn **Uses:** Antioxidant, atopic dermatitis, burns, cardiovascular disease, cirrhosis, common cold, gastric ulcers, HTN, pneumonia; **Preg:** Do not consume more than amounts of sea buckthorn found in food, due to the lack of sufficient evidence; **CIs:** Allergy/hypersensitivity; **ADRs:** insufficient available evidence; **Interactions:** ACE inhibitors/A2RBs (additive effects), anticoagulants/antiplatelets (↑ risk of bleeding), antidiabetic agents (↑ risk of hypoglycemia), antilipemic agents (additive effects), cisplatin (↓ genotoxic effects), immunosuppressants (altered effects); **Dose:** General: berry oil: 5 g PO qd × 4 wk; tea: 1–2 c PO qd; capsules, seed oil: 500 mg PO 1–3 times/day; seed oil: 3–5 mL PO tid. Atopic dermatitis, pulp oil: 5 g PO qd × 4 mo. Cirrhosis, extract: 15 g PO tid × 6 mo; **Monitor:** Blood glucose, coagulation panel; **Notes:** Sea buckthorn may inhibit platelet aggregation and cause bleeding. Discontinue 2 weeks before surgery.

seaweed, kelp, bladderwrack **Uses:** Diabetes mellitus, infection (bacteria, fungus), thyroid disorders; **Preg:** Not recommended during pregnancy and lactation due to potentially high iodine concentrations and frequent contamination with heavy metals; **CIs:** Allergy/hypersensitivity, Heart failure, Thyroid disorders, Iodine allergy, Renal insufficiency; **ADRs:** acne, altered thyroid function (exacerbate/induce hyperthyroidism and hypothyroidism), bleeding, diarrhea, fatigue, nausea/vomiting, nephrotoxicity, ↑ salivation; **Interactions:** Anticoagulants (↑ risk of bleeding), antidiabetic agents (↑ risk of hypoglycemia), antilipemic agents (additive effects), CNS stimulants (additive effects), diuretics (↓ effectiveness), iron (↓ absorption), laxatives (additive effects), nephrotoxic agents (↑ risk of kidney damage), thyroid hormones (altered effects); **Dose:** 200- to 600-mg capsules qd or tid, and gradually increased to 24 capsules/day; **Monitor:** Thyroid function, blood glucose, coagulation panel, weight; **Notes:** Bladderwrack was used in the 18th century as a major dietary source of iodine, and has been used traditionally to treat goiter. In combination with lecithin and vitamins, bladderwrack was not found to be effective in sustaining weight loss.

S

selenium | **Uses:** ALS, antioxidant, arsenic poisoning, asthma, bronchitis, CA prevention/treatment, cardiomyopathy, cardiovascular disease prevention, cataracts, chemotherapy (adjunct), circulation, critical illness, cystic fibrosis, dandruff, dialysis, eczema, epilepsy, esophageal CA, gastric CA, G-6-PD deficiency, HIV/AIDS, hypothyroidism, infection, infertility, intracranial pressure symptoms, Keshan's disease, low birth weight, lymphedema, mortality, prostate CA prevention, postsurgical lymphedema, RA, sepsis, thyroid conditions, tinea capitis, tinea versicolor, ulcerative colitis, uveitis; | **Preg:** Safe when used appropriately; | **CIs:** Allergy/hypersensitivity, Patients at risk for developing nonmelanoma skin cancer or diabetes; | **ADRs:** toxicity symptoms: digestive dysfunction, garlic-like breath odor, hepatorenal dysfunction, irritability, loss or thickening of hair and nails, metallic taste, muscle tenderness, nausea/vomiting, nervous system abnormalities, skin lesions, thrombocytopenia, tremor, weakness; | **Interactions:** Anticoagulants/antiplatelets (↑ risk of bleeding), barbiturates (prolong sedation), chemotherapy (↓ selenium levels), cisplatin (↓ selenium levels), clozapine (↓ selenium levels), corticosteroids (↓ selenium levels), erythropoietin (↑ effectiveness), gold salts (altered effects of selenium), HMG-CoA reductase inhibitors (↓ efficacy of HMG-CoA reductase inhibitors), niacin (↓ efficacy), oral contraceptives (↑ selenium levels), valproic acid (↓ selenium levels), vitamin C (↓ absorption of vitamin C), warfarin (↑ warfarin activity); | **Dose:** Oral, Adult RDA: 80–200 mcg; adult males, 70 mcg; adult females, 55 mcg; pregnant females, 65 mcg; breastfeeding females, 75 mcg; adolescent males, 40–70 mcg; adolescent females, 45–55 mcg. Oral, Adult Tolerable Upper Intake Level: 400 mcg. Oral, pediatric RDA: children 0–6 months, 10 mcg; children 7–12 months, 15 mcg; children 1–6 years, 20 mcg; children 7–10 years, 30 mcg; children 11–14 years, 45 mcg; children 15–18 years, 50 mcg. Oral, Pediatric Tolerable Upper Intake Level: children 0–6 months, 45 mcg; children 7–12 months, 60 mcg; children 1–3 years, 90 mcg; children 4–8 years, 150 mcg; children 9–13 years, 280 mcg. Oral, cancer: 200 mcg qd; | **Monitor:** Selenium levels, thyroid function; | **Notes:** Selenium may reduce thyroxine (T_4) levels. High amounts of selenium may reduce sperm motility. Selenium toxicity can elevate creatinine kinase levels.

senna *(Cassia senna)* | **Uses:** Constipation, bowel preparation; | **Preg:** Most laxatives carry a Pregnancy Category B or C classification and the use of fiber supplements and senna have been supported. The American Academy of Pediatrics has classified senna as usually compatible with breastfeeding;

CIs: Allergy/hypersensitivity; **ADRs:** abdominal pain, arthralgia, bloating, cachexia, ↓ circulating B lymphocytes, colon pigmentation, cramping, diarrhea, discolored urine, finger clubbing, flatulence, hepatitis, hypertrophic osteoarthropathy, hypogammaglobulinemia, hypokalemia, incontinence, intestinal perforation, liver damage, loss of haustral folds in the colon, myalgia, nausea, nephrocalcinosis, neuropathy, portal vein thrombosis, tetany, ↑ urothelial cancer risk, weakened bones or muscles, weight loss; **Interactions:** Digoxin (↑ risk of hypokalemia), laxatives (additive effects), potassium-depleting drugs (↑ risk of hypokalemia), warfarin (↑ INR/↑ risk of bleeding); **Dose:** Oral: Up to 14.8 g senna or up to 180 mg sennoside daily as needed (not to exceed 10 days); 1–2 tablets Senokot daily or every other day, maximum 3 tablets PO bid; **Monitor:** Electrolyte levels; **Notes:** Long-term use should be avoided. Chronic use of laxatives may lead to "lazy-bowel syndrome," in which the stomach and intestines gradually lose the ability to contract without being stimulated by the laxative

shakuyaku-kanzo-to **Uses:** Insufficient available evidence; **Preg:** Not recommended due to insufficient evidence; **CIs:** Allergy/hypersensitivity; **ADRs:** insufficient evidence; **Interactions:** Antihypertensive agents (↓ effects), drugs that alter heart rhythm (interfere with effects); may interact with agents with similar effects or related mechanisms of action (antidepressants); **Dose:** Insufficient evidence; **Monitor:** Insufficient evidence; **Notes:** Shakuyaku-kanzo-to is a Japanese herbal formula that is a part of the ever-evolving system of traditional Japanese medicine, called Kampo. Shakuyaku-kanzo-to is made up of a blend of two crude drugs: shakuyaku (peony root) and kanzo (glycyrrhiza root, or licorice). Shakuyaku-kanzo-to is prescribed in Japan to relieve calf cramps, and menstrual and nonspecific abdominal pain.

shark cartilage **Uses:** Arthritis, cancer, Kaposi's sarcoma, macular degeneration, osteoarthritis, pain, psoriasis, renal cell carcinoma; **Preg:** Not recommended due to insufficient evidence; **CIs:** Allergy/hypersensitivity; **ADRs:** arrhythmias, ↑ blood glucose, ↓ blood pressure, constipation, dizziness, dyspepsia, fatigue, nausea/vomiting, weakness; **Interactions:** Antiangiogenic agents (synergistic effects), calcium (↑ risk of hypercalcemia); **Dose:** Oral: arthritis: 0.2–2 g/kg PO qd 2–3 divided doses; cancer: 80–100 g or 1–1.3 g/kg PO qd in 2–4 divided doses; shark cartilage derivative AE-941 (Neovastat): 30–240 mL daily or 20 mg/kg PO bid. Enema (cancer): 15 g or 0.5–1 g/kg daily, prepared as an enema, in 2–3 divided doses. Psoriasis, topical: 5%–10% preparations applied daily; | **Monitor:** Calcium levels; | **Notes:** AE-941 and U-995 are currently being investigated in several preclinical and phase I to III clinical trials.

shea butter | **Uses:** Anticoagulant, decongestant, hyperlipidemia; | **Preg:** Not recommended due to insufficient evidence; | **CIs:** Allergy/hypersensitivity, Latex allergy; | **ADRs:** insufficient available evidence; | **Interactions:** Anticoagulants/antiplatelets (↑ risk of bleeding); antilipemic agents (additive effects); | **Dose:** Oral, hyperlipidemia: diet consisting of shea butter (42% stearic acid) × 3 wk. Topical: apply daily; | **Monitor:** Lipid profile, coagulation panel; | **Notes:** Shea butter is extensively marketed as a skin and hair moisturizer and as a treatment for a variety of skin-related conditions, including acne, burns, chapped lips, dry skin, eczema, psoriasis, scars, stretch marks, and wrinkles.

shepherd's purse | **Uses:** Insufficient available evidence; | **Preg:** Not recommended due to insufficient evidence and traditional use as an abortifacient; | **CIs:** Allergy/hypersensitivity, History of kidney stones, Pregnancy; | **ADRs:** altered thyroid function, hyper-/hypotension, palpitations, sedation, tachycardia; | **Interactions:** Androgens (additive effects), antihypertensives (alter effects), CNS depressants (additive sedation); thyroid hormones (interfere with therapy); | **Dose:** Dried, above-ground parts: 1–4 g dried PO 3 times/day. Liquid extract (1:1 in 25% alcohol): 1–4 mL PO 3 times/day. Tea: steep 1–4 g dried above-ground parts in 150 mL boiling water 10–15 minutes, strain, consume PO 3 times/day; | **Monitor:** Blood pressure, heart rate, thyroid function; | **Notes:** The seeds, leaves, and flowering shoots of shepherd's purse are edible and may be consumed raw or cooked. Seed oil, seed pods, and dried roots are used as flavorings in food. Shepherd's purse has been used in humans as a folk remedy to treat numerous conditions, including diarrhea and bleeding. It has also been used to stimulate uterine contractions.

shiitake | **Uses:** Chemotherapy (adjunct), genital warts, HIV (adjunct), immunomodulator; | **Preg:** Likely safe when consumed in amounts found in foods; not recommended for medicinal use due to insufficient available evidence; | **CIs:** Allergy/hypersensitivity, Eosinophilia; | **ADRs:** abdominal discomfort, allergic dermatitis, chills, diarrhea, fever, hematologic toxicity (thrombocytopenia, eosinophilia, granulocytopenia, and leukocytosis), hypersensitivity pneumonitis (cough, dyspnea, hypoxia, cyanosis, bibasilar crackles), ↑ LFTs, nausea, pain (back, leg, lumbar); | **Interactions:** Anticoagulants/antiplatelets (↑ risk of bleeding), antilipemic agents (additive effects), antineoplastic agents (↑ risk of hematologic toxicity), BCG vaccine (enhanced response), hepatotoxic agents (↑ risk of hepatotoxicty), photosensitizers (↑ risk of photosensitivity); | **Dose:** IV or IM: 1–4 mg/wk; oral: 6–16 g of mushrooms; | **Monitor:** CBC, CD4 counts (in patients with HIV), coagulation panel, LFTs; | **Notes:** Hypersensitivity pneumonitis (cough, dyspnea, hypoxia, cyanosis, bibasilar crackles) has been reported in a number of case reports following inhalation of shiitake mushroom spores. In clinical study, hematological toxicity, including thrombocytopenia, eosinophilia, granulocytopenia, and leukocytosis, have been reported with oral and intravenous administration of lentinan.

sho seiryu to | **Uses:** Insufficient available evidence; | **Preg:** Not recommended due to insufficient evidence; | **CIs:** Allergy/hypersensitivity, Fever, Extended periods of time (more than 2 wk); | **ADRs:** insufficient available evidence; | **Interactions:** Insufficient available evidence; | **Dose:** Traditionally, the formula is taken as a tea, which has an unpleasant taste and odor. Most Westerners take sho seiryu as capsules or tablets, or other method of administration that somewhat diminishes the odor and taste. Dosages are usually larger than most Western medicines, usually about 72 g; | **Monitor:** Insufficient available evidence; | **Notes:** Sho seiryu to, also known as TJ-19, is a Japanese herbal formula that contains equal proportions (9 g) of licorice root, schizandra fruit, ephedra, cinnamon twig, ginger root, peony root, asarum herb, and pinella. It is used to help speed recovery from colds in the absence of fever.

shuang huang lian | **Uses:** Insufficient available evidence; | **Preg:** Not recommended due to insufficient evidence; | **CIs:** Allergy/hypersensitivity; | **ADRs:** insufficient available evidence; | **Interactions:** Insufficient available evidence; | **Dose:** 4 capsules 3 times daily (capsule: 0.4 g); | **Monitor:** Insufficient available evidence; | **Notes:** Shuang huang lian is a formula composed of three herbs: lonicera, scute, and forsythia. It is traditionally known as an antiviral, and it is most commonly used for the treatment of respiratory infections, including upper and lower respiratory tract infections and acute bronchiolitis.

Siberian cocklebur | **Uses:** Insufficient evidence; | **Preg:** Not recommended due to insufficient evidence; | **CIs:** Allergy/hypersensitivity; | **ADRs:** abdominal pain, ↓ appetite, anorexia, anxiety, bradycardia, constipation, diaphoresis, diarrhea, facial flushing, fatigue, fever, jaundice around nose and mouth, liver failure, restlessness, sleepiness; | **Interactions:** Immunosuppressants (altered effects); | **Dose:** Oral: 2–10 g in water, pill, or powder form; | **Monitor:** LFTs; | **Notes:** Siberian cocklebur is an annual spring weed long used in traditional Chinese medicine (TCM). It contains toxic substances that may cause liver failure.

Siberian ginseng | **Uses:** Adaptogen, cancer, chronic fatigue syndrome, exercise performance enhancement, FMF, genital herpes, hypotension, immunomodulation, menopause, pneumonia, respiratory tract infections; | **Preg:** Not recommended due to insufficient evidence; | **CIs:** Allergy/hypersensitivity, Hormone-sensitive conditions, Children; | **ADRs:** aggression, diarrhea, mastalgia (women), muscle spasm, neuritis, nervousness; | **Interactions:** Anticoagulants/antiplatelets (↑ risk of bleeding), antidiabetic agents (↑ risk of hypoglycemia), antihypertensives (↑ risk of hypotension), antilipemic agents (additive effects), CNS depressants (↑ sedation), CYP450 1A2/2C9/2D6/3A4 substrates (inhibits CYP1A2/2C9/2D6/3A4), digoxin (↑ digoxin levels), diuretics (↑ effects), immunosuppressants (altered effects), photosensitizers (↑ risk of photosensitivity reactions). | **Dose:** General: tea: prepared with 9–30 g of Siberian ginseng in boiling water; 2–3 g of dried, powdered Siberian ginseng root and rhizomes, PO qd. Chronic fatigue syndrome: 500 mg PO qid × 2 mo. Exercise performance enhancement: 800–1,200 mg qd for up to 10 days, 800 mg qd × 14 days; 3.4 mL extract qd × 6 wk, 2 mL qd × 8 days. Genital herpes: standardized extract to contain eleutheroside E 0.3% of 400 mg PO qd. Immunomodulation: 8 mL (35% ethanolic extract of Siberian ginseng equivalent to 4 g of dried root) PO qd × 6 wk; | **Monitor:** Blood glucose, coagulation panel, electrolytes; | **Notes:** Siberian ginseng may alter digoxin levels and can falsely elevate serum digoxin concentrations when fluorescence polarization immunoassay (FPIA) or the Abbott Digoxin III are used. A specific production combination of Siberian ginseng and andrographis (Kan Jang) is used for common cold; start within 72 hours of the onset of symptoms.

S

skullcap (*Scutellaria* spp.) | **Uses:** Anxiety, cancer; | **Preg:** Not recommended due to insufficient evidence; | **CIs:** Allergy/hypersensitivity, Pregnancy, Lactation; | **ADRs:** constipation, diarrhea, fatigue, flatulence, headache, nausea, vomiting; | **Interactions:** 5-fluorouracil (↓ myelotoxicity), CNS depressants (↑ sedation), cyclophosphamide (↑ antimetastatic effect, ↓ myelotoxicity), CYP450 substrates (altered drug levels); **Dose:** 350 mL of BZL101 (an extract of Baikal skullcap) has been used as a sole cancer therapy; **Monitor:** CBC, LFTs, lipid profile, serum IgE levels; **Notes:** Baikal skullcap is an ingredient in PC-SPES, a product that has been recalled from the U.S. market and should not be used.

skunk cabbage **Uses:** Insufficient evidence; **Preg:** Not recommended due to uterine stimulating effects; **CIs:** Allergy/hypersensitivity, Pregnancy; **ADRs:** dyspnea, headache, nausea/vomiting, nyctalopia, renal calculi, vertigo; **Interactions:** Calcium (↓ mineral absorption), iron (↓ mineral absorption), sedatives (additive effects), zinc (↓ mineral absorption); **Dose:** Powdered rhizome/root: 0.5–1 mg PO tid mixed with honey or by infusion or decoction. Liquid extract (1:1 in 25% alcohol): 0.5–1 mL PO tid. Tincture (1:10 in 45% alcohol): 2–4 mL PO tid; **Monitor:** N/A; **Notes:** Skunk cabbage is poisonous when not properly handled or prepared, especially when unprocessed. Its seeds reportedly contain a narcotic.

slippery elm **Uses:** Cancer, diarrhea, gastrointestinal disorders, sore throat; **Preg:** Not recommended due to insufficient evidence and traditional use as an abortifacient; **CIs:** Allergy/hypersensitivity, Pregnancy; **ADRs:** rash, urticaria; **Interactions:** ↓ absorption of oral agents; **Dose:** Oral: 200–500 mg tablets or capsules PO 3–4 times/day; decoction, powdered inner bark (1:8): 4–16 mL PO 3 times/day; alcohol extract (1:1 in 60% alcohol): 5 mL PO 3 times/day; tea: 4 g powdered inner bark in 500 mL boiling water, PO 3 times/day. Topical, poultice: coarse powdered inner bark mixed with boiling water; **Monitor:** N/A; **Notes:** Slippery elm is a component of Essiac tea, which also includes sorrel, burdock root, and Indian rhubarb.

sorbic acid **Uses:** Insufficient evidence; **Preg:** Not recommended due to insufficient evidence; **CIs:** Allergy/hypersensitivity; **ADRs:** skin irritation; **Interactions:** Insufficient evidence; **Dose:** Insufficient evidence; **Monitor:** Insufficient evidence; **Notes:** In the United States, sorbic acid is primarily used in a wide range of food and feed products and to a lesser in certain cosmetics, pharmaceuticals, and tobacco products. Sorbic acid is used as a preservative at concentrations of up to 0.2%.

sorrel **Uses:** Allergic rhinitis, antibacterial, antiviral, bronchitis, cancer, sinusitis; **Preg:** Not recommended due to potential oxalate toxicity; **CIs:** Allergy/hypersensitivity,

Children, Large doses, Liver disease, Kidney disease; | **ADRs:** allergic reactions, corrosive GI effects, dermatitis, hepatotoxicity, RENAL CALCULI; | **Interactions:** Antibiotics (synergistic effects), hepatotoxic agents (↑ risk of liver damage), minerals (↓ mineral absorption), nephrotoxic agents (↑ risk of nephrotoxicity); | **Dose:** Sorrel is most often used medicinally as a part of combination formulas. Sinupret (tablets [combination of sorrel, gentian root, European elderflower, verbena, and cowslip flower]): 1–2 tablets PO tid × 2 wk; Sinupret tincture: 50 drops PO tid; Essiac tea (contains sorrel, burdock root, slippery elm inner bark, and Indian rhubarb): 30 mL PO 1–3 times daily on an empty stomach; | **Monitor:** LFTs, renal function tests; | **Notes:** Sorrel leaves contain oxalic acid. Oxalic acid combines with calcium in plasma, forming insoluble calcium oxalate crystals that may precipitate in the kidneys, blood vessels, heart, lungs, and liver, and lead to hypocalcemia and renal lesions.

soy | **Uses:** Allergies, antioxidant, cancer, cardiovascular health, cholagogue, cognitive function, Crohn's disease, cyclical breast pain, diarrhea (infants/children), diabetes, exercise performance enhancement, gastrointestinal motility, HTN, hyperlipidemia, infantile colic, inflammation, iron-deficiency anemia, kidney disease, menopausal symptoms, menstrual migraine, metabolic syndrome, obesity, osteoarthritis, osteoporosis, protein source, RA, skin aging, skin damage, spinal cord injury, thyroid disorders, tuberculosis, weight gain (infants); | **Preg:** Safe when used in amounts found in food; | **CIs:** Allergy/hypersensitivity, Bladder cancer, Patients at risk for kidney stones; | **ADRs:** bloating, ↑ blood pressure, constipation, diarrhea, eczema, fatigue, gastrointestinal disturbances, growth failure, headache, nausea/vomiting, pancreas damage, ↓ thyroid hormone and ↑ TSH levels; | **Interactions:** Antibiotics (↓ effects of soy), anticoagulants/antiplatelets (↓ INR in patient stabilized on warfarin), antidiabetic agents (↑ risk of hypoglycemia), antihypertensive agents (↑ risk of hypotension), antilipemic agents (additive effects), calcium (inhibits calcium absorption), CYP450 2C9 (soy induces CYP2C9), estrogens (competitively inhibit estrogen effects), iron (altered effects), MAOIs (↑ risk of hypertensive crisis), phosphorus (inhibits absorption), selenium (↓ concentrations of selenium), tamoxifen (interfere with effects), thyroid hormones (need to increase dose of levothyroxine), zinc (↓ concentrations of zinc); | **Dose:** 10–106 g PO qd; isoflavone content has ranged from 60–100 mg PO qd; there is currently an approved health claim for 25 g soy daily for cholesterol reduction in the United States; | **Monitor:** Blood glucose, blood pressure, lipid profile, hormones, thyroid function, electrolytes; | **Notes:** There is controversy regarding whether soy consumption increases or reduces cancer, particularly breast cancer, risk.

spirulina | **Uses:** Allergic rhinitis, arsenic poisoning, blepharospasm, diabetes, hypercholesterolemia, malnutrition, oral leukoplakia, weight loss; | **Preg:** Not recommended due to insufficient evidence; | **CIs:** Allergy/hypersensitivity, Phenylketonuria; | **ADRs:** diaphoresis, facial flushing, headache, hepatotoxicity, myalgia, nausea/vomiting, weight loss; | **Interactions:** ACE inhibitors (additive effects), anticoagulants/antiplatelets (↑ risk of bleeding), hepatotoxic agents (↑ risk of liver damage), immunosuppressants (altered effects), osteoporosis agents (↓ effectiveness); | **Dose:** Allergic rhinitis: 1,000 mg or 2,000 mg PO qd × 12 wk. Diabetes: 1 g PO bid with meals. Hypercholesterolemia: 1.4 g 3 times/day with meals × 8 wk. Oral leukoplakia: 1 g PO qd × 1 year. Weight loss: 200 mg PO tid; | **Monitor:** LFTs; | **Notes:** The term "spirulina" refers to a large number of cyanobacteria or blue-green algae. Use cautiously in patients with phenylketonuria due to phenylalanine content. Spirulina may stimulate the immune system and should be used with caution in patients with autoimmune disorders.

spleen extract | **Uses:** Insufficient evidence; | **Preg:** Not recommended due to insufficient evidence; | **CIs:** Allergy/hypersensitivity; | **ADRs:** altered immune function, enhanced perception of pain; | **Interactions:** Antibiotics (synergistic effects), anticoagulants/antiplatelets (altered effects), antifungals (↑ efficacy), cyclophosphamide (synergistic effects), immunosuppressants (altered effects); | **Dose:** 150–300 mg PO 2–3 times daily; | **Monitor:** WBC count; | **Notes:** There are concerns about contaminated products.

squill | **Uses:** Coronary artery disease; | **Preg:** Not recommended due to toxic effects; | **CIs:** Allergy/hypersensitivity, UNSAFE ORALLY; | **ADRs:** toxic effects: abdominal pain, convulsions, hypothermia, nausea/vomiting; | **Interactions:** Calcium (↑ risk of cardioavascular toxicity), CARDIAC GLYCOSIDES (↑ risk of toxicity), corticosteroids (↑ risk of adverse effects), potassium-depleting agents (↑ risk of cardiovascular toxicity), stimulant laxatives (↑ risk of cardiovascular toxicity); | **Dose:** Extract (1 in 1; prepared by percolation with 70% alcohol): 0.03–0.2 mL PO qd. Syrup (vinegar of squill 45 mL, sucrose 80 g, water to 100 mL): 2–4 mL PO qd. Tincture (1 in 10; prepared by maceration with 60% alcohol): 0.3–2 mL PO qd. Vinegar (1 in 10; prepared by maceration with dilute acetic acid): 0.6–2 mL PO qd; | **Monitor:** Toxic effects (cardiovascular

S

toxicity); | **Notes:** Squill has similar effects to digoxin. It may be TOXIC when ingested.

St. John's wort | **Uses:** Anxiety disorders, atopic dermatitis, ADHD, burning mouth syndrome, depression (children), depression (mild to moderate), nerve pain, OCD, pain relief, perimenopausal symptoms, PMS, SAD, social phobia, somatoform disorders; | **Preg:** Not recommended due to insufficient evidence; | **CIs:** Allergy/hypersensitivity, Concurrent use of antiretroviral agents, immunosuppressants, or MAOIs, Patients with suicidal ideation; | **ADRs:** anorexia, anxiety, constipation, drowsiness, dyspepsia, fatigue, gastrointestinal upset, headache, hypertension, hypertensive crisis, mania, nausea, neuropathy, photosensitivity, restlessness, serotonin syndrome (characterized by rigidity, hyperthermia, delerium, confusion, autonomic instability, and coma), sexual dysfunction, tachycardia, xerostomia; | **Interactions:** AMINOLEVULINIC ACID (phototoxicity), AMITRIPTYLINE (↓ concentrations of amitriptyline), anesthetics (↑ risk of adverse effects), ANTIDEPRESSANTS (↑ risk of serotonergic effects), antidiabetic agents (↑ risk of hypoglycemia), barbiturates (↑ sedation), BENZODIAZEPINES (↓ effectiveness of benzodiazepines), CARDIAC GLYCOSIDES (↓ effects of cardiac glycosides), clopidogrel (↑ activity), CNS DEPRESSANTS (↑ sedation), CONTRACEPTIVES (↓ estrogen and progesterone levels), CYCLOSPORINE (↓ cyclosporine levels), CYP450 1A2 and 2C9 substrates (induces CYP1A2 and 2C9), CYP450 3A4 substrates (SJW induces CYP450 3A4), dextromethorphan (↑ risk of serotonergic effects), fenfluramine (↑ risk of serotonergic effects), fexofenadine (↑ plasma concentrations of fexofenadine), IMATINIB (↓ levels of imatinib), IMMUNOSUPPRESSANTS (↓ levels of immunosuppressants), IRINOTECAN (↓ levels of irinotecan), linezolid (↑ risk of serotonergic effects), MEPERIDINE (↑ risk of serotonergic effects), methylphenidate (↓ effectiveness of methylphenidate), NNRTIs (↓ levels of NNRTIs), MAOIs (↑ risk of adverse effects), PENTAZOCINE (↑ risk of serotonergic effects), P-gp SUBSTRATES (SJW induces P-gp), PHENYTOIN (↑ levels of phenytoin), PHOTOSENSITIZERS (↑risk of photosensitivity reactions), procainamide (↑ bioavailability), PROTEASE INHIBITORS (↓ concentrations), reserpine (antagonizes effects), simvastatin (↓ concentrations of simvastatin metabolite), TACROLIMUS (↓ levels of tacrolimus), theophylline (↑ levels of theophylline), TRAMADOL (↑ risk of serotonergic effects), triptans (↑ risk of serotonergic effects), thyroid hormones (altered effects), WARFARIN (↓ effects of warfarin); | **Dose:** Oral: 300 mg PO tid, standardized to contain 0.3% hypericin and/or 2%–5% hyperforin per dose; minimum of

S

4–6 weeks of therapy is recommended before results may be noted; Topical: Apply 1.5% oil extract as needed to affected area; **Monitor:** Blood glucose levels, drug levels, thyroid hormones; **Notes:** Caution is warranted with bipolar disorder and other psychiatric disorders as cases of mania have been reported with St. John's wort use.

star anise **Uses:** Insufficient evidence; **Preg:** Not recommended due to insufficient evidence; **CIs:** Allergy/hypersensitivity, Hormone-sensitive conditions, Use in infants; **ADRs:** allergic reactions; star anise tea can cause convulsions, hypothermia, nausea/vomiting, nystagmus, seizures, spasms, tremors. It is unclear whether this toxicity is caused by star anise alone or by contamination with Japanese star anise; **Interactions:** Anticoagulants/antiplatelets (↑ risk of bleeding); **Dose:** Ground: 3 g PO qd; essential oil: 300 mg PO qd; tea: 0.5–1 g ground seeds boiled in 150 mL water for 120 minutes, strain; **Monitor:** N/A; **Notes:** In 2003, the FDA issued a consumer warning about consumption of teas containing Chinese star anise (*Illicium verum*) owing to reports of contamination with the toxic Japanese star anise (*Illicium anisatum*). Shikimic acid extracted from the pods (which wraps the seeds) of Chinese star anise is the starting material of Tamiflu.

stevia **Uses:** Diabetes, hypertension; **Preg:** Not recommended due to insufficient evidence; **CIs:** Allergy/hypersensitivity, Cross-allergy to Asteraceae/Compositae family; **ADRs:** Abdominal fullness, allergic reactions, asthenia, dizziness, headache, myalgia, nausea/vomiting, paresthesia; **Interactions:** Antidiabetic agents (↑ risk of hypoglycemia), antihypertensive agents (↑ risk of hypotension), calcium channel blockers (additive effects), diuretics (additive effects), vasodilators (additive effects); **Dose:** 250–500 mg stevioside (constituent of stevia) PO tid × 2 yr; leaves: 5 g PO q6h × 3 days; **Monitor:** Blood glucose, blood pressure; **Notes:** In 2008, stevia became available as a food additive and Generally Recognized as Safe.

S

stinging nettle **Uses:** Allergic rhinitis, arthritis, BPH, insect bites, joint pain, plaque/gingivitis; **Preg:** Not recommended due to abortifacient and uterine stimulating effects; **CIs:** Allergy/hypersensitivity, Pregnancy; **ADRs:** oral: constipation, diarrhea, gastrointestinal complaints, hyperperistalsis, hypotension, sweating; topical: burning, pruritus; **Interactions:** Anticoagulants (warfarin: ↓ the effects); antidiabetes drugs (↑/↓ blood glucose); antihypertensive agents (↑ risk of hypotension); CNS depressants (additive sedation); diuretics (additive effects), finasteride (additive effects); | **Dose:** Allergic rhinitis: freeze-dried nettle: 600 mg PO qd × 1 wk. Arthritis: stewed leaves: 50 mg in combination with 50 mg diclofenac × 13 days. BPH: extract (Bazoton capsules): 300 mg PO bid × 6–9 wk; | **Monitor:** Blood glucose, blood pressure; | **Notes:** Use with caution in individuals with gout or a history of uric acid renal stones.

strawberry | **Uses:** Antioxidant, colorectal cancer prevention; | **Preg:** Safe when consumed as food; | **CIs:** Allergy/hypersensitivity; | **ADRs:** contact dermatitis, pruritus, urticaria; | **Interactions:** Antiplatelet agents (additive effects), iron (enhances absorption); | **Dose:** Insufficient evidence; | **Monitor:** N/A; | **Notes:** Caution is warranted in patients with allergies to the Rosaceae family, including peach, apples, and plums.

suma *(Pfaffia paniculata)* | **Uses:** Insufficient clinical evidence; | **Preg:** Not recommended due to insufficient evidence; | **CIs:** Allergy/hypersensitivity; | **ADRs:** allergic asthma, angina, hormonal effects, mild gastrointestinal complaints; | **Interactions:** Hormonal agents (↑ endogenous hormones estradiol, progesterone, testerosterone), may interact with agents with similar effects or related mechanisms of action (antibacterial, anti-inflammatory, antineoplastic, anti-impotence); | **Dose:** Oral: up to 6 g root powder daily in divided doses; | **Monitor:** Hemoglobin, hormone panel, lipid profile; | **Notes:** Suma has been used historically as a folk remedy for various indications such as for sexual enhancement, menstrual disorders, and as a general tonic.

sundew (*Drosera* spp) | **Uses:** Chronic obstructive pulmonary disease (COPD); | **Preg:** Not recommended due to insufficient evidence; | **CIs:** Allergy/hypersensitivity; | **ADRs:** based on historical use and available research, extracts of *Drosera* have been used for up to 6 months without incident; | **Interactions:** May interact with agents with similar effects or related mechanisms of action (antiasthmatic, antibiotic, anti-inflammatory, antispasmodic); | **Dose:** Oral: dried plant: 1–2 g 3 times/day; liquid extract (1:1 in 25% alcohol): 0.5–2 mL 3 times/day; tea: prepare by steeping 1–2 g dried plant in 150 mL boiling water for 5–10 minutes, strain, consume 1 cup 3 times/day; tincture (1:5 in 60% alcohol): 0.5–1 mL three times/day; | **Monitor:** Insufficient evidence; | **Notes:** *Drosera* species are protected by law in many countries. In the United States, several species, such as *Drosera rotundifolia*, are listed as either threatened or endangered.

S

sunflower oil | **Uses:** Cardiovascular disease, clotting disorders, diabetes, hyperlipidemia, mastitis, tinea pedis; | **Preg:** Not recommended due to insufficient evidence; | **CIs:** Allergy/hypersensitivity; | **ADRs:** abdominal cramps, diarrhea, nausea/vomiting; | **Interactions:** Antineoplastic agents (altered effects), anticoagulants/antiplatelets (↑ risk of bleeding), antidiabetic agents (↑ risk of hypoglycemia), antihypertensives (↑ risk of hypotension), antilipemic agents (additive effects), laxatives (additive effects); | **Dose:** Oral: 15–30 mL PO bid. Topical: ozonized sunflower oil (Oleozon) applied daily; | **Monitor:** Blood glucose; | **Notes:** Sunflower oil can cause an allergic reaction in individuals sensitive to the Asteraceae/Compositae family (ragweed, chrysanthemums, marigolds, daisies).

sweet almond | **Uses:** Anxiety, hyperlipidemia; | **Preg:** Not recommended due to insufficient evidence; | **CIs:** Allergy/hypersensitivity; | **ADRs:** allergic reactions; | **Interactions:** Antidiabetic agents (↑ risk of hypoglycemia), estrogens (additive estrogenic effects); | **Dose:** Hyperlipidemia: 84–100 g PO qd; | **Monitor:** Lipid profile; | **Notes:** Hypersensitivity to almonds is common and may lead to severe reactions. Avoid in patients with known hypersensitivity to almonds, almond constituents, or other nuts. Cross-reactivity to other nuts may occur.

sweet annie | **Uses:** Cancer, malaria; | **Preg:** Not recommended due to insufficient evidence; | **CIs:** Allergy/hypersensitivity, Cross-allergy with Asteraceae/Compositae; | **ADRs:** abdominal pain, allergic reaction, cardiovascular and CNS toxicity, hypoglycemia, QT prolongation; | **Interactions:** Antidiabetic agents (↑ risk of hypoglycemia), chloroquine (added benefit); | **Dose:** Oral, tea, for malaria: prepare 5–9 g/day in 1 L of water (providing 50–100 mg of artemisinin); give in divided doses; | **Monitor:** Blood glucose; | **Notes:** Sweet annie's main active constituent, artemisinin, has shown rapid antimalarial activity.

sweet basil | **Uses:** Insufficient evidence; | **Preg:** Not recommended due to insufficient evidence; | **CIs:** Allergy/hypersensitivity; | **ADRs:** allergic reactions, diarrhea; | **Interactions:** UGT 2B7 and 1A9 substrates; | **Dose:** Insufficient evidence; | **Monitor:** N/A; | **Notes:** Sweet basil is a commonly used medicinal herb in Thailand, India, and Turkey, and has been used as a spice in cooking. The constituent, estragole, is naturally found in sweet basil and is used in fragrances and flavorings. Constituents of sweet basil, including estragole and methyleugenol, pose a danger to humans due to carcinogenic effects.

sweet woodruff | **Uses:** Insufficient evidence; | **Preg:** Not recommended due to insufficient evidence; | **CIs:** Allergy/hypersensitivity; | **ADRs:** headache, somnolence, vertigo; | **Interactions:** Anticoagulants/antiplatelets (↑ risk of bleeding); | **Dose:** Tea: 3 cups of boiled water over herb (1 oz of dry herb or 1½ oz of fresh herb), steep for 10 minutes, strain tea and refrigerate unused portions for up to 24 hours. Tincture: 8 ounces of dried herb mixed with 1½ cups of alcohol and 4 cups of water; | **Monitor:** N/A; | **Notes:** Traditionally, sweet woodruff has been used to help relieve stomach ache. It is also used to flavor wines.

tamanu | **Uses:** Insufficient evidence; | **Preg:** Not recommended due to insufficient evidence; | **CIs:** Allergy/hypersensitivity; | **ADRs:** allergic dermatitis, CNS depression, paralysis, sedation; | **Interactions:** Anesthetics (additive effects), anticoagulants (↑ risk of bleeding), CNS depressants (↑ risk of sedation); NRTIs (synergistic effects); | **Dose:** Insufficient evidence; | **Monitor:** N/A; | **Notes:** Oil of tamanu is appropriate for general skin and cosmetic purposes.

tamarind | **Uses:** Dry eyes, skeletal fluorosis prevention; | **Preg:** Not recommended due to lack of sufficient data. Avoid using in amounts greater than those found in foods; | **CIs:** Allergy/hypersensitivity; | **ADRs:** cough, respiratory reactions; | **Interactions:** Anticoagulants/antiplatelets (↑ risk of bleeding), antidiabetic agents (↑ risk of hypoglycemia), aspirin (↑ aspirin absorption), ibuprofen (↑ ibuprofen absorption), laxatives (additive effects), topical ophthalmic antibiotics (synergistic effects), vasoconstrictors (additive effects); | **Dose:** 10 g PO qd × 3 wk; | **Monitor:** N/A; | **Notes:** Tamarind powder can be used as a condiment or flavoring agent. It is also used for chutneys and curries.

S

tangerine | **Uses:** Insufficient evidence; | **Preg:** Safe when used in food; | **CIs:** Allergy/hypersensitivity; | **ADRs:** contact dermatitis, phytobezoar, small intestine obstruction; | **Interactions:** CYP450 3A4 substrates (altered drug levels); | **Dose:** Insufficient evidence; | **Monitor:** N/A; | **Notes:** Tangerine is a fruit and a good source of vitamin C, folate, and beta-carotene.

tansy | **Uses:** Insufficient evidence; | **Preg:** Not recommended due to insufficient evidence and traditional use as an abortifacient; | **CIs:** Allergy/hypersensitivity, Cross-allergenicity to Asteraceae/Compositae family (ragweed, chrysanthemums, marigolds, daisies, etc.); **ADRs:** contact dermatitis; symptoms of toxicity (thujone toxicity): abdominal pain, gastroenteritis, hallucinations, hepatotoxicity, seizures, tachypnea, vomiting; **Interactions:** ALCOHOL (↑ the effects); **Dose:** Insufficient evidence; **Monitor:** N/A; **Notes:** Tansy contains thujone, which is known to be toxic.

tarragon **Uses:** Insufficient evidence; **Preg:** Not recommended due to insufficient evidence and possible hormonal effects; **CIs:** Allergy/hypersensitivity; **ADRs:** ↑ risk of liver cancer; **Interactions:** CYP450 1A2 and 2A6 substrates (altered effects), hepatotoxic agents (↑ risk of liver damage); **Dose:** Tea: boil 1 tsp of dried tarragon in a cup of water, strain and drink the extract twice daily for a month; **Monitor:** LFTs; **Notes:** Tarragon has a long tradition in the West and in Asia for successfully treating dyspepsia. The essential oil of tarragon contains 172–7,000 ppm estragole, a hepatocarcinogen; the German Institute for Consumer Health Protection and Veterinary Medicine warned consumers about tarragon's potential dangers in 2001.

taurine **Uses:** CHF, cystic fibrosis, diabetes, energy, epilepsy, hypercholesterolemia, HTN, iron-deficiency anemia, liver disease, myotonic dystrophy, nutritional supplement (infant formula), obesity, surgery adjunct, TPN, vaccine adjunct, vision problems; **Preg:** Not recommended due to insufficient evidence; **CIs:** Allergy/hypersensitivity, Surgery; **ADRs:** ataxia, ↓ blood pressure, drowsiness; **Interactions:** Anesthetics (altered effects), anticoagulants/antiplatelets (↑ risk of bleeding), anticonvulsants (altered effects), antidiabetic agents (↑ risk of hypoglycemia), antihypertensives (↑ risk of hypotension), diuretics (additive effects), glutamine (altered effects), iron (altered effects), tamoxifen (altered effects), tyrosine (altered effects); **Dose:** Oral: 1–6 g PO qd; cystic fibrosis (children): 30–40 mg/kg body weight PO qd × 6 months. Injection, epilepsy: 200 mg/kg intravenously for 15 days, then once a week for 6 weeks; TPN: 10 mg/kg taurine per day added to TPN × 24 mo; surgery: 5 g intravenously as a single rapid dose has been used 1–3 hours before surgery; **Monitor:** N/A; **Notes:** Taurine is a constituent of some energy drinks, including Red Bull. Use cautiously in patients with bipolar disorder because taurine may exacerbate this condition.

tea tree oil **Uses:** Acne, allergic skin reactions, antibacterial, antifungal, bad breath, dandruff, dental plaque/gingivitis, eye infections, lice, MRSA, onychomycosis, herpes labialis, thrush, tinea pedis, vaginal infections; | **Preg:** Safe when used topically; unsafe when ingested; | **CIs:** Allergy/hypersensitivity, INGESTION; | **ADRs:** topical: contact dermatitis, local irritation, ototoxicity (after instilled in the ear), skin dryness; oral: abdominal pain, CNS depression, diarrhea, dysgeusia, halitosis, nausea; | **Interactions:** CYP450 substrates (altered drug levels), topical drying agents (additive skin dryness), tretinoin (additive skin dryness), vancomycin (additive effects); | **Dose:** Oral, mouthwash: Dilute a few drops of oil in a cup of water, gargle, and expectorate; DO NOT INGEST. Topical: apply 5%–100% oil to affected area as needed; | **Monitor:** N/A; | **Notes:** UNSAFE when used orally.

theanine | **Uses:** Anxiety, HTN, mood; | **Preg:** Not recommended due to insufficient evidence; | **CIs:** Allergy/hypersensitivity; | **ADRs:** altered mental status; | **Interactions:** Antihypertensives (↑ risk of hypotension), antineoplastic agents (altered effects), stimulants (↓ effects of stimulants); | **Dose:** 200 mg/day PO; | **Monitor:** Blood pressure; | **Notes:** Theanine is one of the predominant amino acids ordinarily found in green tea.

thiamin | **Uses:** Acute alcohol withdrawal, Alzheimer's disease, atherosclerosis, athletic performance, CA, cataract prevention, Crohn's disease, DIDMOAD (diabetes insipidus, diabetes mellitus, optic atrophy, and deafness; or Wolfram) syndrome, heart failure, hypothermia, leg cramps (during pregnancy), metabolic disorders, thiamin deficiency, TPN; | **Preg:** Likely safe; RDA: 1.4 mg/day; | **CIs:** Allergy/hypersensitivity; | **ADRs:** burning at injection site, dermatitis, drowsiness (large doses), hypersensitivity reactions, muscle relaxation (large doses); | **Interactions:** Drugs that can cause depletion of thiamin: 5-FU, antibiotics, contraceptives, diuretics, metformin, phenytoin; | **Dose:** RDA: Men 14 yr and older: 1.2 mg/day; boys 9–13 yr: 0.9 mg/day; women older than 18 yr: 1.1 mg/day; women 14–18 years: 1 mg/day; girls: 9–13 yr, 0.9 mg/day; pregnancy: 1.4 mg/day; lactation: 1.5 mg/day; children 4–8 yr: 0.6 mg/day; children 1–3 years: 0.5 mg/day; infants 7–12 months: 0.3 mg/day; infants 0–6 mo: 0.2 mg/day; | **Monitor:** Thiamin levels; | **Notes:** Thiamin (also spelled "thiamine") is a water-soluble B-complex vitamin, previously known as vitamin B_1. Dietary sources of thiamin include beef, brewer's yeast, legumes (beans, lentils), milk, nuts, oats, oranges, pork, rice, seeds, wheat, whole grain cereals, and yeast. Consumption of seafood may increase the risk of thiamine deficiency. Thiamine may interfere with theophylline laboratory tests. Thiamine can cause false-positive results in uric acid laboratory testing and urine spot test for urobilinogen.

thundergod vine | **Uses:** Anti-inflammatory, asthma, CA, contraceptive (male), Grave's ophthalmopathy, kidney disease, organ transplant, RA, skin disorders, SLE; | **Preg:** Not recommended due to insufficient evidence and possible teratogenic effects; | **CIs:** Allergy/hypersensitivity, Immunocompromised, Osteoporosis, Pregnancy; | **ADRs:** alopecia, amenorrhea, ↓ bone density, cardiac adverse effects (diastolic hypertension, ventricular tachyarrhythmia), diarrhea, gastrointestinal upset, headache, infertility, ↑ LFTs, menstrual irregularities, nephrotoxicity, skin reactions; | **Interactions:** Antihypertensive agents (altered effects), DMARDs (synergistic effects), immunosuppressants (enhanced effects); | **Dose:** Asthma: 40–60 mg PO qd × 4 wk. Grave's ophthalmopathy: 30–60 mg PO qd × 4 wk. Organ transplant: 1 mg/kg or 2 mg/kg body weight PO daily × 5 years. RA: 180–570 mg PO qd or tincture applied topically over affected joints. Kidney disease, children: 1 mg/kg body weight PO qd. SLE: 15 g crude extract 3 times daily × 5 years; | **Monitor:** Renal infection; | **Notes:** Thundergod vine may have both immunosuppressive and immunostimulant properties.

thyme, thymol | **Uses:** Alopecia, antifungal, bronchitis, cough, dental plaque, inflammatory skin disorders; | **Preg:** Safe when used in amounts commonly found in food; | **CIs:** Allergy/hypersensitivity; | **ADRs:** asthenia, contact dermatitis (topical), dyspepsia, gastrointestinal upset, hypotension, nausea/vomiting; | **Interactions:** 5-FU (altered effects), anticoagulants/antiplatelets (↑ risk of bleeding), estrogens (altered effects), progesterone (altered effects), thyroid hormones (altered effects); | **Dose:** Extract: 1–2 g PO qd in divided doses or 20–40 drops (liquid extract 1:1 w/v fresh leaf or 1:4 w/v dried leaf) 3 times/day in juice or beverage. Tea: 1–2 g dried herb in 150 mL boiling water for 10 minutes, strain, and drink several times a day until symptoms subside; | **Monitor:** Coagulation panel, estrogens, thyroid function panel; | **Notes:** Cross-sensitivity to oregano and other Lamiaceae species has been noted in patients allergic to thyme.

T

thymus extract | **Uses:** Allergy, alopecia, anxiety, arthritis, asthma, burns, CA, chemotherapy adjunct, cardiomyopathy, COPD, dermatomyositis, diabetes, eczema, encephalitis, food allergies, gastritis, glaucoma, HIV/AIDS, human papillomavirus, immunostimulant, keratitis, liver disease, myelodysplastic syndrome, psoriasis, respiratory tract infections, skin conditions, systemic lupus erythematosus, tuberculosis, UTI, warts; | **Preg:** Not recommended due to insufficient evidence; | **CIs:** Allergy/hypersensitivity, Immunocompromised; | **ADRs:** potential contamination; | **Interactions:** Immunosuppressants (↑ risk of infection); | **Dose:** Oral: 250–500 mg 3 times/day. IM: Thymostimulin 70–150 mg daily; | **Monitor:** N/A; | **Notes:** Thymus extract has immunomodulatory effects. Thymus extract that is produced from animals such as cows may be contaminated.

thyroid extract | **Uses:** Hypothyroidism, infertility, thyroid cancer; | **Preg:** Insufficient evidence; however, thyroid hormones are considered safe during pregnancy (FDA Pregnancy Category A); however, there is limited available evidence regarding the safety of thyroid extract; | **CIs:** Allergy/hypersensitivity, Eating disorders; | **ADRs:** atrial fibrillation, fever, gastrointestinal complaints, hair loss, headache, insomnia, irregular menstruation, irritability, leg cramps, ↑ risk of osteoporosis, tremors, weight loss; | **Interactions:** Amiodarone (altered effects), antacids (prevent absorption of thyroid extract), anticoagulants/antiplatelets (↑ risk of bleeding), antidepressants (altered effects), barbiturates (↓ response to thyroid extract), calcium (↓ absorption of thyroid extract), carbamazepine (↓ response to thyroid extract), corticosteroids (altered effects), CYP450 substrates (altered effects), digoxin (altered effects), estrogens (↓ response to thyroid extract), garlic (↓ effects of thyroid extract), green tea (altered effect), holy basil (altered effects), immunosuppressants (altered effects), iron (↓ absorption of thyroid extract), ketamine (↑ risk of hypertension and tachycardia), magnesium (↓ absorption of thyroid extract), olive leaf (additive effects), phenytoin (↓ response to thyroid extract), rifamycin (↓ response to thyroid extract), seaweed (altered effects), sucralfate (↓ absorption of thyroid extract), theophylline (altered effects), thyroid hormones (additive effects); | **Dose:** 60 mg PO 1–3 times/day; | **Monitor:** Thyroid panel; | **Notes:** Thyroid extracts are derived from animal thyroid tissue, usually bovine (beef) sources.

toki-shakuyaku-san | **Uses:** Menstrual irregularity; | **Preg:** Not recommended due to insufficient evidence; | **CIs:** Allergy/hypersensitivity; | **ADRs:** insufficient evidence; | **Interactions:** ANTICOAGULANTS/ANTIPLATELETS (↑ risk of bleeding), phenytoin (↓ levels of phenytoin); | **Dose:** 2.5 g PO tid; | **Monitor:** Coagulation panel; | **Notes:** Toki-shakuyaku-san (Tsumura TJ-23) is a Chinese medicine that contains soujyutsu, shakuyaku, takusha, toki, and senkyu. It is traditionally used to treat dysmenorrhea, a disorder in women that involves painful menstrual periods.

tree tobacco **Uses:** Insufficient evidence; **Preg:** Avoid use; may cause deformities; **CIs:** Allergy/hypersensitivity, ORAL USE; **ADRs:** DEATH, hallucinations, nausea/vomiting, respiratory depression, seizures; **Interactions:** Cholinergic drugs (additive effects); **Dose:** UNSAFE when used orally; **Monitor:** N/A; **Notes:** Smoking or ingesting tree tobacco is not safe and has caused death.

tribulus **Uses:** Angina, atopic dermatitis, CAD, exercise performance enhancement, infertility (male and female); **Preg:** Not recommended due to insufficient evidence and traditional use as an abortifacient; **CIs:** Allergy/hypersensitivity, Prostate conditions (prostate CA, BPH); **ADRs:** insomnia, menorrhagia, photosensitivity, pneumothorax; **Interactions:** Antidiabetic agents (↑ risk of hypoglycemia), antihypertensive agents (↑ risk of hypotension), beta blockers (↑ risk of hypotension), calcium channel blockers (↑ risk of hypotension), digoxin (additive effects), diuretics (additive effects), steroids (additive effects); **Dose:** 85–250 mg of 40% furostanol saponins extract in 3 divided doses with meals has been used; **Monitor:** Blood glucose, blood pressure, electrolytes; **Notes:** Spine-covered fruit is unsafe when used orally.

true unicorn root **Uses:** Insufficient evidence; **Preg:** Not recommended due to insufficient evidence and possible hormonal effects; **CIs:** Allergy/hypersensitivity, GI disorders; **ADRs:** colic, diarrhea, loss of balance, nausea/vomiting, sedation, stupor, vertigo; **Interactions:** Antacids/H2 blockers/PPIs (↓ effectiveness of antacids/H2 blockers/PPIs), CNS depressants (additive sedation), hormonal agents (altered effects); **Dose:** Dried powdered root: 5–10 grains. Saturated tincture: 5–15 drops in water. Fluid extract: ½–1 drachm. Root: 0.3–0.6 g PO tid; **Monitor:** N/A; **Notes:** True unicorn root is unsustainable owing to habitat destruction. It is thought that, in large doses, the fresh root may act as a narcotic, emetic, and cathartic. These properties may be lost when the root is dried. Dried root is commonly used for flatulence, colic, hysteria, and to tone up the stomach. It may also have a tonic influence on female organs. Use cautiously in patients with hormone-sensitive conditions.

T

trumpet tree **Uses:** Diabetes; **Preg:** Avoid use; **CIs:** Allergy/hypersensitivity; **ADRs:** ↓ blood pressure,

↑ heart rate, ↑ salivation; | **Interactions:** Antidiabetic agents (↑ risk of hypoglycemia), antihypertensives (↑ risk of hypotension), antilipemic agents (additive effects), diuretics (additive effects); | **Dose:** 13.5 mg dried and milted leaves, boiled for 5 minutes in 1 L of water to create an aqueous leaf extract containing 2.91 mg of chlorogenic acid and 2.4 mg of isoorientin PO qd; | **Monitor:** Blood glucose, blood pressure, electrolytes, heart rate, lipid profile; | **Notes:** Traditionally, trumpet tree has been used by the Palikur indigenous tribes in Guyana and the Amazon basin, as well as by traditional healers in Cuba and other parts of Central and South America for various ailments, including arteriosclerosis, asthma, bone fractures, bruises, diarrhea, fever, genitalia disinfection, gonorrhea, herpes, kidney disorders, liver disorders, mouth and tongue sore, obesity, Parkinson's disease, rheumatic inflammation, skin diseases, warts, and wounds. Trumpet tree is generally avoided in pregnancy due to its anecdotal ability to promote menstruation and childbirth.

turmeric, curcumin *(Curcuma longa)* | **Uses:** CA, cholagogue, cognitive function, dyspepsia, hepatoprotection, HIV/AIDS, hyperlipidemia, inflammation, IBS, oral leukoplakia, osteoarthritis, PUD, RA, scabies, thrombosis prevention, uveitis, viral infection; | **Preg:** Generally considered to be safe when used as a spice in foods; not recommended in high doses due to emmenagogue or uterine stimulant effects; | **CIs:** Allergy/hypersensitivity, Bile duct obstruction, Gallstones; | **ADRs:** alopecia, contact dermatitis, epigastric burning, gastrointestinal disturbances, giddiness, hepatotoxicity (high doses), hypotension, nausea, pruritus; | **Interactions:** Anticoagulants/antiplatelets (↑ risk of bleeding), antidiabetic agents (↑ risk of hypoglycemia), antihypertensives (↑ risk of hypotension), hepatotoxic agents (↑ risk of liver damage); | **Dose:** Root: 1.5–7 g in divided doses. Tea: 1–1.5 g of dried root steeped in 150 mL of water for 15 minutes, bid; | **Monitor:** Coagulation panel, LFTs; | **Notes:** Used to flavor and color foods. The active constituent of turmeric is curcumin.

T

tylophora *(Tylophora indica)* | **Uses:** Asthma; | **Preg:** Not recommended due to insufficient evidence and traditional use as an abortifacient; | **CIs:** Allergy/hypersensitivity, Immunocompromised patients; | **ADRs:** abdominal pain, diarrhea, dysgeusia, mouth soreness, nausea/vomiting, ↑ salivation; | **Interactions:** CNS depressants (additive sedation), immunosupressants (additive effects); | **Dose:** 250 mg 1–3 times daily, standardized to 0.1% of tylophorine per dose;

30–60 mg twice daily standardized to 0.15% of tylophorine; **Monitor:** N/A; **Notes:** May have laxative and purgative properties.

tyrosine **Uses:** ADD/ADHD, Alzheimer's disease, cocaine addiction, depression, energy, HTN, hypothyroidism, narcolepsy, PKU, Rett's syndrome, schizophrenia, sleep deprivation, stress, substance abuse, wrinkles; **Preg:** Not recommended due to insufficient evidence; **CIs:** Allergy/hypersensitivity, Grave's disease, Hyperthyroidism; **ADRs:** arthralgia, dyspepsia, fatigue, headache, nausea, ↑ thyroid hormone levels; **Interactions:** Levodopa (↓ effectiveness of levodopa), MAOIs (↑ risk of hypertensive crisis), thyroid hormones (additive effects); **Dose:** 1,000–5,000 mg PO qd, 30 minutes before meals; **Monitor:** Thyroid panel; **Notes:** Tyrosine is a nonessential amino acid vital to the structure of proteins. It can be synthesized from phenylalanine in the body.

umckaloabo ***(Pelargonium sidoides)*** **Uses:** Bronchitis, common cold, pharyngitis, sinusitis; **Preg:** Not recommended due to insufficient evidence; **CIs:** Allergy/hypersensitivity; **ADRs:** conjunctivitis, gastrointestinal irritation, rash; **Interactions:** Antibiotics (altered effects), anticoagulants/antiplatelets (↑ risk of bleeding), immunosuppressants (altered effects); **Dose:** 30 drops of EPs 7630 solution (4.5 mL per day) (Umckaloabo, EPs 7630, Schwabe GmBh, Germany), PO tid × 7 days; **Monitor:** Coagulation panel; **Notes:** Umckaloabo has been used in traditional South African folk medicine for the treatment of respiratory diseases.

usnea **Uses:** Human papillomavirus, oral hygiene; **Preg:** Not recommended due to insufficient evidence; **CIs:** Allergy/hypersensitivity; **ADRs:** usnea is not well tolerated in humans except as a topical preparation or homeopathic agent; contact dermatitis (topical), hepatotoxic (oral); **Interactions:** Anticoagulants/antiplatelets (↑ risk of bleeding), CYP450 3A (induces CYP3A); **Dose:** No safe internal dosage of usnea has been clinically established. Dosages are based on historical evidence or expert opinion, except for oral lozenge, which is approved by the German Commission E for use in humans. All dosages are based on short-term use only. One lozenge (equivalent of 100 mg powdered usnea lichen) 3–6 times daily for oral irritation has been used; **Monitor:** Coagulation panel, LFTs; **Notes:** Usnic acid, a metabolite of usnea, is found in dietary supplements, including Lipokinetix, marketed as a weight loss agent. It was been reported that ingestion of Lipokinetix was

U

responsible for causing hepatotoxicity and acute liver failure in several individuals.

uva ursi *(Arctostaphylos uva-ursi)* | **Uses:** Hyperpigmentation, urinary tract infection; | **Preg:** Avoid use; oxytocic effects; | **CIs:** Allergy/hypersensitivity, Kidney disease, Pregnancy; | **ADRs:** arrhythmias, bull's eye maculopathy, convulsions, cyanosis, dyspnea, gastrointestinal disturbances, greenish-brown urine color, hepatotoxicity, insomnia, nausea/vomiting, retinal thinning, seizures, tachycardia, tinnitus; | **Interactions:** Anti-inflammatory agents (additive effects), diuretics (additive effects); | **Dose:** 1 cup of infusion (3 g of uva ursi steeped in 150 mL of cold water for 12–24 hours, then strained) taken 3 or 4 times daily has been used. Urinary tract infection: 250–500 mg powdered extract (20% arbutin, uva ursi glycoside) PO tid × 4 days. Hyperpigmentation: 3% arbutin topically daily × 12 weeks; | **Monitor:** Uva ursi can interfere with colorimetric urine tests and can turn urine greenish-brown; | **Notes:** Arbutin, the main chemical constituent of uva ursi, is a phenolic glycoside that becomes hydrolyzed to hydroquinone.

valerian *(Valeriana officinalis)* | **Uses:** Anxiety, depression, insomnia, menopausal symptoms, panic disorder; | **Preg:** Not recommended due to concerns over the teratogenic effects of valeprotriates; | **CIs:** Allergy/hypersensitivity, Pregnancy, Surgery; | **ADRs:** ataxia, cardiovascular disturbances, delayed reaction time, excitability, headache, hepatotoxicity, hypotension, hypothermia, insomnia, tachycardia, uneasiness; | **Interactions:** ALCOHOL (↑ sedative effects); antidepressants (↑ sedative effects); antihypertensive agents (↑ risk of hypotension); BENZODIAZEPINES (↑ sedative effects); caffeine (antagonizes effects); CNS depressants (↑ sedative effects); CYP450 3A4 substrates (valerian inhibits CYP3A4); hepatotoxic agents (↑ risk of liver damage); tamoxifen (↑ risk of breast CA); | **Dose:** Anxiety: 80–300 mg PO qd. Insomnia: 400–900 mg 30–60 minutes before bedtime; | **Monitor:** LFTs, sedation; | **Notes:** Valerian is generally well tolerated for up to 4–6 weeks.

U

vanilla | **Uses:** Insufficient evidence; | **Preg:** Insufficient evidence; | **CIs:** Allergy/hypersensitivity; | **ADRs:** atopic dermatitis, tooth decay, vertebral osteomyelitis; | **Interactions:** Anticoagulants (vanilla products have been reported to be adulterated with coumarin); | **Dose:** Insufficient evidence; | **Monitor:** Insufficient evidence; | **Notes:** Vanilla has been shown to exacerbate several medical conditions, such as eczematous reactions and Quincke's edema in children with atopic dermatitis, gastrointestinal symptoms, and allergy.

verbena *(Verbena officinalis)* | **Uses:** Insufficient evidence; | **Preg:** Not recommended due to insufficient evidence and possible contraceptive effects; | **CIs:** Allergy/hypersensitivity; | **ADRs:** insufficient evidence; | **Interactions:** Anticoagulants (verbena contains vitamin K), estrogens (additive effects), iron (inhibits absorption), progestins (additive effects); | **Dose:** Insufficient evidence; | **Monitor:** Coagulation panel, estrogen levels, progesterone levels; | **Notes:** Verbena may have estrogen and progestin activity. When combined with gentian root, elderflower, cowslip flower, and sorrel (SinuComp, Sinupret), verbena may be useful for treating acute or chronic sinusitis.

vetiver *(Chrysopogon* spp.*)* | **Uses:** Insufficient evidence; | **Preg:** Avoid use due to potential abortifacient and uterine stimulating effects; | **CIs:** Allergy/hypersensitivity, Pregnancy; | **ADRs:** insufficient evidence; | **Interactions:** Insufficient evidence; | **Dose:** Insufficient evidence; | **Monitor:** Insufficient evidence; | **Notes:** Vetiver is closely related to fragrant grasses such as lemongrass. It is commonly used in high-end perfumes.

vitamin A | **Uses:** Acne, acute promyelocytic leukemia, AIDS, breast CA, CA prevention, cataracts, cervical dysplasia, chemotherapy adverse effects, Crohn's disease, diarrhea, esophageal CA, fibrocystic breast disease, gastric CA, goiter, hemorrhoids, immune function, infant mortality, iron-deficiency anemia, lung CA, malaria, measles, menorrhagia, norovirus, nyctalopia (night blindness), pancreatic CA, photorefractive keratectomy, pneumonia, polyp prevention, pregnancy-related complications, PMS, psoriasis, respiratory infection, retinitis pigmentosa, rosacea, skin aging, sore throat, ulcerative colitis, UTI, weight loss, wound healing, xerophthalmia, vitamin A deficiency ; | **Preg:** Likely safe when used appropriately; avoid use above RDA due to risk of birth defects. Excessive doses of vitamin A have been associated with CNS malformations. RDA: pregnancy 14–18 years, 750 mcg/day (2,500 units); 19 years and older, 770 mcg/day (2,600 units). Tolerable Upper Intake Levels (UL): pregnancy and lactation, 2,800 mcg/day (9,000 units); | **CIs:** Allergy/hypersensitivity, Alcoholism, Liver disease; | **ADRs:** toxicity symptoms: alopecia, amenorrhea, anorexia, arthralgia, blurred vision, bone pain, epistaxis, fatigue, headache, hepatomegaly, hydrocephalus (transient), nausea, rash, splenomegaly, weakness, vomiting, weight loss, xeroderma; symptoms of deficiency: defective tooth and bone formation, immunosuppression, nyctalopia, reduced synthesis of steroid hormones; | **Interactions:** Anticoagulants (high doses, ↑ risk of bleeding), hepatotoxic agents (↑ risk of hepatotoxicity), measles vaccine (↓ effectiveness), RETINOIDS (↑ risk of toxic effects), tetracyclines (↑ risk of benign intracranial hypertension), vitamin E (interferes with absorption of vitamin A), vitamin D (vitamin A antagonizes action of vitamin D); drugs that decrease the absorption of vitamin A include antacids, bile acid sequestrants (cholestyramine and colestipol), estrogens, mineral oil, neomycin, orlistat; | **Dose:** Recommended Dietary Allowance (RDA): men 14 years and older, 900 mcg/day (3,000 units); women 14 years and older, 700 mcg/day (2,300 units); 9–13 years, 600 mcg/day (2,000 units); 4–8 years, 400 mcg/day (1,300 units); children 1–3 years, 300 mcg/day (1,000 units). Tolerable Upper Intake Levels (UL): adults age 19 and older (including pregnancy and lactation), 3,000 mcg/day (10,000 units); children 14–18 years (including pregnancy and lactation) 2,800 mcg/day (9,000 units); children 9–13 years, 1,700 mcg/day (6,000 units); children 4–8 years, 900 mcg/day (3,000 units); infants and children from birth to 3 years, 600 mcg/day (2,000 units); | **Monitor:** Vitamin A levels; | **Notes:** Vitamin A supplementation has been shown in one study to increase the risk of HIV transmission between mother and newborn. Caution is warranted.

vitamin B_6 | **Uses:** Adverse effects of cycloserine (prevention), akathisia, Alzheimer's disease, angioplasty, arthritis, asthma, ADHD, autism, birth outcomes, cardiovascular disease, carpal tunnel syndrome, CHD risk reduction, coronary restenosis, depression, diabetic peripheral neuropathy, epilepsy, headache, hereditary sideroblastic anemia, homocysteine reduction, hyperkinetic syndrome, immune function, insomnia, kidney stones, lactation suppression, lung CA, monosodium glutamate (MSG) sensitivity, nausea/vomiting, PUD, PMS, pyridoxine deficiency, pyridoxine-dependent seizures in newborns, renal calculi, tardive dyskinesia, vincristine-induced neuropathy; | **Preg:** Likely safe when used in appropriate amounts; | **CIs:** Allergy/hypersensitivity; | **ADRs:** toxicity symptoms: prolonged, excess use can cause neuropathy; symptoms of deficiency: anemia, depression, immunosuppression, irritability, nausea, premenstrual tension (females), renal calculi, smooth tongue, vomiting; | **Interactions:** Drugs that can cause depletion of vitamin B_6: antibiotics, cycloserine, estrogen-containing

V

medications (oral contraceptives and estrogen replacement therapy), hydralazine, isoniazid, loop diuretics, penicillamine, theophylline; amiodarone (pyridoxine exacerbates amiodarone-induced photosensitivity), levodopa (pyridoxine enhances the metabolism of levodopa), phenobarbital/phenytoin (pyridoxine ↓ levels of phenobarbital and phenytoin); **Dose:** Oral: RDAs of vitamin B_6: men older than 50 years, 1.7 mg/day; women older than 50 years, 1.5 mg/day; men 14–50 years, 1.3 mg/day; women 19–50 years, 1.3 mg/day; women 14–18 years, 1.2 mg/day; children 9–13 years, 1 mg/day; children 4–8 years, 0.6 mg/day; children 1–3 years, 0.5 mg/day; infants 7–12 months, 0.3 mg/day; infants 0–6 months, 0.1 mg/day; pregnant women, 1.9 mg/day; lactating women, 2 mg/day. Toxic dose: 250–1,000 mg/day; **Monitor:** Vitamin B_6 levels; **Notes:** Vitamin B_6 is present in many foods, including cereal grains, legumes, vegetables, liver, meat, and eggs. Pyridoxine can yield a false-positive result in the spot test with Ehrlich's reagent.

vitamin B_{12}

Uses: AIDS, Alzheimer's disease, angioplasty, asthma, atherosclerosis, atopic dermatitis, breast CA, CHD, circadian rhythm sleep disorders, cognitive function, coronary restenosis, Crohn's disease, depression, diabetic peripheral neuropathy, fatigue, homocysteine reduction, hyperhomocysteinemia, hypertriglyceridemia, Imerslund-Grasbeck disease, male infertility, megaloblastic anemia, memory loss, multiple sclerosis, orthostatic tremor (shaky leg syndrome), pernicious anemia, radiation-induced mucosal injury, shaky leg syndrome, sickle cell disease, stroke, sulfite sensitivity; **Preg:** Safe when used appropriately; RDA: 2.6 mcg/day; **CIs:** Allergy/hypersensitivity, Cobalamin or cobalt hypersensitivity, Leber's disease; **ADRs:** symptoms of deficiency: fatigue, hypersensitivity, insomnia, irritability, loss of coordination, megaloblastic anemia; **Interactions:** CHLORAMPHENICOL (delay or interrupt the reticulocyte response to supplemental vitamin B_{12}); drugs that can cause depletion of vitamin B_{12}: aminosalicylic acid, antibiotics, biguanides (e.g., metformin), bile acid sequestrants, cobalt irradiation, colchicine, ethanol, H2 blockers, nicotine, nitrous oxide, oral contraceptives, phenytoin, proton pump inhibitors, potassium chloride (time-release), zidovudine; **Dose:** RDAs: Children 14 years and older and adults, 2.4 mcg/day; children 9–13 years, 1.8 mcg/day; children 4–8 years, 1.2 mcg/day; children 1–3 years, 0.9 mcg/day; infants 7–12 months, 0.5 mcg/day; infants 0–6 months, 0.4 mcg/day; pregnant women, 2.6 mcg/day; lactating women, 2.8 mcg/day; **Monitor:** Vitamin B_{12} levels; **Notes:** Frequently combined with other B vitamins.

vitamin C | **Uses:** AIDS, albuminuria, alkaptonuria, allergies, Alzheimer's disease, asthma, atherosclerosis, athletic performance, CA prevention/treatment, cardiovascular disease, cataracts, cervical dysplasia, chromosome damage, circulation, common cold, complex regional pain syndrome, constipation, CHD, Crohn's disease, diabetes, erythema, exercise recovery, gallbladder disease, gastroprotection, gingivitis, glaucoma, gout, *Helicobacter pylori* infection, HIV transmission, hypertension, immune support, infertility, iron absorption, ischemic heart disease, lead toxicity, leukemia, LDL oxidation, macular degeneration, metabolic abnormalities, multiple sclerosis, MI risk reduction, nitrate tolerance, nonalcoholic steatohepatitis, osteoarthritis, pain, Parkinson's disease, PUD, pregnancy, radiation proctitis, reflex sympathetic dystrophy, sickle cell disease, skin damage, stress, stroke prevention, sunburn, tyrosinemia, UTI, vaginitis, vitamin C deficiency, wound healing, wrinkled skin; | **Preg:** Safe when used appropriately; Tolerable Upper Intake Level (UL): 2,000 mg per day; | **CIs:** Allergy/hypersensitivity; | **ADRs:** toxicity symptoms: most common side effects of large doses are abdominal cramps, diarrhea, nausea, and skin rashes; excess intake in diabetics may give falsely elevated blood glucose readings; symptoms of deficiency: allergies, anemia, arthralgia, atherosclerosis, bleeding gums, bone fragility, immunosuppression, slow wound healing; | **Interactions:** Drugs that can cause depletion of vitamin C: aspirin and other salicylates, barbiturates, diuretics, estrogens, indomethacin, oral contraceptives, nicotine, proton pump inhibitors, tetracyclines; acetaminophen (vitamin C ↑ adverse effects associated with acetaminophen), aluminum-containing antacids (↑ aluminum levels), antineoplastic agents (↓ efficacy of some antineoplastic agents such as doxorubicin), calcium channel blockers, dihydropyridine (inhibit uptake of vitamin C), copper (↓ copper levels), estrogens (vitamin C ↑ estrogen levels), fluphenazine (↓ fluphenazine levels), HMG-CoA reductase inhibitors (reduces the rise in HDL), protease inhibitors (vitamin C ↓ levels of these drugs), iron (↑ iron levels), niacin (reduces the rise in HDL), warfarin (high doses, lowers prothrombin time); | **Dose:** Oral: RDI: men: 90 mg/day; women: 75 mg/day; ODA: 250–1,000 mg/day; should not exceed 2,000 mg/day in men or women; | **Monitor:** Vitamin C levels; | **Notes:** The use of vitamin C in the prevention/treatment of the common cold and respiratory infections remains controversial.

V

vitamin D | **Uses:** Cardiovascular disease, CA, CHF, colorectal cancer, corticosteroid-induced osteoporosis, Crohn's disease, diabetes, epilepsy, fall prevention, familial hypophosphatemia, Fanconi's syndrome, hearing loss, hepatic osteodystrophy, hyperparathyroidism, hypocalcemia, immune response, mortality, multiple sclerosis, muscle weakness, myelodysplastic syndrome, nutritional status, osteogenesis imperfecta, osteoporosis, periodontal disease, physical performance, pigmented lesions, prostate CA, proximal myopathy, psoriasis, renal osteodystrophy, RA, rickets, scleroderma, SAD, senile warts, tooth retention, warts, weight loss; **Preg:** Safe when used appropriately; Tolerable Upper Intake Level (UL): 50 mcg (2,000 units) per day; **CIs:** Allergy/hypersensitivity; **ADRs:** toxicity symptoms: anorexia, arterial calcium deposits, constipation, dehydration, headache, hypercalcemia, nausea, polydipsia, renal calculi, vomiting, weakness, weight loss; symptoms of deficiency: bone and tooth disorders, osteomalacia, rickets; **Interactions:** Drugs that can cause depletion of vitamin D: anticonvulsants, bile acid sequestrants, corticosteroids, H_2-receptor antagonists, isoniazid, laxatives, mineral oil, rifampin; aluminum (↑ aluminum absorption), calcipotriene (↑ risk of hypercalcemia), calcium and phosphorus (↑ absorption of calcium and phosphorus), calcium channel blockers, nondihydropyridine (hypercalcemia caused by vitamin D can ↓ effectiveness of calcium channel blockers), cimetidine (inhibits enzyme involved in conversion of vitamin D to active form), CYP450 3A4 substrates (induces CYP450 3A4/↓ levels of CYP 3A4 substrates), digoxin (↑ risk of hypercalcemia), magnesium-containing antacids (↑ the risk of hypermagnesemia), thiazide diuretics (↓ vitamin D levels), vitamin A (antagonizes the effects of vitamin D); **Dose:** Oral: RDI: 400 IU/day; ODA: 400 IU/day; should not exceed UL of 50 mcg (2,000 IU)/day; children younger than 1 year should not exceed the UL of 25 mcg (1,000 IU)/day; **Monitor:** Vitamin D levels; **Notes:** Vitamin D may increase calcium levels; use with caution in patients with hypercalcemia, hyperparathyroidism, lymphoma, renal disease, sarcoidosis, and tuberculosis. Overuse of sunscreens may contribute to vitamin D deficiency.

vitamin E **Uses:** Acne, allergic rhinitis, altitude sickness, Alzheimer's disease, anemia, angina, arterial elasticity, asthma, ataxia associated with vitamin E deficiency, atherosclerosis, beta-thalassemia, BPH, bladder CA, breast CA, CA treatment/prevention, cardiovascular disease, cataracts, cervical dysplasia, chromosome damage, colon CA prevention, CHF, diabetes, dyslipidemias, dysmenorrhea, eczema, endometriosis, epilepsy, esophageal CA, fibrocystic breast disease, G6PD deficiency, gallbladder, gastric CA, glomerulosclerosis, hemorrhoids, hepatitis C, hyperlipidemia, immune support, infertility, intermittent claudication, LDL oxidation, macular degeneration, mucositis, multiple

V

sclerosis, neurotoxicity, Parkinson's disease, PUD, peripheral circulation, photorefractive keratectomy, platelet aggregation, PMS, prostate CA prevention, psoriasis, respiratory infection prevention, RA, scleroderma, seizure disorder, steatohepatitis, sunburn, SLE, tardive dyskinesia, ulcerative colitis, uveitis, venous thromboembolism; vitamin E deficiency; | **Preg:** Safe when used in amounts that do not exceed the RDA; | **CIs:** Allergy/hypersensitivity, Active bleeding; | **ADRs:** abdominal pain, blurred vision, diarrhea, fatigue, gonadal dysfunction, headache, intestinal cramps, ↑ RISK OF MORTALITY (HIGH DOSES, with history of severe cardiovascular disease such as stroke or myocardial infarction), symptoms of deficiency: cataracts, dry hair, eczema, hot flashes, impaired wound healing, psoriasis, xeroderma; | **Interactions:** Drugs that interfere with the absorption of vitamin E include anticonvulsants, bile acid sequestrants, carbamazepine, isoniazid, mineral oil, olestra, orlistat, phenobarbital, phenytoin, sucralfate; amprenavir (may ↑ vitamin E levels), anticoagulants/antiplatelets (↑ risk of bleeding), chemotherapy (interfere with effectiveness), cyclosporine (↑ absorption of cyclosporine), gemfibrozil (↓ vitamin E levels), iron (impairs absorption of vitamin E), HMG-CoA reductase inhibitors (reduce the rise in HDL), niacin (reduce the rise in HDL), vitamin C (possible ↑ risk of adverse effects); | **Dose:** RDI: Adults: 22.5 IU/day; lactating women: 28.5 IU/day; ODA: 400 IU/day; maximum dose: 1,500 IU/day; Adequate Intake (AI): healthy breastfeeding infants 0–6 months, 4 mg/day (6 IU); infants 7–12 months, 5 mg/day (7.5 IU); RDA: children 1–3 years, 6 mg/day (9 IU); children 4–8 years, 7 mg/day (10.5 IU); children 9–13 years, 11 mg/day (16.5 IU); children 14 years and older, 15 mg/day (22.5 IU); | **Monitor:** Coagulation panel (with high doses), vitamin E levels; | **Notes:** Discontinue use before dental or surgical procedures (generally at least 14 days before).

vitamin K | **Uses:** Bleeding disorders, coronary artery disease, hemorrhagic disease, hypercholesterolemia, hypoprothrombinemia, osteoporosis prevention, vitamin K deficiency, warfarin anticoagulation; | **Preg:** Category: C, safe when used in recommended amounts; | **CIs:** Allergy/hypersensitivity; | **ADRs:** dizziness, dysgeusia, pain and swelling at injection site; | **Interactions:** Antacids (↓ vitamin K efficacy), antibiotics (↑ risk of vitamin K deficiency), ANTICOAGULANTS (antagonizes the effects of anticoagulants such as warfarin), anticonvulsants (↑ risk of vitamin K deficiency), bile acid sequestrants (↓ absorption of vitamin K), coenzyme Q10 (additive effects, ↑ risk of clotting), dactinomycin (↓ vitamin K efficacy), hemolytics (↑ risk of toxic adverse effects), orlistat (↓ absorption

V

of vitamin K), primaquine (↑ risk of toxic adverse effects), quinidine (↑ risk of vitamin K deficiency), quinine (depress hepatic enzymes that synthesize vitamin K–dependent clotting factors), rifampin (↑ risk of vitamin K deficiency), salicylates (↑ need for vitamin K), sucralfate (↓ vitamin K efficacy), sulfa drugs (↑ risk of vitamin K deficiency), vitamin A (antagonizes vitamin K effects), vitamin E (antagonizes vitamin K effects); | **Dose:** Adequate intake (AI) recommendations: men older than 19 years, 120 mcg/day; women older than 19 years (including those pregnant and lactating), 90 mcg/day; adolescents 14–18 years (including those pregnant or lactating), 75 mcg/day; children 9–13 years, 60 mcg/day; children 4–8 years, 55 mcg/day; children 1–3 years, 30 mcg/day; infants 6–12 months, 2.5 mcg/day; infants 0–6 months, 2 mcg/day; | **Monitor:** Coagulation panel, vitamin K levels; | **Notes:** Vitamin K_1 (phytonadione) is obtained from dietary sources, such as leafy green vegetables. Vitamin K_2 is a group of menaquinones obtained from meat, cheese, and eggs.

vitamin O *(oxygen)* | **Uses:** Insufficient evidence; | **Preg:** Insufficient evidence; | **CIs:** Allergy/hypersensitivity; | **ADRs:** headache; | **Interactions:** Sodium chloride (additive effects); | **Dose:** Insufficient evidence; | **Monitor:** N/A; | **Notes:** Also known as liquid oxygen (saltwater liquid). Use cautiously in patients with hypertension due to sodium chloride content.

wasabi | **Uses:** Insufficient evidence; | **Preg:** Insufficient evidence; | **CIs:** Allergy/hypersensitivity; | **ADRs:** painful cold sensations; | **Interactions:** Analgesics (interfere with effects); anticoagulants/antiplatelets (↑ risk of bleeding), NSAIDs (interfere with effects); | **Dose:** Insufficient evidence; | **Monitor:** N/A; | **Notes:** Wasabi is frequently associated with fresh fish in Japanese cuisine, because its antibacterial qualities may keep the fish fresh longer.

water hemlock *(Cicuta spp.)* | **Uses:** Not safe for human use; | **Preg:** Avoid use due to toxic effects; | **CIs:** Allergy/hypersensitivity; ORAL USE; | **ADRs:** toxic effects: ACUTE RENAL FAILURE, COMA, CONVULSION, DEATH, METABOLIC ACIDOSIS, ORTHOSTATIC HYPOTENSION, SEIZURES, TACHYCARDIA, VOMITING; | **Interactions:** Diuretics (additive effects); | **Dose:** Avoid use, unsafe when ingested; | **Monitor:** Toxic effects; | **Notes:** According to the United States Department of Agriculture (USDA), "water hemlock is the most violently TOXIC plant that grows in North America." Water hemlock is toxic, and death can occur a soon as 15 minutes after ingestion.

watercress *(Nasturtium officinale* R. Br.*)* | **Uses:** Insufficient evidence; | **Preg:** Not recommended due traditional use as an abortifacient; | **CIs:** Allergy/hypersensitivity, Kidney disease, Ulcers (gastric or duodenal); | **ADRs:** contact dermatitis, dyspnea, gastrointestinal distress, nephrotoxicity; | **Interactions:** Acetaminophen (additive effects), chlorzoxazone (↑ effects of chlorzoxazone), cytochrome P450 2A substrates (altered drug levels), diuretics (additive effects), warfarin (antagonistic effects); | **Dose:** Dried herb: 4–6 g daily; fresh herb: 20–30 g daily; | **Monitor:** INR; | **Notes:** Watercress contains high amounts of vitamin K and may antagonize the effects of warfarin.

wheatgrass *(Triticum aestivum)* | **Uses:** Beta-thalassemia; ulcerative colitis; | **Preg:** Avoid use due to lack of evidence; caution is warranted due to possible bacterial or mold contamination; | **CIs:** Allergy/hypersensitivity; | **ADRs:** allergic reactions, edema; | **Interactions:** Insufficient evidence; | **Dose:** Normal health maintenance: 1–4 oz of juice daily. Beta-thalassemia: 100 mL of juice daily. Ulcerative colitis: 100 mL of juice daily for 1 month as an adjunct to standard therapy. Colon cleansing: 8–32 oz of juice administered via enemas, rubber bulb syringes, or colonics; | **Monitor:** N/A; | **Notes:** Wheatgrass is gluten free.

white horehound *(Marrubium vulgare)* | **Uses:** Antispasmodic, atherosclerosis, cough, diabetes, dyspepsia, pain; | **Preg:** Not recommended due to traditional use as an abortifacient; | **CIs:** Allergy/hypersensitivity; | **ADRs:** ARRHYTHMIAS (large amounts), asthenia, contact dermatitis (topical), diarrhea, edema, hypokalemia, purgative effects; | **Interactions:** Anesthetics (additive effects), antidiabetic agents (↑ risk of hypoglycemia), antihypertensive agents (↑ risk of hypotension), diuretics (additive effects), estrogen (additive effects), penicillin (altered effects), SSRI antidepressants (additive effects), vasodilators (additive effects); | **Dose:** For gastrointestinal disorders, 4.5 g per day of cut white horehound herb, 2–6 tablespoons of fresh white horehound juice. For respiratory disorders, 10–40 drops of extract in water 3 times a day; | **Monitor:** Blood pressure, EKG, electrolytes; | **Notes:** May be found in herbal cough remedies such as Ricola.

white oak *(Quercus alba)* | **Uses:** Insufficient evidence; | **Preg:** Insufficient evidence; avoid use; | **CIs:** Allergy/hypersensitivity, Cardiovascular conditions, Eczema, Hepatic dysfunction, Hypertonia, Infectious disease, Renal dysfunction;

W

ADRs: gastrointestinal complaints, hepatotoxicity, nausea/vomiting, nephrotoxicity; **Interactions:** Hepatotoxic agents (↑ risk of liver damage), iron (may precipitate iron salts due to tannin content), nephrotoxic agents (↑ risk of kidney damage); **Dose:** Oral: tea: 1 cup of tea up to 3 times daily for up to 3–4 days; prepare tea by adding 1 g coarsely powdered bark to 150 mL cold water, boil and strain; do not use for more than 3–4 days. Topical: mix 2 tsp of powder bark in 500 mL of water, strain; do not use for more than 2–3 weeks. Rinse: prepare 20 g of bark in 1 L of boiling water and gargle; **Monitor:** Kidney and liver function; **Notes:** Do not use for extensive periods of time.

white water lily *(Nymphaea odorata)* **Uses:** Insufficient evidence; **Preg:** Insufficient evidence; **CIs:** Allergy/hypersensitivity; **ADRs:** hallucinations; **Interactions:** Antipsychotic agents (↑ risk of adverse effects), CNS depressants (additive sedation); **Dose:** Decoction/infusion: 30–60 mL of an infusion 3–4 times daily, between meals; prepare infusion with 30 g of the powdered root, macerated, and boiled in 300 mL of water for 30 minutes or 1–2 g dried root steeped in 150 mL boiling water for 5–10 minutes and strained. Fluid extract: 1–5 mL of a 1:1 extract in 25% ethanol daily. Powder: 1–2 g daily given in milk or sweetened water. Tincture: 1–10 drops of tincture daily made from 240 g of the root in 76% ethanol; **Monitor:** N/A; **Notes:** May act as a narcotic.

wild arrach *(Chenopodium vulvaria)* **Uses:** Insufficient evidence; **Preg:** Insufficient evidence; **CIs:** Allergy/hypersensitivity; **ADRs:** insufficient evidence; **Interactions:** Insufficient evidence; **Dose:** Insufficient evidence; **Monitor:** N/A; **Notes:** Wild arrach has a rotten fish smell owing to its trimethylamine content.

wild indigo *(Baptisia australis)* **Uses:** Respiratory tract infections; **Preg:** Avoid use orally or topically due to its toxic potential; **CIs:** Allergy/hypersensitivity, Gastrointestinal disorders; Oral or topical use (TOXIC); **ADRs:** diarrhea, gastrointestinal complaints, nausea/vomiting, spasms; **Interactions:** Immunomodulators (altered effects); **Dose:** Avoid; wild indigo is toxic; **Monitor:** N/A; **Notes:** Wild indigo is considered TOXIC and is on the FDA's list of toxic plants.

wild yam *(Dioscorea villosa)* **Uses:** Hyperlipidemia, menopausal symptoms; **Preg:** Insufficient evidence; **CIs:** Allergy/hypersensitivity, Hormone sensitivity conditions, Protein S

W

deficiency; | **ADRs:** contact dermatitis, gastrointestinal upset; | **Interactions:** Antidiabetic agents (↑ risk of hypoglycemia), antilipemic agents (additive effects), hormones (altered effects); | **Dose:** Oral: dried root: 2–4 g or 1–2 tsp daily in 2–3 divided doses; capsule: 250 mg of wild yam taken 1–3 times or 450–900 mg daily of dioscorea extract from wild yam; liquid (1:1 in 45% alcohol): 2–4 mL daily in 3 divided doses; tincture, 4–12 drops or 2–4 mL taken 3–5 times daily. Topical: available in vaginal creams; | **Monitor:** Menopausal symptoms, potassium; | **Notes:** Wild yam possesses DHEA-like properties and acts as a precursor to human sex hormones.

willow bark *(Salix spp.)* | **Uses:** Osteoarthritis, headache, lower back pain; | **Preg:** Not recommended, willow bark contains salicylates; | **CIs:** Allergy/hypersensitivity including salicylates, Dengue fever, Glucose-6-phosphate dehydrogenase deficiency (G6PD), Pregnancy/lactation; | **ADRs:** allergic reactions, gastrointestinal distress, headache, hypertriglyceridemia; | **Interactions:** May displace various drugs, including tolbutamide, chlorpropamide, methotrexate, phenytoin, probenecid, valproic acid; acetazolamide (↑ risk of adverse effects), alcohol (reduced risk of hangover), anticoagulants/antiplatelets (↑ risk of bleeding), aspirin/salicylates (additive effects), diuretics (additive effects), methotrexate (altered effects), spironolactone (altered effects), sulfonylureas (altered effects), valproic acid (↑ risk of adverse effects); | **Dose:** 120–240 mg daily; | **Monitor:** Creatinine, triglycerides; | **Notes:** Willow bark contains salicylates. Discontinue willow bark 2 weeks before surgery because willow bark has antiplatelet effects and ↑ may risk of bleeding. Avoid or use cautiously in individuals with aspirin hypersensitivity, asthma, dengue fever, diabetes, gout, hemophilia, hypoprothrombinemia, kidney or liver disease, peptic ulcers, or glucose-6-phosphate dehydrogenase (G6PD) deficiency.

witch hazel *(Hamamelis virginiana)* | **Uses:** Eczema, hemorrhoids, insect bites, perineal discomfort after childbirth, skin irritation, UV damage, varicose veins; | **Preg:** Not recommended due to lack of sufficient evidence; | **CIs:** Allergy/hypersensitivity; | **ADRs:** ↓ blood glucose, hepatotoxicity, nephrotoxicity, skin irritation (topical); | **Interactions:** Antidiabetic agents (↑ risk of hypoglycemia), hepatotoxic agents (↑ risk of liver damage), nephrotoxic agents (↑ risk of kidney damage); | **Dose:** Oral: infusion: 2–3 g dried plant material in 150 mL boiled water for 10–15 minutes; fluid extract: prepared with 2–4 g dried plant material or 2–4 mL of a 1:1 extract in 45% alcohol; tincture: 0.4–0.8 g dried plant material.

Topical, powder: 2–3 g in 150 mL cold water, brought to boil and simmered 10–15 minutes, or 5–10 g leaves boiled in 250 mL water, apply 6 times daily. Suppositories: 0.1–1 g leaves or bark in combination with cocoa butter, use rectally or vaginally; | **Monitor:** Blood glucose, LFTs, renal function tests; | **Notes:** Leaves contain 8%–10% tannins; bark contains 12% of tannins.

yarrow *(Achillea millefolium)* | **Uses:** Plaque/gingivitis; | **Preg:** Not recommended due to insufficient evidence and traditional use as an abortifacient; | **CIs:** Allergy/hypersensitivity; Cross-allergic reaction with Asteraceae/Compositae family (including ragweed, chrysanthemums, marigolds, and daisies); | **ADRs:** dermatitis (topical), diuresis, photosensitivity, sedation; | **Interactions:** Antacids (↓ effectiveness), anticoagulants/antiplatelets (↑ risk of bleeding), antihypertensives (↑ risk of hypotension), barbiturates (additive sedation), diuretics (additive effects), H2 blockers (↓ effectiveness), photosensitizers (↑ risk of phototoxicity), proton pump inhibitors (↓ effectiveness); | **Dose:** A rinse with 10 mL of mouthwash twice a day for a period of 3 months; | **Monitor:** Coagulation panel, electrolytes; | **Notes:** Discontinue yarrow 2 weeks before any surgical procedures because yarrow may ↑ risk of bleeding.

yellow dock *(Rumex crispus)* | **Uses:** Insufficient evidence; | **Preg:** Avoid use; anthraquinones may be unsafe; | **CIs:** Allergy/hypersensitivity, Intestinal obstruction, Lactation, Pregnancy; | **ADRs:** diarrhea, hepatotoxicity, hypokalemia, nephrotoxicity; | **Interactions:** DIGOXIN (↑ risk of hypokalemia), estrogens (additive effects), hepatotoxic agents (↑ risk of liver damage), laxatives (additive effects), minerals (↓ mineral absorption), nephrotoxic agents (↑ risk of kidney damage), POTASSIUM-DEPLETING DIURETICS (thiazides, loop; ↑ risk of hypokalemia), warfarin (↑ INR, ↑ risk of diarrhea); | **Dose:** Tincture of the fresh roots: 20 drops, 2 or 3 times a day. Fresh root vinegar preparation, tea: 1–2 tablespoons or 30 mL, no more than 1 cup daily; | **Monitor:** LFTs, potassium, renal function tests; | **Notes:** Yellow dock contains anthraquinones, which act as laxatives. A fatal poisoning from yellow dock has been reported. Yellow dock may discolor urine and interfere with colorimetric tests.

yerba mate *(Ilex paraguariensis)* | **Uses:** Obesity/weight loss; | **Preg:** Avoid use; | **CIs:** Allergy/hypersensitivity; | **ADRs:** abdominal bloating, arrhythmias, constipation, eczema (large amounts), flatulence, gastrointestinal upset, headache, hypertension, hypoglycemia, IBS, ↑ intraocular pressure, irritability, nausea, nervousness, renal calculi, sleep disturbances, tachyarrhythmias, tremor; | **Interactions:** Most interactions are based on the caffeine content: alcohol (↑ caffeine concentrations), AMPHETAMINES (additive CNS effects), anticoagulants/antiplatelets (↑ risk of bleeding), antidiabetic agents (altered glucose control), antihypertensives (altered effects), beta agonists (↑ inotropic effects of beta agonists), caffeine (additive effects), cimetidine (↑ effects of caffeine), clozapine (↑ effects of clozapine), CNS depressants (interfere/counteract with effects), CNS STIMULANTS (↑ stimulatory effects), dipyridamole (inhibits dipyridamole-induced vasodilation), disulfiram (↑ effects of caffeine), ergot derivatives (↑ the absorption of ergotamine), estrogens (↑ effects of caffeine), fluconazole (↑ effects of caffeine), grapefruit juice (↑ effects of caffeine), inotropes (↑ inotropic effects), iron (inhibit iron absorption), lithium (↑ risk of lithium toxicity), mexiletine (↑ effects of caffeine), MAOIs (↑ risk of hypertensive crisis), nicotine (additive CNS effects), phenylpropanolamine (↑ blood pressure), quinolones (↑ effects of caffeine), terbinafine (↑ caffeine concentrations), theophylline (↑ risk of theophylline toxicity), verapamil (↑ effects of caffeine); | **Dose:** Liquid extract (1:1 extract in 25% alcohol): 2–4 mL PO tid. Tea: 2–4 g dried leaf in 1 cup of water (150 mL), steeped for 5–10 minutes and then strained, PO tid; | **Monitor:** Blood pressure, calcium levels, heart rate; | **Notes:** Yerba mate is a beverage used as a stimulant and diuretic. Caution is warranted in patients with anxiety disorders, cardiovascular conditions, diabetes, glaucoma, HTN, osteoporosis. Consuming alcohol and smoking with yerba mate greatly increases the risk of cancer.

yerba santa *(Eriodictyon californicum)* | **Uses:** Respiratory disorders; | **Preg:** Not recommended due to lack of safety data and presence of ethanol; | **CIs:** Allergy/hypersensitivity, Ophthalmic use; | **ADRs:** insufficient evidence; | **Interactions:** CYP450 substrates (may inhibit/altered drug levels); diuretics (additive effects); | **Dose:** Oral: 2–4 g of dried herb or as a tea; liquid extract: 2–4 mL PO tid; | **Monitor:** Insufficient evidence; | **Notes:** Insufficient evidence.

yew *(Taxus baccata, Taxus brevifolia)* | **Uses:** Insufficient evidence; | **Preg:** Avoid use; | **CIs:** Allergy/hypersensitivity; AVOID INGESTION/POISONOUS; | **ADRs:** Toxic symptoms: abdominal pain, arrhythmia, bradycardia, coma, DEATH, dyspnea, hypotension, involuntary shaking/tremor, mydriasis, myocardial infarction, nervousness, pale/cyanotic skin, red lips, xerostomia; | **Interactions:** Antineoplastic agents (additive effects); | **Dose:** Insufficient evidence; | **Monitor:** For toxic symptoms; **Notes:** All parts of the yew plant are poisonous. Pacific yew bark contains 0.01% paclitaxel.

yi zhu **Uses:** Hepatitis; **Preg:** Insufficient evidence; **CIs:** Allergy/hypersensitivity; **ADRs:** insufficient evidence; **Interactions:** Insufficient evidence; **Dose:** Insufficient evidence; **Monitor:** Insufficient evidence; **Notes:** The herbal decoction, yi zhu, is a compound of 10 herbs: *Artemisia capillaris*, black ants, *Bupleuri chinensis*, *Glycyrrhiza uralensis*, *Ligustrum lucidum*, *Paeonia lactiflora*, Phyllanthus species, *Polygonum cuspidatum*, *Salviae miltiorrhizae*, *Scutellariae baicalensis*.

yohimbe *(Pausinystalia yohimbe)* **Uses:** Athletic performance, depression, erectile dysfunction, libido (women), orgasm improvement (men), orthostatic hypotension, sexual dysfunction due to antidepressant drugs, xerostomia; **Preg:** Avoid use due to possible uterine relaxant effects and fetal toxic effects; **CIs:** Allergy/hypersensitivity, Angina, Anxiety, BPH, Cardiovascular disease, Concurrent use with MAOIs or phenothiazines, Depression, Diabetes, Hyper-/hypotension, Liver disease, Kidney disease, Post-traumatic stress disorder (PTSD), Pregnancy; **ADRs:** agranulocytosis, anxiety, headache, HYPERTENSION (low doses), HYPOTENSION (high doses), insomnia, impulsivity, irritability, lupus-like syndrome, nausea/vomiting, polyuria, psychosis, renal failure, salivation, tachycardia, tremor; **Interactions:** Antihypertensives (interfere with blood pressure control), clonidine (antagonistic effects), guanabenz (antagonistic effects), MAOIs (additive effects; ↑ risk of hypertensive crisis), phenothiazines (↑ risk of toxic effects), stimulants (↑ risk of hypertensive crisis), tricyclic antidepressants (↑ risk of adverse effects); **Dose:** For erectile dysfunction, 5–50 mg in divided doses; **Monitor:** Blood pressure, heart rate; **Notes:** Avoid tyramine-containing foods, due to the risk of hypertensive crisis.

yucca *(Yucca schidigera)* **Uses:** Hypercholesterolemia; **Preg:** Not recommended due to insufficient evidence; **CIs:** Allergy/hypersensitivity; **ADRs:** allergic rhinitis, urticaria; **Interactions:** Antifungal agents (additive effects), anti-inflammatory agents (additive effects), antilipemic agents (additive effects), antineoplastic agents (additive effects), antiviral agents (additive effects); **Dose:** Traditionally 380–490 mg of powdered yucca stalk or root 2–3 times daily; decoction by boiling ¼ oz of root in 16 oz of water for 15 min, 3–5 cups daily; **Monitor:** Insufficient clinical evidence; **Notes:** Insufficient clinical evidence.

Z **Zemaphyte** | **Uses:** Immunomodulator, inflammation, skin damage; | **Preg:** Insufficient clinical evidence; | **CIs:** Allergy/hypersensitivity; | **ADRs:** diarrhea, ↑ LFTs, urticaria; | **Interactions:** Methotrexate (↓ adverse effects), vincristine (↓ adverse effects); | **Dose:** One or two packets mixed in hot water and drunk once a day; | **Monitor:** LFTs; | **Notes:** Zemaphyte is a Chinese herbal remedy produced in the UK that contains siler (fangfeng; *Ledebouriella seseloides*), potentilla (baitougweng; *Potentilla chinensis*), akebia (mutong; *Clematis armandii*), rehmannia (dihuang; *Rehmannia glutinosa*), red peony (chishao; *Paeonia lactiflora*), lophatherum (danzhuye; *Lophatherum gracile*), dictamnus (baixianpi; *Dictamnus dasycarpus*), *Tribulus terrestris* (baijili), licorice (gancao; *Glycyrrhiza glabra*), schizonepeta (jingjie; *Schizonepeta tennuifolia*).

zinc | **Uses:** Acne vulgaris, ADHD, alopecia, anorexia, athletic performance, beta-thalassemia, blood disorders, boils, burns, cirrhosis, cognitive impairment (children), common cold, Crohn's disease, dandruff, diabetes (types 1 and 2), diabetic neuropathy, diaper rash, diarrhea (children), Down syndrome, eczema, fungal infections (scalp), gastric ulcers, Gilbert's syndrome, growth/development (infants), halitosis, head injury, hepatic encephalopathy, hepatitis C, herpes simplex virus, HIV/AIDS, hyperlipidemia, hypothyroidism, immunostimulant, kwashiorkor, leg ulcers, leprosy, lower respiratory tract infections, macular degeneration, malaria, menstrual cramps, parasites, plaque/gingivitis, poisoning (arsenic), pregnancy, prostatitis (chronic), psoriasis, radiation-induced mucositis, renal impairment, respiratory papillomatosis, rheumatoid arthritis, sickle cell anemia, skin damage, stomatitis, taste alterations, tinnitus, trichomoniasis, viral warts, Wilson's disease, wound healing, zinc deficiency; | **Preg:** Likely safe when used orally and appropriately; do not exceed the Tolerable Upper Intake Level (UL) of 34 mg/day for pregnant women 14–18 years, and 40 mg/day for pregnant women age 19–50; | **CIs:** Allergy/hypersensitivity; | **ADRs:** abdominal cramping, acute tubular necrosis, benign prostatic hyperplasia/urinary retention, bleeding, dermatitis, diarrhea, dysgeusia, gastric erosion, hepatitis, hypersensitivity pneumonitis, interstitial nephritis, intestinal bleeding, leukopenia, ↓ levels of HDL cholesterol, liver failure, loss of smell (zinc gluconate [Zicam]), metallic taste, microcytic anemia, nausea/vomiting, neutropenia, reduced immune responses, respiratory infections, ↑ risk of BPH and prostate disease, sideroblastic anemia, skin conditions, slight tingling or burning sensation in the nostril, urinary complications, urinary lithiasis, urinary tract infection, worsening of an acne condition;

Interactions: Drugs that can cause depletion of zinc: caffeine, calcium, captopril, cholestyramine, copper, corticosteroids, deferoxamine, diuretics (loop, thiazide), EDTA, estrogens, ethambutol, D-penicillamine, H_2-receptor antagonists, iron, oral contraceptives, penicillamine, phenytoin, propofol, proton pump inhibitors, valproic acid, zidovudine (AZT); zinc can cause ↓ effectiveness of the following drugs: fluoroquinolone antibiotics, tetracycline antibiotics; amiloride (↓ urinary zinc excretion), cisplatin (interfere with cisplatin therapy); **Dose:** RDA, adults: 11 mg/day for men 19+ years old; 8 mg/day for women 19+ years old; 11 mg/day for pregnant women 19+ years old; 12 mg/day for lactating women 19+ years old. RDA, children: 3 mg/day for infants and children 7 months to 3 years old; 5 mg/day for children 4–8 years old; 8 mg/day for children 9–13 years old; 11 mg/day for men 14–18 years old; 9 mg/day for women 14–18 years old; 13 mg/day for pregnant women 14–18 years old; and 14 mg/day for lactating women 14–18 years old; **Monitor:** HbA_{1c}, lipid profiles **Notes:** Elemental zinc may increase HbA_{1c}; zinc supplementation may reduce HDL and increase LDL. Toxic dose: Prolonged intake at levels >150 mg/day may be associated with toxicity. Use zinc cautiously in patients with HIV infection.

INDEX

C

W

Y

Z